THE IDEOLOGY OF WORK

TAVISTOCK

The International Behavioural and Social Sciences Library

ORGANIZATIONAL BEHAVIOUR
In 10 Volumes

THE IDEOLOGY OF WORK

P D ANTHONY

First published in 1977 by
Tavistock Publications Limited

Reprinted in 2001 by
Routledge
11 New Fetter Lane, London EC4P 4EE

Transferred to Digital Printing 2002

Routledge is an imprint of the Taylor & Francis Group

Printed and Bound in Great Britain

British Library Cataloguing in Publication Data
A CIP catalogue record for this book
is available from the British Library

The Ideology of Work
ISBN 0-415-26463-4
Organizational Behaviour: 10 Volumes
ISBN 0-415-26513-4
The International Behavioural and Social Sciences Library
112 Volumes
ISBN 0-415-25670-4

The Ideology
of Work

P. D. ANTHONY

TAVISTOCK PUBLICATIONS

First published in Great Britain 1977
By Tavistock Publications Limited
11 New Fetter Lane, London EC4
Photoset by Red Lion Setters
Holborn, London
Printed in Great Britain at
J.W. Arrowsmith Ltd.,
Bristol BS3 2NT

ISBN 0 422 74310 0

To Irene and David Anthony,
my Mother and Father.

Contents

Preface

I must thank Professor G.F. Thomason for encouraging the development of studies at University College, Cardiff, which made the preparation of the material for this book possible. I also want to thank Mrs Mair Price for her patience and skill in typing and re-typing many disorderly manuscripts: she demonstrated a commitment to work for which I have good reason to be grateful, a commitment which will not, I hope, be reduced by anything she has read hereafter. Finally, I must thank my wife, Nia, for her help with the first chapter and for enduring many tedious discussions about a subject for which she maintains a decent and classical disrespect.

Introduction

The purpose of this book is to examine ways in which our ideas about work have developed and the values that underlie our assumptions about its importance. Some part of this examination will concern the development of ideas from classical and Christian origins to a capitalist framework of theory and to the radical alternatives, as they appear to be, of anarchism and communism. The rest will be occupied with contemporary views about work, reviewing attempts directed at overcoming what is often described as the problem of the alienated worker in industrial society. If the worker is to be spoken of as a problem then there is already an implication that work and its attendant values may be perceived differently by those who control it and by those who do it.

The inferences to be drawn from this distinction are important because in discussing the ideology of work I am not concerned simply with ideas about work but, rather, with the various exhortations that have been made for its efficient or enthusiastic performance. These appeals contain two elements: the first directed at the subordinate and intended to engage his co-operation; the second, emphasized whenever there is a challenge to authority, intended to legitimate the authority and also, thence, both the force of its appeal and the appropriateness of the subordinate's relationship to it. Professor Bendix, defining management ideologies as 'those ideas which are espoused by or for those who exercise authority in economic enterprises' (Bendix 1956 : 55) implies that ideologies function to support authority and are directed at those who are subordinate. The function of much of business ideology is to legitimate authority, it has the 'manifest purpose of influencing the sentiments and actions of others' (Sutton *et al.* 1956). The 'others' are subordinates, workers, and the influence is intended to promote work and its effective control by their bosses.

Professor Bendix has given Andrew Ure's *Philosophy of Manufacturers* and General Motors' pamphlet *Man to Man on the Job* as examples, and he added 'The serious analysis of such documents is at variance with the prevailing tendency to discuss them as obviously

biased and hence unworthy of consideration on their own terms ...
Accordingly, ideologies of management might be dismissed because
they *merely* express a class-interest or because they disguise *actual*
exploitative practices' (Bendix 1970 : 195). Professor Bendix regretted
this contemptuous dismissal of valuable evidence for achieving an
understanding of social structure: 'each ideological position may be
examined in terms of its logical corollaries as these relate to the
authority of the employer and in a wider sense to the class position of
employers and workers in the society' (Bendix 1970 : 196). True, and
no doubt this is a deserved rebuke to sociologists, but the present
examination of the ideology of work is not intended as a contribution
to sociological study. To put it more simply, I am not a sociologist and
have neither the equipment nor ambition to engage in a comparative
study of social structures. I am not so much concerned with the social
implications of ideological statements about work as with the exposure
of statements about work as being ideological. In other words, I wish
to try to establish that many historical and, more to the point,
contemporary views about work which have been regarded as
axiomatic are ideological in that they are intended to influence the
behaviour of subordinates.

Ideologies of management, says Professor Bendix, 'are attempts by
bodies of enterprises to justify the privilege of voluntary action and
association for themselves, while imposing upon all subordinates the
duty of obedience and the obligation to serve their employers to the
best of their ability' (Bendix 1956 : xx); they 'interpret the facts of
authority and obedience so as to neutralize or eliminate the conflict
between the few and the many in the interest of a more effective
exercise of authority' (Bendix 1956 : 13). The intention is often, as he
illustrates with a quotation from GEC's (USA) *Employee Communication: Executive Summary*, 'to endow this mythical personality which
the employee calls "the Company" with the qualities of friendliness,
consideration, fairness, and competence' (Bendix 1956 : 321).

Business or management ideologies are not the same as ideologies of
work. Business and management ideologies function to support those
in control in a given system, the ideology justifies their membership of
a group with power and it explains the activities of the members.
Ideologies of work and ideologies of management are related, of
course. Ideologies of management often appear to be subordinate
parts, if that is not a contradiction, of ideologies of work. Ideologies of
management express a particular and a necessary requirement to

defend or disguise the authority of those in whose interest work is controlled. Ideologies of work, on the other hand, are primarily directed at subordinates; their function is to explain the relative position of the subordinate and to influence his beliefs and his behaviour concerning the activities he is required to perform. An ideology of work is a defence of subordination and it entails an ideology of management upon which it is dependent.

Ideologies may be more effective when their appeal is covert and their intentions are disguised. For this reason we are going to be much more concerned with the discussion of meanings than with social consequences or social measurements. The analysis of meaning is essentially a philosophical preoccupation and if in pursuing it the lack of sociological apparatus may be an advantage, the absence of a philosopher's skill is a grave weakness. While I do not apologize for attempting something that social scientists have not always done well (to the extent that their obfuscations have sometimes appeared to be deliberate and their argument has often been eristic), I have to apologize for philosophical incompetence. My excuse is that the rest of us must be allowed to do the best we can when philosophers show little interest in helping us in the analysis of practical affairs which seem to us to be important. We can only follow the example of Hannah Arendt, when she states that in the face of 'heedless recklessness, or hopeless confusion or complacent repetition of "truths" which have become trivial and empty ... What I propose, therefore, is very simple: it is nothing more than to think what we are doing' (Arendt 1958 : 5).

Before setting out on a venture of any length, particularly if others are to be persuaded to join it, it is worth asking whether the journey is likely to be worthwhile. There are some grounds for doubt in this case. Work, in a sense, is a joke and, like some other basic functions, very difficult to take seriously unless its performance breaks down. There is, in any case, something ironic about devoting some time and effort to a task that is concerned with the study of work when readers are also expected to participate. It suggests the fascination that activity holds for the idle spectator, the absorbing occupation of watching other men's efforts from the comfort of an observation platform.

The advantages of this study are obvious: this most universally performed activity has received scant attention directed at the examination of its surrounding beliefs and its fundamental values. Perhaps it is *because* work is so general and commonplace that we believe it to be a matter of common sense and general agreement; our assumptions about it are so basic that we do not even recognize them as assumptions.

This is a persuasive explanation of the long silence concerning the ideology of work. The most successful ideology is one which is not recognizable as such, a system of beliefs and assumptions so much a part of everyday life that it is not even identifiable, much less open to question. Yet, it is surprising that while the examination and analysis of political theory have formed a traditional, necessary, and respectable intellectual activity, the equally important relationships of authority and subordination involved in work have been given much less attention. There are signs that they are beginning to attract attention, perhaps because our relationship to work is changing. Alasdair Clayre (1974) has produced an interesting contrast between received theories of the importance of work and statements of the way it is perceived by those who do it. The autobiographical record of workers themselves has been provided with two recent and distinguished additions, one American and the other British. The opening of Studs Terkel's *Working* (1975) reveals a bitter aspect of work which is not new but which has been newly recorded. 'This book, being about work, is by its very nature, about violence — to the spirit as well as to the body'. Professor Burnett has provided historical autobiographies which, apart from their vividness, show that the resignation of those 'who lead lives of hard work but rarely expect to find fulfilment from it' (1974 : 18) contrasted strongly with the ideology which would have them regard their work as of central importance rather than 'the family, interpersonal relationships, and relationship with God'. These accounts suggest that it is not so much the attitude of the worker which has changed but the expectation of what those attitudes should be which has recently been transformed.

In another sense, there has always been a great deal of attention to work. There has never been a shortage of advice as to how it should be done or how seriously its performance should be taken. More recently this attention has been lifted to a higher level of generalization, achieving the status of academic studies of the motivation and organization of work. But all this is concerned with how to get it done, or with the study of theories about how to get it done. What we are asking here is *why* it should be done, or why people believe it should be done, or how they have been persuaded that it should be done.

These questions have been raised, of course, but not often in respectable quarters. If the ideology of work has never been regarded as a subject of study and if its assumptions have rarely been criticized in intellectual terms, it has never been entirely protected from criticism. It was not only two nations which emerged so clearly in the nineteenth century but also, possibly, two ideologies of work. Perhaps there is a consistent, broad, and unofficial view, shared among workers, a kind of underground theory shared by the cognoscenti, by those who work in occupations that only a fool could regard as important in themselves. Dull and repetitive tasks are most frequently the target of the ·personnel technologist intent on job-enlargement and job-enrichment. What is the purpose of this attention? Is it to promote the social and psychological health of workers, or is it to make changes in work which will at last make it conceivable to extend an ideology of work to those most recalcitrant, or alienated, workers who have been so far exempted from its appeal by the patent absurdity of its application to their own jobs. A great deal of the ideology of work is directed at getting men to take work seriously when they know that it is a joke.

If a man in such a job is asked why he works he answers, after recovering from surprise at the apparent stupidity of the question, that he works in order to live. Obviously so! But men have not always given this answer and some who do not have to work in order to live are among those who work hardest. In complicated modern industrial societies the relationship between work and survival becomes more and more tenuous, yet we generally subscribe to an economic theory of work: that people work in order to provide goods and services in return for money which they spend on goods and services, and that they generally work harder to get more. But this explanation is not sufficient in itself: it has not always been held, it does not explain the behaviour of everyone at the present time, it does not explain the behaviour of the indigent or the criminal, and it does not explain less extreme problems of withdrawal from work (such as absenteeism). Even at the high tide of economic theory or, rather, particularly at the high tide of economic theory, work has been regarded as a moral or religious duty. Some part of the activities of contemporary behavioural scientists seems to be directed at the restoration of a sense of transcendental purpose in work.

There are likely to be many different answers to the question 'what is work for?'. Some certainly concern the economic element in work; in the long run we do work to survive or prosper. In complex industrialized societies work, as Alan Fox argues, 'embodies a preference for consumer rather than producer values' (Fox 1971 : 14). Some kinds of work can still be regarded as satisfying in themselves, and those whose work involves a 'craft ethic' may be tempted to transpose their own attitudes to those whose relationship to employment is entirely instrumental and whose jobs afford purely extrinsic satisfactions. Some answers to the question concern moral or even theological elements. There is an apocryphal tale of the chronic absentee colliery-worker who was asked by his exasperated manager why he worked only four shifts every week, 'because' replied the man 'I can't live on three'.

When this tale is told the aim of the storyteller is not to illustrate and applaud the precise calculation of which the worker is capable (a facility of which we should surely be proud if we were all truly economic men). It is told, rather, with a moral shudder at the degradation of the working classes. We all believe or, rather, some of us believe sometimes, that work is not a precise contract to be nicely calculated in detail (although managers have often made it that), but something to be undertaken as a whole, with a good heart. There is a very strong element of 'ought' about work. Not only do we think that work ought to be undertaken but that, for the most part, it should be done well, with enthusiasm, even with devotion. The notion of a concert pianist or a doctor, or a house painter, working with the deliberate intention of turning out a performance just good enough to pass as adequate (in Elliot Jaques's terms, to avoid the judgement of marginally sub-standard performance) is repulsive to most of us. The vague moral element in our attitude to work may relate to a more consistent theological account. Many contemporary attitudes are founded in the Bible and we shall be examining the accounts given by Weber and Tawney of fundamental changes in the ideology of work which accompanied the reformation, and which have been embodied in the concept of the protestant ethic.

The relationship of political theory to ideologies of work and their development has been so important and obvious as to need no advertisement here. Political theory divides broadly, since Karl Marx, between accounts that stress the co-operative aspects of work in a consensual framework of society and those that see work as an aspect of exploitation. But while the political theories receive consistent attention the implication of those theories in terms of work is more frequently ignored. Political theory has concerned itself with classic questions concerning the relationship of the citizen to the state, the forms of authority and its legitimate functions, the relationship and distribution of power within the state. These have always been questions of absolute importance, but for the majority of the citizenry the most immediate and urgent questions of power and authority are likely to arise in work. Indeed, the most significant and immediate differences between tyrannies and democracies, as far as the citizen is concerned, are likely to first manifest themselves in work.

If we begin by adopting a work perspective as compared to a social or political perspective, if we try to look at work as a worker might do, then we get a rather unusual view of some hitherto familiar theories. Political theories no longer seem so concerned with advocating harmony on the one hand or resistance to exploitation on the other. If we could submit political theory to reclassification in terms of its implications for the ideology of work we might emerge with two new classes of theory: those theories which support an economic emphasis, which stress work and authority and those theories which emphasize non-economic values and which do not value work. Quite distinct traditions of political theory can be seen to emerge from this classification and the division between the two has nothing in common with any traditional division between conservative and radical, left and right, progressive or reactionary. The fact that economic institutions, the intensification of work, and the specialization of industrial processes have been carried to their present high level of development may, in this way, explain the increasingly apparent irrelevance of those traditional distinctions. The organization of work now matters more than the organization of the state.

If we classify political theories by their new principle of division we find, on the one hand, a European tradition established in Greece, kept alive in some parts of the Catholic Church, dimly perceptible in some aspects of fascism, maintained by anarchists and now most strongly represented by the new left and the counter-culture. Opposing it we can find another tradition, the official tradition, established with the protestant ethic and entrenched by the spirit of capitalism, and now divided by the awful challenge of its product, industrialism, into an eastern and a western orthodoxy. The western branch, represented by American managerialism recognizes that an effective ideology of work can only be realistically maintained if work itself is changed. Work must be rehabilitated before anyone can be persuaded to take it seriously. The eastern branch, confronted by the same problem looks to changing society in order to maintain the reality of work. Society must be rehabilitated before anyone can be persuaded to take work seriously.

Looked at in this way, the division between capitalism and communism seems narrower than it is usually supposed to be. Their mutual hostility may be the result of the kind of bitter conflict which is often generated between two sects of the same faith. This hostility has forced almost everyone to join one camp or the other so that we all stereotype our opponents as enemies of our own values. In fact, in terms of values, there is very little between us.

There are recent signs of a true opposition of values emerging, however. After centuries of neglect, there is some evidence of a revival of the old European anti-economic outlook. The old view takes new forms which give it the appearance of a left-wing movement and which tempt us to associate it with communism in our simple and out-dated political spectrum of left and right. It is, as Paris showed in May 1968, anathema to communism. This new threat to orthodox economic ideology is an enemy equally to communism and to capitalism.

When both sets of the same orthodoxy are subjected to an attack from outside, they are likely to draw together in the defence of what they had forgotten they held in common. This process may well be the explanation of the current convergence which seems to be taking place between the Soviet Union and the United States of America. While this is commonly put down to the emergence of the same patterns of behaviour in the face of the same problems of scale, management, and technology, it is equally likely that this is no mere recent phenomena, that it represents the practical convergence of policies conditioned by what were always almost identical ideologies and value structures. In this sense, communist and capitalist policies have always revealed basic similarities of outlook which were concealed by their very sameness. The recent attack on the values of both by the counter-culture enables them both to engage in a common defence.

Basic to both is a deep commitment to an ideology of work, in the communication of appeals that work should be undertaken willingly by those who are subordinate to superordinates whose authority over them is legitimate. The success of these exhortations largely depends upon the validation of the claim to legitimacy. This has been the major problem in getting work done in any industrialized society since Marx dwelt on alienation. We shall see, finally, that both communist and capitalist societies are actively concerned with its solution. The fact that the means are different should not conceal the unity of their beliefs.

There are signs, however, that this convergence is occurring at a time when the 'problem' of work begins to recede. Perhaps, just as societies and institutions are said to build their most magnificent monuments when they are in decline, so the ideology of work reaches its most refined state when it becomes redundant. There are clear signs that society is becoming more uncertain and disturbed about the relevance of purely economic theories of work. Economic analysis and explanations are now constantly confronted with the challenge of views expressed in terms of environmental issues and the 'quality of life', to an extent that their expression has reached the level of the inescapable cliché. To regard an outlook as being generally expressed in clichés is not simply to criticize it, however, for the status of a cliché may be the mark of an ascendent ideology and, to this extent, the new challenge to economics could conceivably represent the first major shift in social values for several centuries.

In more immediate and more practical terms, work itself appears to be shedding some significance in our lives. The simple equation between work and production is no longer so obvious; machines, rather than human effort, produce goods; chemical plants, rather than their human occupants, refine and synthesize materials; sensing equipment, rather than human senses, supervise and inspect production processes; computers, rather than managers, control and direct manufacture and assembly. While the concepts of collective bargaining have been widened by the implications of productivity bargaining, it is very doubtful that any significant proportion of wages is paid for 'work' in a traditional sense. Higher wages are expected to be financed from higher productivity, but it is social rather than productive considerations that determine the rewards of the worker.

There is also some worrying negative evidence concerning the declining significance of work. We hear more and more about leisure, sometimes as a reward to be conferred on us, sometimes as a major social problem that must be met by investment and training, a problem which may lead, if it is not solved, to civil discord, delinquency, even revolution. We hear new things being said about redundancy, which was once regarded as a dreadful and undeserved deprivation associated with throwing embittered men on to the scrap-heap but which is now more frequently described in neutral

terms as the inevitable and even the beneficial consequence of
technical change. Managers are likely to be less enthusiastic in the
transmission of appeals for work to be made the basis of life when they
themselves are becoming redundant and unemployable in their
mid-forties in increasing numbers. We are all likely to become a little
more sceptical about the creative possibilities of work when we see
engineers, consultants, and scientists discarded because their devotion
to their work has been so absolute that they are deemed incapable of
adaptation to changes in technology. More important than changes in
our own attitudes as recipients of ideological appeals, the nature of the
ideological appeal begins to set up dissonance among its promoters as
its unreality becomes apparent.

We shall begin by looking at a different world, two thousand years
away, in which work was clearly perceived as a tedious activity which
no man of culture could take seriously. Ideological appeals for hard
work begin to emerge with its organization on a larger scale, at least in
circumstances in which the organization of labour is not based upon
coercion and slavery. The perception of a need to direct ideological
appeals at workers is clearest with the capitalist organization of
manufacturing process and the requirements associated with it for
orderly, disciplined, and committed workers. But capitalism breeds
dissent, at least it is by definition based upon competition, and it
engenders conflict. The greatest need for committed workers is
produced in conditions that make their commitment impossible.

Until this point the development of the foundations of an ideology
of work has been fairly straightforward and unitary. But the
paradoxical obstacles to the simple ideological appeals of capitalism
are inescapable. The simple development of an ideology of work now
divides into a radical and an orthodox wing. The purpose of our
tracing this development is to argue that the function of radical
statements concerning work is not to challenge its foundations or the
appeals based on them but to reinforce them. The effect, if not the
intention, is to make the world a place in which work can be restored,
that is, in which the obstacles to zealous work created by capitalism
can be removed. This intention often requires operations beyond the
immediate environment of work so that we are taken, willy-nilly, into
an examination of programmes for political reform, because a
preoccupation with problems associated with the 'alienated worker'
have often seemed to require the reconstruction of political society.
From this perspective, politics becomes a subordinate branch of the

study of work.

The orthodox stream re-emerges with minimum disturbance to capitalism and to associated forms of political government. It comprehends a different attempt to change the environment of work because it now asserts that problems of non-co-operation are the result of mismanagement or faulty organization. In this way we end the examination of the development of an ideology of work with an inquiry into some characteristics of contemporary management as the current repositories of the orthodox view.

Part 1
Foundations of an Ideology

1. Work as Slavery

The greatest contrast with our own attitude to work comes from the classical roots of our society. We know that a great part of our intellectual equipment, the basic fabric of our culture, comes from classical Greece. But Athenian ideas of work are probably more remote than any in the history of Europe from a contemporary attitude; they are not only remote in time but they represent values that are, in some measure, the reverse of our own. We are going to begin here not because of an established contemporary relevance, but because the Athenian outlook is a construct of attitudes of a particular type, a type that contrasts with our own and has had little influence in the economic history of Europe. It is a type, however, which may deserve re-examination at the present time.

Work was not taken seriously in classical Greece, it 'was not assigned the moral value which it has gained from twenty centuries of Christianity, and from the birth of the Labour movement'. Mossé (1969 : 25) quotes one of the earliest examples of the Greek's contempt for some kinds of work in Xenophon 'to be sure, the illiberal arts ... are spoken against, and are, naturally enough, held in utter disdain in our states. For they spoil the bodies of the workmen and the foremen, forcing them to sit still and live indoors, and in some cases to spend the day at the fire. The softening of the body involves a serious weakening of the mind'.

Let us begin with Plato and Aristotle. Some elements in Plato's thought are deceptively near to a modern economic view. He recognizes, he may even have invented, the notion of the division of labour, first by the division of the people in a community into rich and poor, and second by the division among them of different kinds of work. The division into rich and poor, he says, is a constant source of conflict in a community. In *The Republic* he argues that this conflict can only be avoided by (and that it therefore warrants) the abolition of private property or, at least, the avoidance of extremes of poverty and wealth existing in a society at the same time.

One of the functions of the state in *The Republic* is to facilitate the exchange of goods and services between individuals. 'What the state takes cognisance of is the mutual exchange, and what it tries to arrange is the most adequate satisfaction of needs and the most harmonious interchange of services. Men figure in such a system as the performers of a needed task and their social importance depends upon the value of the work they do' (Sabine 1951 : 55). Plato saw that the advantages of the specialization of labour were because the aptitudes of men differ and because their skills are improved by application to work for which they have special aptitude.

So far we have a rudimentary exposition of a theory that would be approved by Adam Smith and by any contemporary industrial training officer. Plato is distinguished by the relative value that he attaches to work in the community. There are three essential activities in his state: the provision of necessary services, the protection of the state, and the government of the state. The first is to be undertaken by workers, the second and third by two classes of 'guardians', or by guardians and a philosopher-king. Plato's educational system was devoted to the production of a guardian class. Work, the production of goods and services, was not regarded as of any great importance and neither was the education of workers. It could hardly be otherwise; the purpose in *The Republic*, was, after all, an examination of the ideal, the good, and the beautiful.

The distinction between social functions and their values emerges even more clearly in *The Laws*. Plato here re-admits private property along with the family (he was not the only commentator on society to see these institutions as inseparable) but, more relevant to our purpose, he decides that citizens of the state are to be prevented from engaging in industry or trade, from pursuing a craft, or promoting a business. It would not be possible to conceive of a clearer illustration of the distance separating us from Plato in this respect than to consider his recommendation that these commercial activities, among the most highly rewarded in our own society, should be limited to resident immigrants in his. Sabine describes his attitude thus: 'Agriculture is the special function of slaves, trade and industry of freemen who are not citizens, all political functions are the prerogative of citizens ... What he arrives at is a state in which citizenship is frankly restricted to a class of privileged persons who can afford to turn over their private business — the sordid job of earning a living — to slaves and foreigners' (Sabine 1951 : 81).

This inversion of our own values, or perhaps we should put it the other way about, our inversion of classical values, is shown still more clearly in Aristotle, more particularly in the *Politics*. To begin with, Aristotle's discussion is even more exclusively preoccupied with the content of a liberal education for rulers 'and shows, far more than Plato's an actual contempt for the useful' (Sabine 1951 : 95). Aristotle regarded work not only as inferior but as debased and debasing: 'in the best governed states ... none of them [citizens] should be permitted to exercise any mechanic employment or follow merchandise as being capable and destructive to virtue; neither should they be husbandman, that they may be at leisure to improve in virtue and perform the duty they owe to the state' (*Politics* : 1328b).

Aristotle has no doubt about private property or about the virtue that seems to be attached to wealth and, by contrast the vice associated with the lack of it. 'It is also necessary that the landed property should belong to these men; for it is necessary that the citizens should be rich and these are the men proper for citizens, for no mechanic ought to be admitted to the rights of a citizen, nor any other sort of people whose employment is not entirely noble, honourable and virtuous' (*Politics* : 1329b).

Work, as Aristotle sees it, gets in the way of the more proper pursuits of a citizen, not only wasting his time in inferior activities but corrupting him and making his pursuit of virtue more difficult. Aristotle's advice is concerned more with what should be than with the actual state of affairs that existed in his way. It is probable that most Athenian citizens were tradesmen, artisans, or farmers, engaged in those very activities of which Aristotle so strongly disapproved in citizens. But their occupations were indeed interruptions of what Aristotle considered to be superior activities '... their political activities had to take place in such time as they could spare from their private occupations. It is true that Aristotle deplored this fact and thought it would be desirable to have all normal work done by slaves, in order that citizens might have the leisure to devote themselves to politics ... Aristotle was not describing what existed but was proposing a change for the improvement of politics' (Sabine 1951 : 18).

This 'contempt for the useful' characterized Aristotle's outlook also to the commercial aspects of work and his view was to become very influential. It grew out of the distinction he made between proper and improper usage 'it is not therefore proper for any man of honour, or any citizen, or anyone who engages in public affairs, to learn these servile employments without they have occasion to them for their own use' (*Politics* : 1277b). This idea of use was developed specifically into a critical view of the charging of interest and of usury, and this application was to achieve great significance in late scholastic teaching and thence in the mediaeval attitude to commerce. Bertrand Russell (1946 : 209) paraphrases Aristotle's view in this way:

> 'There are two uses of a thing, one proper, the other improper; a shoe, for instance, may be worn, which is the proper use. It follows that there is something degraded about a shoemaker who must exchange his shoes in order to live. Retail trade, we are told, is not a natural part of the art of getting wealth. The natural way to get wealth is by skilful management of home and land ... Wealth derived from trade is justly hated, because it is unnatural. The most hated sort, and with the greatest reason, is usury, which makes a gain out of money itself, and not from the natural object of it. For money was intended to be used in exchange, but not to increase an interest ... Of all modes of getting wealth this is the most unnatural.'

The proper and improper use of a thing distinguished, more precisely, between what the Greeks regarded as proper and improper work. To work for oneself was praiseworthy, even for a soldier and a gentleman to engage in what we would regard as menial manual labour was perfectly honourable. It was not the nature of the task which was significant, it was rather the purpose of the task:

> 'In order to understand the contempt attached to manual labour two ... factors must be taken into consideration. First the ties of dependence which were created by labour, and secondly, the growth of a slave economy ... to work for another man in return for a wage of any kind is degrading ... for the ancients, there is really no difference between the artisan who sells his own products and the workman who hires out his services. Both work to satisfy the needs of others, not their own. They depend upon others for their livelihood. For that reason they are no longer free.' (Mossé 1969 : 27, 28).

Arendt (1958): 31) writes that, in Greece 'a poor free man preferred the insecurity of a daily-changing labour market to regular assured work, which, because it restricted his freedom to do as he pleased every day, was already felt to be servitude (*douleia*), and even harsh, painful labour was preferred to the easy life of many household slaves'. Work as such was not despised by the Athenian because, when carried out upon one's land, it was a natural and necessary activity. Zimmern (1915 : 270) specifically refutes

> 'the false idea that the Greeks of the great age regarded manual labour as degrading ... In truth they honoured manual work far more than we do ... But they insisted, rather from instinct than from policy, on the duty of moderation, and objected, as artists do, against doing any more work than they needed when the joy had gone out of it. Above all they objected to all monotonous activity, to occupations which involved sitting for long periods in cramped and unhealthy postures ... It was these occupations,' those of our respectable clerks and secretaries of all grades, rather than our rough-clad artisans, which they regarded as "menial".'

Work was not despised, because it was natural and it was necessary and because it could contribute to use, beauty, and happiness, but it was subordinated to these ends; an Athenian would have thought it absurd to regard it as an end in itself. All work seems to have been regarded in much the same light; doctors, and sculptors, and schoolmasters were all paid 'like masons and joiners and private soldiers, at the customary standard rate' although they worked for wages only rarely and when their city needed them for some public work; generally to work for wages would put the craftsman in the position of the slave whereas his 'aim in life was very different: to preserve his full personal liberty and freedom of action, to work when he felt inclined and when his duties as a citizen permitted him ... to participate in the government, to take his seat in the courts, to join in the games and festivals, to break off his work when his friends called ... — all of them things which were incompatible with a contract at a fixed rate' (quoted by Zimmern 1915 : 270).

Aristotle systematized and, therefore, exaggerated what was probably the ordinary Athenian view. Aristotle was quite clear that 'the aim of the state ... is to produce cultivated gentlemen — men who combine the aristocratic mentality with love of learning and the arts' (Russell 1946 : 216). The principle of specialized production, recognized by Plato, has in a sense been exchanged by Aristotle for the principle of specialized corruption. While Plato saw that a degree of productive specialization was required by the unequal distribution of abilities and by the need for the development of skill, Aristotle substituted the single end of the production of gentlemen. He argued that, because work was corrupting, the continued existence of cultured citizens required the corruption of a special class of producers; slaves and foreigners. There are, thus, two strands in his doctrine: that leisure is more valuable than work and that the existence of a leisured class was incompatible with the general spread of education and leisure. Aristotle wanted the citizens to become aristocrats but their existence was to depend upon slaves.

It was not only the classical economy but also the classical ideology of work which depended on slaves. Aristotle's attitude to slavery is straightforward: 'A slave is an animated instrument' (*Politics* : 1253b). This was not the most callous view of slavery that was to be put forward in the ancient world but, for Athens, it was probably once again an exaggerated abstraction. In Athens it was not uncommon for free men and slaves to undertake the same work side by side for much the same wages. In the Athenian household slaves were often on close terms with their masters and were treated with humane consideration. But generally, the close association of free man and slave in the same work did not point to the latter's advantage, rather the reverse. 'When the free man and the slave shared the same toil, the tendency was for them both to incur the same contempt' (Mossé 1969 : 29). The dependence of Athenian and Roman society upon slaves did not honour them in the eyes of their superiors, and certainly invoked no feeling of gratitude or debt towards them. We have become used to paying a certain respect to workers upon whose efforts our economic structure may rest, but in a society in which economic values were subordinated to cultural and political ends, to be at the bottom of the economic structure was to be at the bottom of the dung heap.

Slavery was an integral part of the ancient world but the employment of slaves was probably much more extensive and widely organized in the Roman Empire than it had been in the Greek city states. To begin with the condition of the slaves seems to have been moderately good, but it deteriorated. Roman works on estate management advised the employment of slaves in moderate numbers (comparable with their earlier employment on Greek farms) and with due consideration; out of both humanity and the self-interest of the landowner. Small-scale cultivation or business no doubt depended on and promoted some degree of personal relationship between slaveowner and slave. But the economies of scale and extensive landowning changed this: 'The economy of the Latifundia was quite different' as it developed in the South of Italy, in Sardinia, Sicily, and

North Africa (Mossé 1969 : 64). Large-scale grain production from estates of hundreds of acres owned by aristocratic or imperial absentee landlords who owned hundreds or thousands of slaves changed conditions for the worse.

'There was no longer any question of considering them as human beings, of treating them with a compassionate but strict justice, nor was there any question of encouraging them to hope for freedom in return for loyal service. They were many and therefore to be feared. They had to be treated as a vanquished foe if they were to be forced into obedience. At the same time, the fact that it was very easy to procure them and that their cost was extremely low had the effect of positively depriving them of any personal value. They were cattle and were treated as such. Chains and branding irons were common-place, as were the most deplorable corporal punishments — torture and crucifixion. The harshness with which they were treated accounts for the great slave revolts which broke out in Sicily and in the south of Italy in the second century BC.' (Mossé 1969 : 68)

If slaves continued to be regarded as animated instruments the fact of their animation could become bothersome (as it has often been throughout the history of employment). It could, at worst, lead to revolution; the Empire lived in almost perpetual fear of its own overthrow by the vast mass of the slave population which it had created. At best the slaves' 'animation' meant that they had to be treated with a consideration which was not necessary towards tools or even animals. But the difference of treatment did not always work to the slaves' advantage. Cato the Elder, a comparatively humane authority in these matters, believed that slaves were to be treated like animals, although because the ox was not so good at taking care of itself it needed to be tended more carefully than the slave. In Cato's view 'the best principle of management is to treat both slaves and animals well enough to give them the strength to work hard' (Grant 1960 : 112). This principal of management was stated in a form more recognizable to us in contemporary terms by Varro (116 - 27 BC) who 'looked upon slaves as articulate implements — differing from their voiceless counterparts such as a pitchfork in that they need psychological study and sensible, unbrutal handling' (Grant 1960 : 115).

Changes, for better or worse, in the conditions of slaves, depended in part on the manner of and the potential for their economic exploitation. Work begins to be taken seriously as slavery declines:

> 'it is significant that the glorification of labour (in the poems of
> Hesiod or of Virgil and in certain writings of such Fathers of the
> Church as St Basil of Caesarea) and laws against idleness ... only
> occurred either at a time when slavery was still in its very first stages,
> or when it was declining, when the scarcity of labour of any kind
> and the rise in prices put a premium on free and individual labour,
> thereby creating suitable conditions for an anti-slavery ideology to
> develop and for a partial rehabilitation of the idea of work.' (Mossé
> 1969 : 29)

An ideology of work is redundant when the labour force can be
conscripted and coerced at will. In conditions of a freer labour market
an ideology has to be developed in order to recruit labour and then in
order to motivate it by persuading it that its tasks are necessary or
noble. In conditions of a free market and a chronic shortage of labour,
the manufacture and communication of an ideology of work becomes
a central preoccupation of society. We shall argue later that the process
reaches its highest development in advanced capitalism and in state
socialism.

It has also been suggested that non-economic developments
contributed to the end of slavery. One, rather metaphysical,
explanation is that the breakdown of the city state accompanied by the
growth of the vast Alexandrian and Roman empires so dwarfed the
individual as a political entity that the compensating development of
reassuring religions was inevitable; assurance of importance after death
was necessary to make up for man's palpable insignificance before it.
The individual, it has been said, was driven within himself to 'claim
his own unsharable inner life as the origins from which all other values
grow. In other words he could set up the claim of an inherent right,
the right to have his own personality respected' (Sabine 1951 : 131).

Equality, previously a claim confined to members of a privileged
elite of citizens, began to be thought of, if not actually shared, by all
men — citizens, foreigners, and slaves. This development depended
upon the conception of a law beyond the law, some universal system of
law greater than the law of the state and against which the law of the
state could be compared. In this process of development 'the twin
conceptions of the rights of man and of a universally binding rule of
justice and humanity were built solidly into the moral consciousness of
the European peoples' (Sabine 1951 : 131).

The vehicle of this process of development was the Stoic group of philosophers, heirs of the last of the Athenian schools and influencing both Roman political thought and Christian teaching. Some of the Stoic characteristics are those generally evoked by the name today, the stern virtues of duty and self-sufficiency fostered by a discipline of the will which promotes contempt for the attractions of pleasure. Stoicism also contained a religious element which, Sabine (1951 : 135) suggests, was close, in some respects to Calvinism. Stoic philosophers stressed 'the duty of every man to play well the part for which he is cast, whether it be conspicuous or trifling, happy or miserable'. This notion of a role which is predetermined and which carries with it the duties of acceptance and performance was to become an important part of later church teaching and of the general justification of feudal society.

Other elements in Stoic philosophy were to cast a very long shadow. Stoics believed that although nature was one, both man and God were distinguished from animals by their possession of reason, while animals had instincts and abilities appropriate to their species. Because men and God share in the power of reasoning there is an affinity between them; men are the children of God therefore they are brothers. Because they are brothers all men are equal, except for innate differences, between wise men and fools (in practice, Sabine (1951 : 136)) suggests that 'the Stoics, like most rigorous moralists, were impressed by the number of fools'). If all men were essentially equal, the older attitude to slavery could hardly be tolerated.

The idea of men as equal, reasoning beings grew from the conception of man as a citizen of a world society (which, in a sense, he had literally become). Even if men did not share a common political or judicial constitution they could be envisaged as governed by a common law, the law of right reason, which was the same everywhere for all men, teaching what to do and what to avoid doing. 'Right reason is the law of nature, the standard everywhere of what is just and right, unchangeable in its principles, binding on all men whether ruler or subjects, the law of God' (Sabine 1951 : 136).

The idea of natural law, persistent and unchanging, was to become an inseparable part of mediaeval thinking and was to become influential in political and legal thought long after the middle ages; it is still significant today. But to acknowledge a natural law is to pose problems about statute law and its apparent deficiencies. How do we reconcile the inevitable conflicts between right reason and the law of men?

One unequivocal answer came from Cicero. He accepted the development of a universal law emerging from the rational and social character of man and he concluded that any piece of legislation that contradicted it did not merit the respect due to law. An effective state, he said, was bound to respect the mutual recognition of rights between its citizens and was itself subject to the natural law. His egalitarian teaching was difficult to reconcile with the institution of slavery; perhaps he avoided rather than achieved the reconciliation by advocating personal warmth and sympathy towards slaves. The despotism was at least becoming enlightened.

Other reconciliations were attempted, including the justification through necessity; as civilized society depended upon the existence of slaves the employment of slaves must be acceptable to the moral law. Slaves were, in fact, the most intractable and irreconcilable element in the co-existence of natural and civil law because slavery was necessarily acceptable to every legal code and unacceptable in any statement of natural law. Roman lawyers finally accepted a distinction in which legality could be established according to the appropriate law to which reference was being made. By distinguishing *ius civile*, the customary law of the state; *ius gentium*, municipal law; and *ius naturale*, natural law, it was possible for a particular case to be both legal and illegal at the same time. Thus, 'by nature all men are born free and equal but slavery is permitted according to the *ius gentium*' (Sabine 1951 : 152). This kind of ambivalence has been called upon since the Romans whenever economic practice has contradicted ethical teaching; perhaps ambivalence is preferable to the total subjection of ethics to economic practice.

Stoic teaching, the influence of humane Romans, and the recognition of the natural deficiencies of Roman law all contributed to an improvement in the condition of slaves. The condition of those who employed them was less easily improved. The reverse effects of slavery were probably disastrous from an economic point of view. The fact that work was done by slaves had established the circular argument for despising both slaves and work; the experience of the one contaminated attitudes to the other. Grant (1960 : 75) explaining the Romans' apparent inability to apply their scientific theory suggests that science and industry continued to be despised and excluded from education. Cicero apparently approved entirely of the Aristotelian view that 'all mechanics are engaged in vulgar trades; for no workshop can have anything liberal about it'. If this view strikes us as laughable we must remember that we often approach it in reverse, that 'all mechanics are engaged in vulgar trades; for no liberals can have anything mechanical about them'; at least one modern American text seriously advises business managers to avoid the selecting of liberal-minded university graduates (Miner 1963).

Grant (1960 : 75) explains that Roman prejudice largely resulted from the employment of slaves; slavery 'both allowed techniques to stagnate and caused social prejudice against the manual efforts which might have improved them'. 'Slavery', he concluded, 'ruined Italian agriculture, exhausted the soil, and stagnated techniques' (Grant 1960 : 118).

One other aspect of slavery deserves some attention. The Greeks regarded human activity as arranged hierarchically so that superior activities were reserved for cultivated and superior men. In the purest form of this view, citizens were to be exempted from work so that they could be educated to engage in the government of their state. Work was assigned to slaves and foreigners so that gentlemen could avoid the demands it would make on their time and the corruption of its menial character. So, the cultural, political, and economic strata of this society coincided; those at the bottom have least culture, least authority, and least economic power, and vice versa.

This coincidental stratification was not always true of late societies. In first and second century Rome, a good part of the intellectual life of society was carried on by slaves, often of Greek origin. It is as though, today, the . civil service and the professions (particularly teaching and the universities) were largely dependent on the lowest order of society. It suggests that slavery is not necessarily and indissolubly identified with the most menial or manual kinds of work. Where any activity becomes specialized and is divorced from the possession of power, it becomes possible to regard it as a subordinate activity, subordinate even to the point of slavery. Where political power is in the hands of an oligarchy it is possible to regard culture as the activity of specialists.

The distinction between manual and intellectual specialist work becomes important again in the nineteenth and twentieth centuries. It became commonplace to assume that the intellectual specialist was privileged by virtue of his greater authority, economic resources, and culture. He was also believed to be fortunate in the pursuit of satisfying and enjoyable work. Karl Marx finally suggested that as functionaries of the bourgeois, intellectual specialists were not significantly different from other members of the proletariat. Perhaps George Gissing was one of the first to clothe this insight in imaginative reality when he showed the intellectual worker as reduced in effect to the position of a slave.

But the re-appearance of intellectual functionaries or slaves is some two thousand years removed from the period we have been discussing. The most immediate and potent legacy of Stoic philosophy was a theme of egalitarianism. The egalitarian tradition began in an even earlier classical myth of a golden age in which all were equal, there were no rich or poor, there was complete sexual promiscuity and work was not necessary. The golden age had vanished when 'the wary surveyor marked out with long boundary lines the earth which hitherto had been a common possession like the sunshine and the breezes' (Ovid : *Metamorphoses*), and when covetousness had produced private property. 'At least by the third century AD, Christian doctrine had assimilated from the extraordinary influential philosophy of Stoicism the notion of an egalitarian State of Nature which was irrecoverably lent' (Cohn 1962 : 201).

The distinction between natural law and the law of man was reflected in the distinction between the state of nature and the existing conditions of man.

'It was agreed by most of the later Fathers that inequality, slavery, coercive government and even private property had no part in the original intention of God and had come into being only as a result of the Fall. Once the Fall had taken place, on the other hand, a development began which made such institutions indispensable. Corrupted by Original Sin, human nature demanded restraints which could not be found in an egalitarian order; inequalities of wealth, status and power were, thus, not only consequences of but also remedies for sin. The only recommendations which could be authorised by such a view were recommendations directed towards individuals and dealing solely with problems of personal conduct. That a master ought to behave fairly reasonably towards his slave who is as dear to God as he is himself ... such were the practical conclusions which were drawn, within the limits of orthodoxy, from the doctrine of the prime egalitarian State of Nature.' (ibid.)

St. Augustine in *The City of God*, held that man had been created as a rational being and was intended to be set above animals, not above other men. But sin had created servitude 'by which man is subjected to man by the bonds of his condition'. This was orthodox Christian teaching. St Ambrose pronounced that nature 'created a common right, but use and habit created private right' that 'The Lord God specially wanted this earth to be the common possession of all, and to provide fruits for all; but avarice produced the rights of property'.

Cohn (1962 : 206) suggests that the myth of an egalitarian state of nature was popularized by Jean de Meun in the *Roman de la Rose*, about 1270, which, he says, was a forecast by some five hundred years of Rosseau. Once upon a time, runs the story, society was simple, all were equals and there was no private property. They knew well the maxim that love and authority never yet dwelt companionably together. But the vices of Deceit, Pride, Covetousness, and Envy promoted discord and distrust, men 'became false and began to cheat; they fastened on properties, they divided the very soil and in doing so they drew boundaries, and often in settling their boundaries, they fought and snatched whatever they could from one another, the strongest got the biggest share.' The resultant anarchy led to a search for order, men chose 'a big villein as lord and the lords needed taxes to pay them to enforce order. Men fortified cities and castles ... for those who held these riches were much afraid lest they should be taken from them either by stealth or by force.'

The Church advised a communal life of voluntary poverty but as an ideal possible only for the elite (another startling illustration of the inversion of our own values). This advice led to the establishment of the religious orders of monks and friars and, after the eleventh century, to the creation of lay communities sharing all property together. 'But to imitate this imaginary version of the primitive Church was not yet to restore, or even attempt to restore, the last Golden Age of all humanity which had been portrayed for the ancient world by Seneca and for medieval Europe by Jean de Meun' (Cohn 1962 : 208).

The myth of a golden age was a picturesque representation of the difference between the ideal and the actual, the distinction that was recognized in a plurality of laws, natural and civil. The contradictions involved in this dualism challenged solution. One response (by St Thomas Aquinas) was to resolve the contradictions by a higher synthesis, to build them into a bigger system. Another response was to try to create the ideal and to substitute it for the actual. The attempt to recreate a golden age again on earth 'produced a doctrine which became a revolutionary myth as soon as it was presented to the turbulent masses of the poor and fused with ferocious phantasies of popular eschatology' (Cohn 1962 : 210).

Cohn suggests that the myth of a golden age began to be considered as a plan for the immediate future around 1380 in Flanders and northern France, and in England in the Peasants' Revolt of 1381. Froissart repeats a sermon attributed to John Ball: 'They [the lords] have beautiful residences and manors, while we have the trouble and the work, always in the fields under rain and snow. But it is from us and our labour that everything comes, with which they maintain their pomp. Good folk, things cannot go well in England nor ever shall until all things are in common and there is neither villein nor noble, but all of us are of one condition.' Power and wealth came under general attack; partly on theological grounds concerning their threat to salvation, partly emanating from a less spiritual injunction to revolt by a lower clergy eager to assume the role of divinely inspired prophets. Cohn adds that 'it must really have seemed that all things were being made new, that all social norms were dissolving and all barriers collapsing ... Certainly it was a situation in which it must have been easy enough to proclaim and to believe that the path lay wide open to an egalitarian, even a communistic millenium' (Cohn 1962 : 216).

The construction of utopias, past or present, here on earth, is a process to which the upper orders can give only limited approval. The church hierarchy attempted to solve the contradictions of the dualism by looking in the opposite direction, by searching for a synthesis. The architect of this construction was St Thomas Aquinas. The synthesis incorporated classical foundations: 'The Catholic ideal of economical life finds condensed expression in the principles of the Gospels, which were elaborated successively by St Paul, the Fathers, and the Doctors till ... St Thomas Aquinas, prince of Catholic philosophers, grafted Catholic principles on the old, all but forgotten trunk of Aristotelianism' (Fanfani 1935 : 119). Aquinas created a complete and consistent conception of a Christian universe in which human law was a part of the system of divine law. The system contained three parts, a hierarchy of knowledge, a hierarchy of nature, and human society, 'a system of ends and purposes in which the lower serves the higher and the higher directs and guides the lower'. Following Aristotle, Aquinas described society as a mutual exchange of services for the sake of a good life. Many callings contribute to it, the farmer and artisan by supplying material goods, the priest by prayer and religious observance, each class by doing its own proper work, 'rulership is an office or trust for the whole community. Like his lowest subject the ruler is justified in all that he does solely because he contributes to the common good' (Sabine 1951 : 219).

Human society is governed by the same principles of reason and order that permeate the whole universe, principles of which human law is a manifestation. 'Since all things which are subject to divine providence are measured and regulated by the external law ... it is clear that all things participate to some degree in the external law ... This participation in the eternal law by rational creatures is called the natural law' (D'Entrèves 1970 : 115). Human law derives from eternal law and the ruler is as bound by it as is his subject. The power of the ruler, if it is just, is the power needed to maintain the common good, no more. This notion of sufficiency is applied also to property and to wealth. They are provided and justified by need.

'Material goods are provided for the satisfaction of human needs. Therefore the division and appropriation of property, which proceeds from human law, must not hinder the satisfaction of man's necessity from such goods. Equally, whatever a man has in superabundance is owed, of natural right, to the poor for their sustenance .... But because there are many in necessity, and they cannot all be helped from the same source, it is left to the initiative of individuals to make provision from their own wealth, for the assistance of those who are in need ... [But] if a person is in immediate danger of physical privation, and there is no other way of satisfying his need, — then he may take what is necessary from another person's goods, either openly or by stealth. Nor is this, strictly speaking, fraud or robbery.' (D'Entrèves 1970 : 171)

Aquinas stressed the virtue of civil obedience but allowed that if tyranny went beyond the point where it threatened the free moral nature of the subordinate, the subordinate had a right to resist it. In modern times we might say that Aquinas conceived of society as a closed system in stable equilibrium. He regarded Christian society as eternal and the universal application of his theory with its interdependent and interlocking parts reinforced any tendency within it to resist change. Aquinas was concerned 'to construct a rational scheme of God, nature, and man within which society and civil authority find their due place. In this sense his philosophy expresses most maturely the convictions, moral and religious upon which mediaeval civilization was founded' (Sabine 1951 : 225).

Mediaeval civilization was founded on an agricultural economy and its society for the most part was composed of small, local, self-sufficient communities. But local villages and farms could not, in times of great disorder, be self-sufficient for the purpose of the protection of life and property, and a relatively weak central government was prevented by primitive communications from exercising a policing function. In the circumstances the weak had to seek the defence of the strong; a hierarchical system of landowning was reflected in a system of protective dependency and of obligation, service was returned for protection and the system extended from the king to the serf. At the bottom of the system various services and dues went to the lord of the manor — merchet in payment for getting a daughter married, chevage for permission to leave the manor, week-work of two to three days a week on the lord's land. These activities which once might have been voluntary, had been turned. by long practice into customary and therefore unquestionable obligations. Some of these obligations tended to preserve the stability of the system. The villein could not sell or exchange his land and needed his lord's consent to sell his cattle. He would also seek his lord's agreement before his children could enter holy orders or take up a trade.

The network of obligations, rights, and protections ran through the whole society. The economic relationships were such as to stress not effort or zeal or initiative, but the simple performance of obligations. Work was necessary in order to ensure the survival of the family, and as a kind of tax due to the lord. There could be little point in working harder or more productively because, as the market economy was rudimentary, there would be nothing to do with a surplus. The taskmaster was, as is always the case with those at work on the land, not so much a man as nature itself; what was done had to be done according to a rhythm dictated by the natural cycle.

But there was a primitive management system, and in it the subordinate exercised a measure of control. The management of the strips of land cultivated by the village was communally exercised. The management of the lords' demesnes, at least the largest of them, was conducted by officials who superintended the farming of vassals and tenants. The chief official was the bailiff, the lord's man, but he was assisted by the reeve. The duties of the two officers were sometimes confused and they were often amalgamated but the reeve was sometimes a representative of the peasants, chosen from among them from a list which they might have nominated; he was not necessarily a free man.

The economic structure was an expression of Aquinas's view that society was 'a mutual exchange of services for the sake of a good life ... The common good requires that such a system shall have a ruling part, just as the soul rules the body'. The functioning of such a system would depend upon obedience, on the correct carrying out of duties, upon respect for custom and constituted authority, virtues emphasized by the early Christian fathers. It was a society which might last for ever — as long as it did not change.

But in the twelfth and thirteenth centuries it did change. Lords of the manor found that wage-labour paid them better than the services provided for them by peasants, so the lords began to take annual payments in the place of the services. The villeins often left for work in towns or for wage-work on other demesnes, severing their feudal obligations by a payment or, simply, by absconding. 'By the 1370's and 1380's great lords in most places were finding it an unsupportable burden to administer the old "manorial system". It was difficult when the price of produce was low to pay for a whole system of bailiffs, reeves and servile workers ... labour was hard to get; expensive if it had to be bought, and unobtainable if the old cheap labour services were demanded. Men simply ran away' (Du Boulay 1970 : 54). In order to retain those peasants who remained, the lords made concessions, relieving them of many of the customary personal obligations. Nabholtz suggests that, by the beginning of the fourteenth century, half the dependent 'cultivators were free. Sometimes the lord gave over the whole of his demesne for complete cultivation by peasants in return for rents, fixed payments in place of the old obligation. In this way the lord not only [got] the money that he wanted, but he saved the expense of officials by leaving everything to the tenant. If the tenant paid regularly, his lord no longer worried about the details of his farming' (in Clapham and Power 1941 : 511).

Work could begin to be taken seriously, particularly as markets began to develop. Nabholtz argues that it was becoming both possible and worth-while for the tenant to put more work into his own holding because increasing mobility made it easier for him to sell his surplus produce in a town market; the transition from a self-sufficient to an exchange economy was taking place. With the growth of markets and a money economy came new cleavages in the old stable social order. Trevelyan (1944 : 10) describes the filling-in of the great distance that

separated the land and the villein: 'Indeed the villein serf is in process
of extinction. He is becoming a yeoman farmer, or else a landless
labourer. And between these two classes enmity is now set. The
peasantry are divided among themselves as employers and employed'.

Between 1348 and 1368 change was tragically accelerated by the
Black Death, which, in an economy experiencing falling wages,
contributed a labour shortage and a rise in wages of up to fifty per
cent. In consequence conflict of interest between lords and peasants
led to an attempt to control prices and incomes. An ordinance of 1350
said that the labour shortage had led to demands for excessive wages
which it pegged to the level of 1346. Like most attempts at an incomes
policy it was unsuccessful and like some more recent attempts it may
have made things worse; wages 'rose highest, not immediately after
the plague, but in the fifties and sixties. So the stiffening of the law
had results exactly opposite to what was intended' (Clapham and
Power 1941 : 515). In a situation of inherent advantage to the
peasantry the lords were attempting to restore crumbling feudal
structures and to reinforce their own position.

There is great debate about the causes of the Peasants' Revolt of
1381 but it succeeded widespread protest and violence, by labourers
against the suppression of wages, by villein farmers against irksome
feudal restrictions, by townsmen seeking greater municipal liberties,
by parish priests against the power of the church. Feudal society, in
which each man's position was carefully prescribed and in which the
prescription was given the authority of theological doctrine, was being
subjected to considerable stress. To the pressures of economic change,
revolt, and plague two new movements added their weight: 'the first,
the subject between 1485 and 1640 of twelve statutes, seven Royal
Commissions, and endless pamphleteering, concerned the tenure of
land. The second ... related to credit and was described as that of
usury' (Tawney 1925 : 19).

The problem of land tenure concerned the enclosure of land for
sheep-farming. The effects of enclosure may have been exaggerated,
even in contemporary accounts.[1] One reason for doubting the extent
of the movement up to Tudor times is that so much land remained to
be enclosed in the eighteenth and nineteenth centuries. But, 'the
amount of noise made over economic and social change is determined,
not by the extent and importance of the changes that actually occur,
but by the reaction of contemporary opinion to the problem.'
(Trevelyan 1944 : 117) And the reaction was vociferous. Here, for

example, is Sir Thomas More (*Utopia* : 24):

'Therefore that on covetous and unsatiable cormaraunte and very plage of his natyve contrey maye compasse aboute and inclose many thousand akers of grounde together within one pale or hedge, the husbandmen be thrust owte of their owne ... For one Shephearde or Heardman is ynoughe to eate up that grounde with cattel, to the occupiyng whereof aboute husbandrye manye handes were requisite. And this is also the cause why victualles be now in many places dearer. Yea, besides this the price of wolle is so rysen, that poore folkes, which were wont to worke it, and make cloth thereof, be nowe hable to bye none at all ... And though the number of shepe increase never so faste, yet the price falleth not one myte, because there be so fewe sellers. For they be almooste all comen into a fewe riche mennes handes, whome no neade forceth to sell before they lust, and they luste not before they maye sell as deare as they luste.'

Attitudes and practice concerning both enclosure and usury were confused. The outcry against both was considerable but both were widely practised and for different purposes. The enclosure of arable or common land for sheep pasture was detested but some enclosure was carried out by peasants to bring about a more rational distribution of their open field strips. Usury, the making of money out of money without an advantage to both parties, was proscribed by theological doctrine, but lending was necessary to maintain a rudimentary economy and the lenders were often yeomen. But the extension of practices which were condemned led to wider social acceptance, a diminished doctrinal attack, and, finally, to the incorporation of practice in preaching; old ideologies cannot survive new worlds. To begin with, 'to live by usury as the husbandman doth by his husbandry' had commonly been treated as ignominious, immoral, or positively illegal: when it evolved, money-lending was on the way to enjoying the legal security of a recognized and reputable profession. But the change itself was part of a larger revolution which

'set a naturalistic political arithmetic in the place of theology, substituted the categories of mechanism for those of theology and turned religion itself from the master interest of mankind into one department of life with boundaries which it is extravagant to over-step ... the issue at stake was not merely the particular question, but the fate of the whole scheme of medieval economic thought which had attempted to treat economic affairs as part of a hierarchy of values embracing all human interests and activities, of which the apex was religion.' (Tawney 1925 : 106)

The question was determined neither quickly nor decisively. The distinction between preaching and practice survived for a long time, as it always does.

'In the matter of trade ... canon law in the early twelfth century still spoke of it as an occupation scarcely compatible with Christianity. But as the growing needs of society produced more elaborate forms of commercial organization, the ecclesiastical lawyers began to have other thoughts. They modified some principles and interpreted others until a large field was cleared for commercial enterprise, and the restrictions that remained were largely ignored or circumvented.' (Southern 1970 : 40)

There is an inescapable danger of settling this particular issue summarily by simply concluding that the feudal system gave way to the development of a market economy in preparation for the emergence of capitalism. Any such perfunctory simplifications must be qualified by the understanding that the changes so described developed over some four hundred years, were the result of a variety of enormous and complex social forces, and are the subject of considerable disagreement among specialist historians. The middle ages did not come to an end abruptly and there is a wide range of emphasis over the characteristics which marked significant change. Sombart 'if he were forced to give a single date for the "beginning" of modern capitalism ... would choose 1202, the year in which appeared the *Liber Abbaci* a primer of commercial arithmetic' (Heilbroner 1968 : 55f); Spengler emphasized the invention of double-entry bookkeeping in 1494; Tawney concentrated upon changes in the sixteenth century as marking the 'rise of capitalism'. It is easy to oversimplify. There is a danger of suggesting that the Aquinian objection to usury and to trade as base 'in that it has not of itself any honest or necessary object' was briskly overcome by the protestant ethic. We shall follow this argument in the next chapter but it is worth remembering that Catholic theologians in France, well into the eighteenth century, continued to thunder that usury was 'a vice detested by God and condemned by the Church', that usury is 'a species of robbery and derives from it as a stream from its source' (Groethuysen 1968 : 202, 203).

Change on this scale is the result (if that is not, already, too deterministic a conclusion) of a conjunction of a variety of forces which themselves took hundreds of years to develop. The scale of events is not that of ordinary history but must be compared with the change from one geological period to its successor; a change so slow that it cannot be perceived, but which undeniably took place because the world was transformed by it. The reduction of Europe's population by plague contributed to the end of feudalism because it encouraged the commutation of feudal services for money, which itself helped to promote a money economy and the development of free labour (and, therefore, of the concept of labour itself). These changes encouraged changes in agriculture which are summarized in the movement for enclosure. The development of a money economy was assisted by increasing supplies of gold and silver from German and Austrian mines and by the influx of treasure following Spanish conquests in the New World. These conquests indirectly assisted the independence and commercial freedom of the Low Countries which was to help 'to make Antwerp the base for financial operations of unexampled magnitude and complexity' (Tawney 1948 : 84). On a lesser scale the development of towns demanded and made profitable the organization of markets and the growth of industries. At the same time the protectionist attitude of the towns to 'foreign' trade 'forced the territorial State to the fore as the instrument of ''nationalization'' of the market and the creator of internal commerce ... Deliberate action of the state in the fifteenth and sixteenth centuries foisted the mercantile system on the fiercely protectionist towns and principalities' (Polanyi 1944 : 65).

Positive forces of development may help to explain the transformation of the mediaeval world; negative forces of decay may help to explain its decline. There is some argument among historians as to whether the later middle ages were poor or prosperous. The disagreement seems partly to be resolved by a tendency for English historians to concentrate upon expansion and for French historians to dwell upon decline after the Hundred Years' War, but a less chauvinistic explanation suggests that both development and decline were taking place in different regions at the same time. Mediaeval Europe certainly suffered from a sequence of cataclysms which might have been enough in themselves to end one world in preparation for the development of the next: 'from the beginning or second quarter of the fourteenth century until the second quarter or middle of the fifteenth, a series of disasters occurred which led the economy and society through many crises towards the forms which they assumed in modern times'. Du Boulay (1970 : 170-2) goes on to catalogue these disasters following the plagues:

'There were deadly famines causing villages to be abandoned by the thousand ... Cultivated land which had been won from waste and woodlands by centuries of effort, reverted to fallow and pasture. The Bordeaux vineyards exported only a tenth of their early fourteenth century production. The countryside was continually overrun by bands of adventurers ... There were sudden peasant risings sparked off by distress, an unmistakable stiffening of the exploitation of the peasants by the lords and a continual fall in agricultural prices. Industries declined or disappeared ... trading or banking companies failed, the currency was debased and monetary stocks exhausted.'

It is not our purpose to attempt some superficial explanation or summary of mediaeval economic history because such an attempt would be ridiculous and ill-informed. It is necessary, on the other hand, to take some account of descriptions of changes in the economic background of the middle ages which transformed a stable agricultural society so that a 'naturalistic political arithmetic' came to replace theology.

'When the age of the Reformation begins, economics is still a branch of ethics, and ethics of theology; all human activities are treated as falling within a single scheme, whose character is determined by the spiritual destiny of mankind; the appeal of theorists is to natural law, not to utility; the legitimacy of economic transactions is tried by reference, less to the movements of markets, than to moral standards derived from the traditional teaching of the Christian Church.' (Tawney 1948 : 272)

The destruction of this transcendence of spiritual over economic values and of the emergence of a high regard for the virtues of work will occupy us in the next chapter. During our excursion into mediaeval economic history, precious little has been said about work. This is because, as with the Greeks, there is very little available concerning the attitudes to work adopted by any level of society, by lords, or guildsmen, or peasants. There is a great deal about the content of work, about the extent of week-work, about artisans' changes of occupation at harvest time, about food, drink, and clothing. But there is no evidence of an ideology.

The explanation lies in the ground that has been covered. It grows out of St Thomas's doctrine of the harmony of the Christian commonwealth in which every class did its own 'proper work'. The social, political, and spiritual system are harmonious as long as each member plays the part allotted to him. No aspect of human affairs could be isolated for special attention, especially one which, at the base of a theological system and still carrying Aristotelian connotations of contempt, seemed furthest from spirituality. The Church had elevated work and the worker from the base position accorded to him by Aristotle, but there were limits to how seriously they should be taken. The worker might contribute to the mutual exchange of services for the sake of a good life, but the good life was the end and it was not to be measured in ergonomic or economic terms. The church developed a new doctrine of the importance of work but strictly as an instrument of spiritual purpose. The Benedictine rule emphasized the spiritual danger of idleness and ordered regular work at fixed times of the day in order to reduce it. The church also recommended labour as a penance on good scriptual authority emanating from man's fall. Work was a discipline, it contributed to the Christian virtue of obedience. It was not seen as noble, or rewarding, or satisfying, its very endlessness and tedium were spiritually valuable in that it contributed to Christian resignation. The distinction between labour as a spiritual discipline and labour as a means was made clearly by Groote in the fourteenth century, 'labour is wonderfully necessary to mankind in restoring the mind to purity ... Labour is holy, but business is dangerous' (Southern 1970 : 348).

Work was not a special subject, it was a part of the general social and spiritual framework. Work was done out of necessity, because it was ordered so by a natural cycle and by God. The popular agitations of the time were probably not radical in any contemporary sense and did not aim at a different order in which workers would take a different place: 'to be told that social disorders take place because an envious proletariat aims at seizing the property of the rich would seem to them a very strange perversion of the truth. They want only to have what they have always had. They are conservatives, not radicals or levellers, and to them it seems that all the trouble arises because the rich have been stealing the property of the poor' (Tawney 1912 : 333).

Until the speed of economic change became so great as to carry all along with it, until it revealed the irrelevance of traditional doctrine and demanded the construction of a new ideology, the agitators could draw support from their betters. They could ask for the assistance of authority because authority was under attack and authority could respond with a passionate defence of the poor (like Sir Thomas More) or with attempts to slow down the rate of change (by acts against enclosure). Both reformers and conservatives had custom and authority on their side; 'In the middle of the sixteenth century the English peasants accepted the established system of society with its hierarchy of authorities and division of class functions, and they had a most pathetic confidence in the crown' (Tawney 1912 : 339).

What we have done so far is to sketch out a background which, as it includes the distinct civilizations and histories of Greece, Roman and mediaeval Europe, contains many different and irreconcilable features. But it is possible to speak of some kind of cultural inheritance which related the three. Roman culture borrowed heavily from Greek: translated Greek theology and employed Greek teachers. Christian doctrine and mediaeval theory looked back to Roman law and to Aristotle. And there was an element noticeably absent through this development, an element which we cannot imagine as separate from our own outlook; economic calculation, the concept of material value, its production and measurement.

There always have been economic men, of course. The Roman empire was a monument to material acquisition and display. But perhaps what divided the Greeks and the Romans was that Greeks did not care about what they did not have, and Romans did not have to care about what they had (by conquest) in such abundance.

2. The Protestant Ethic

I *The Foundation of the Official Ideology*

We are concerned here with the construction of economic man. Economic men, as we have concluded, have always existed but the construction of economic man as a concept was new. The concept and its survival explains why the boundaries of our own perception and the values which underlie our own society are almost entirely set in economic terms, why even the most radical critics and the most conservative advocates of capitalism have, for the most part, no difficulty in understanding each other because they share an economic vocabulary and economic values. Communists and capitalists merely disagree about control of the machine and the distribution of its product. The transcendence of economic man required an enormous shift in attitudes and beliefs. It required the almost total dismantling of the mediaeval and classical system of thinking, their concepts, understanding, and perceptions. In order to change the world it was necessary to change men's understanding of it.

There is, in fact, a considerable dispute as to which changed first, the world or men's understanding. The materialist view taken by Marx is that all thought is correlative and dependent upon economic relationships, in which case capitalist theory, and religious beliefs appropriate to capitalist development, follow changes in economic structure and behaviour.

The alternative view, of which Max Weber is probably the most distinguished representative, is that the explosion of economic activity signifying the development of capitalism required, and was partially caused by, the emergence of a spirit of capitalism which emanated from the protestant reformation. Like all debates concerning the precedence of chicken or egg, the discussion always seems interminable because it must be inconclusive. It is important for us to examine Weber's account, however, because although we do not have to accept his explanation of the development of capitalism, an important subsidiary part of his argument concerns changes in the ideology of work. It might be more accurate to say that the argument concerns not so much changes in as the construction of an ideology of work.

Like all important and influential works, Weber's *The Protestant Ethic and the Spirit of Capitalism* has often been misinterpreted. Weber specifically refuted the idea that it is catholic other-worldliness that suppresses the spirit of capitalism, and protestant materialism that encourages it. He also denied that he was attempting to establish protestantism as the sole cause of the development of capitalism. The spirit of capitalism involves, he says, a philosophy of avarice 'which appears to be the ideal of the honest man of recognised credit, it is an ethic rather than a mere rule of business, in which the increase of capital is assumed as an end in itself, in which economic acquisition is no longer subordinated to man as the means for the satisfaction of his material needs' (Weber 1967 : 50).

Opposition to the new ethos comes from traditionalistic attitudes which can be found even in some forms of business enterprise. Weber describes with nostalgic affection the life of a putter-out in the textile trade. He led a comfortable existence, he worked from five to six hours a day, his earnings were moderately high, he led a respectable life enjoying good relationships with his competitors. 'A long daily visit to the tavern, with often plenty to drink, and a congenial circle of friends, made life comfortable and leisurely' (Weber 1967 : 67). This kind of business was destroyed by the new man who either turned peasants into labourers, changed their methods of marketing, adapted the quality of the product to meet the needs and wishes of the customers, introduced low prices for a large turnover. The old life, says Weber, gave way 'to a hard frugality in which some participated and came to the top, because they did not wish to consume but to earn' (Weber 1967 : 68).

Traditionalist qualities reside also in the worker. Early in the nineteenth century, Gaskell gave an idealized account of the typical domestic manufacturer that could have been written as partner to Weber's description of the merchant. He

'commonly lived to a good round age, worked when necessity demanded, ceased his labour when his wants were supplied, according to his character, and if disposed to spend time or money in drinking, could do so in a house as well conducted and as orderly as his own "belonging to a publican" whose reputation depended upon good ale and good hours ... who, in nine cases out of ten, was a freeholder of some consequence in the neighbourhood.' (Gaskell 1836 : 29)

But traditionalistic qualities in the worker are obstacles in the way of the development of capitalism. The purpose of piecework payment is to maximize output, but improvements in the piece-rate may result in less rather than more work because, says Weber,

'the opportunity of earning more was less attractive than that of working less. He did not ask: how much can I earn in a day if I do as much work as possible? but, how much must I work in order to earn the average ... which I earned before and which takes care of my traditional needs ... Whenever modern capitalism has begun its work of increasing the productivity of human labour by increasing its intensity, it has encountered the immensely stubborn resistance of this leading trait of pre-capitalist labour.' (Weber 1967 : 60)

One solution to the problem is to reduce rates to make the worker work harder in order to stand still. [2] But low wages, as every manager knows, are not necessarily cheap wages. Where skill is required 'labour must be performed as if it were an absolute end in itself, a calling'. This is not a natural state of affairs, however, it 'can only be the product of a long and arduous process of education' (Weber 1967 : 62).

The concept of a calling, of a life-task set by God, is the product of the reformation. There is no direct authority in the Bible for such an idea, says Weber. The notion of a calling is, if anything, refuted by Jesus in the Prayer 'Give us this day our daily bread'. The New Testament, at least, regarded worldly activity with indifference or hostility. This, says Weber, was also Luther's initial position, he regarded the pursuit of material gain beyond the level of need as a sign of the absence of grace. But, as Luther became more involved in temporal affairs, 'he came to value work in the world more highly' although he never abandoned a traditional view that we should work well in the station in which God has placed us.

It was Calvin, says Weber, who supplied the interpretation of a calling that was essential to the development of capitalism and has become symbolized in the phrase 'the protestant ethic' of work. Lutherans believed that a state of grace could be lost and won back again. Calvinists believed that some men, a minority, 'are predestined unto everlasting life, and others are ordained to everlasting death'; to assume otherwise would entail the contradiction that God's eternal decrees were open to reversal by human influence. There was no means of knowing, according to Calvin, whether anyone was of the elect or doomed because there were no external and visible differences that could be perceived in this life.

If we stopped here, of course, we would still be at some distance from the steps necessary to establish a work ethic. So, at this point, Weber has to ascribe to Calvinism characteristics of belief that were specifically denied by Calvin. His doctrine was altogether too difficult to be applied in practice and, says Weber, it was changed by pastoral advice, so that it was held to be an absolute duty to regard oneself as chosen and to regard doubts on the matter as temptation. The Calvinist was also enjoined to a life of discipline and good works, not as a means of attaining salvation, for nothing could do that, but partly in order to reduce doubt and partly as a sign to others of salvation. If one could do nothing to improve one's chance in the next world one could at least convince others and oneself that the chances were good.

Weber goes on to take as an example of puritanism in general, rather than Calvinism in particular, the seventeenth-century English Presbyterian and author of the *Christian Directory*, Richard Baxter. Baxter thundered against the danger of wealth — that it led to idleness — against 'loss of time through sociability, idle talk, luxury or more sleep than is strictly necessary'. 'Along with a moderate vegetable diet and cold baths, the same prescription is given for all sexual temptations as is used against religious doubts ... Work hard in your calling'. Work is no longer a necessity, as it was to Catholics and even to Luther, it is a positive thing to be done well for the glory of God and the preservation of the individual's soul (Weber 1967 : 158, 159).

While puritanism emphasized work and gave religious sanction to the pursuit of profit, it prohibited the enjoyment of the wealth which it encouraged, 'when the limitation of consumption is combined with this release of acquisitive activity, the inevitable practical result is obvious: accumulation of capital through the ascetic compulsion to save'. So, Weber concludes, the puritan outlook favoured the development of a rational bourgeois economic life, 'it was most important, and above all the only consistent influence in the development of that life. It stood at the cradle of modern economic man' (Weber 1967 : 172, 174).

It performed one other important function, it contributed to the recruitment and to the education of a willing labour force. Religious asceticism, apart from enabling the businessman to make money with a good conscience, also provided him 'with sober, conscientious, and unusually industrious workmen, who clung to their work as to a life purposed willed by God' (Weber 1967 : 177). Baxter specifically recommended the employment of godly servants, 'a truly Godly servant will do all your service in obedience to God, as if God himself had bid him do it', the less godly are inclined 'to make a great matter of conscience of it' (Weber 1967 : 281f). The engagement of God as the supreme supervisor was a most convenient device; a great part of the efforts of modern management has been aimed at finding a secular but equally omnipotent equivalent in the worker's own psyche.

The same alternatives, between external coercion and internal motivation, presented themselves as solutions to what Walzer (1966 : 203) describes as one of the main social problems in the transformation of feudal to modern society, 'how were men to be reorganised, bound together in social groups, united for co-operative activity'. Hill (1964 : 124) sees the problem of the seventeenth century as that of any backward economy — 'failure to use the full human resources of the country'. If the country was to begin an economic advance, he continues, an ideology advocating regular systematic work was required (op.cit. : 125). Walzer suggests there were alternative approaches to the general disorder (1966 : 204), Hobbes looked for absolute power to curb what would become a war of all against all, 'Puritans searched instead for obedient and conscientious subjects'.

Economic, religious, and political considerations seemed to converge on requiring a new man to emerge. Conservatives continued to look back nostalgically upon a mediaeval age, becoming more golden as it became more distant. Puritans condemned it and its aftermath. Richard Morison recommended hard work as 'a remedy for sedition' (Hill 1964 : 127). Work and its many virtues were often identified with the industrious (and Calvinist) Dutch, and even more frequently identified with puritanism. Popery drew people to idleness while protestantism and a multitude of beggars were mutually exclusive.

Hill argues that a new discipline of work was necessary to solve the problems of the seventeenth-century society. Walzer suggests that one method by which puritans created a new discipline was by stressing vocation as a means of social contract.

'The new view of work and the rhetorical violence of the accompanying critique of idleness formed the concrete basis of the Puritan repudiation of the old order. God honoured men as he honoured angels; in proportion to their serviceableness — that is, to their zealous application, their skill, and their effectiveness. And he organised men as he organised angels, through a division of labour, in a chain of command. *All men must work*, gentlemen and commoners alike.' (Walzer 1966 : 209)

Times had changed, Hill (1964 : 141) quotes a contemporary writer's command that 'no one should live merely in the calling of a gentleman. This was a profession so abused to advance sin and Satan's Kingdom as nothing more'.

Work had every advantage. It was good in itself. It satisfied the selfish economic interest of the growing number of small employers or self-employed. It was a social duty, it contributed to social order in society and to moral worth in the individual. It contributed to a good reputation among one's fellows and to an assured position in the eyes of God. Work was becoming a standard, cliché, cure-all. It was even said to have that supreme moral advantage peculiarly attractive to the English and found in their long tradition of hard work and cold baths; according to Walzer (1966 : 211) William Whately stressed the importance of keeping busy if one was to avoid committing adultery (and, presumably, one was to so avoid it), 'for pains in a calling will consume a great part of that superfluous nourishment that yields matter to this sin. It will turn the blood and spirits another way.'

Puritans stressed the great importance of contracts and of order in business. They also, says Hill (1964 : 130) began to develop and to emphasize the importance of time: 'The Puritan horror of waste of time helped not only to concentrate effort, to focus attention on detail, but also to prepare for the rhythms of an industrial society, our society of the alarm clock and the factory whistle'. One seventeenth-century writer, after carefully accounting for the amount of time wasted in sleep every week, recommended its reduction by the avoidance of mid-day snoozes. Even thoughts had to be disciplined: 'thoughts' said Thomas Goodwin 'are vagrants, which must be diligently watched for, caught, examined, whipped and sent on their way' (Hill 1964 : 131).

Some of the consequences of this new ideology of work would have surprised its proponents. Once work is dignified, it is a short and almost inevitable step to dignifying the worker, and when work is set up for enthusiastic comparison with idleness it is difficult to avoid admiration for the worker and contempt for the idle. This meant an inversion of established values, in the context of the times; to have got so far is to entail democracy, even revolution. Hill quotes seventeenth-century writers who point in this direction: 'they that apply themselves to labour for their living do eat their own bread and are profitable to others, whereas those stately idle persons are driven to put their feet under other men's tables and their hands into other men's dishes'. Since God 'doeth prefer the poor, despised, industrious, laborious and giveth His voice for their precedence, why should we give titles to ruffians and roisterers' (Hill 1964 : 140).

Hill concludes that the emphasis on work was likely to lead to the final conclusion that property was justified by work and was not justified without it, so that idleness' should be followed by expropriation.

This radical notion grows out of the protestant ethic as surely as does the spirit of capitalism. The new doctrine of the importance of work could develop in two directions. The first development, the official doctrine, emphasized effort in a calling, abstinence, and thrift; it led to capitalist acquisition and the spread of business enterprise. The second, the radical doctrine, emerges in socialism and communism. Although these doctrines are usually presented as extreme alternatives to capitalism they are not as different as may be supposed. Although demanding the absolute rejection of capitalism they differ from it largely in the extent to which they exaggerate, rather than deny, those characteristics of the protestant ethic from which capitalism springs.

The first is abstinence from display and from self-indulgence. The moderation in personal expenditure so necessary to capitalist accumulation of savings becomes, in the alternative doctrine, the abolition of private property and the total negation of self-indulgence. The second, the ascendancy of rational economic calculation, reaches a level in socialist thinking which exceeds its achievement in capitalism. The third, the primacy of work, becomes, in the alternative ideology, the central pivot of the conceptual system, carrying with it the idealization of the worker; in capitalism it remains an instrumental necessity. If we look at the radical ideology as developing from the same source and if we look at it in terms of those essential characteristics, we see it not so much as the opponent of capitalism but as its idealization; in the later forms the radical ideology sought changes in society in order to facilitate a pure expression of characteristics which could find only imperfect expression in capitalism. So, we shall argue later that socialist versions of the work ideology are capitalism set free of its impurities.

The truly revolutionary change came with the emergence, first, of an ideology of work accompanying the development of the protestant ethic. If we regard this as the major cleavage between the traditionalistic, classical outlook and the new puritan ideology, the subsequent conflict between incipient capitalism and incipient communism appears as a minor schism within the new orthodoxy.

II *The Foundation of the Radical Ideology of Work*

It is certainly possible to see the roots of communism as well as capitalism in the seventeenth century. Two groups in seventeenth-century England, the Levellers and the Diggers, are often presented as 'companion pieces' representing democratic and socialist radicalism. They can equally well be seen as standing for the two sides in the division opening within protestantism.

The existence of two trends within protestantism has been noted before. The first, stern tradition comes down from Calvin, is associated with predestination, prizes work and thrift as signs of election, and is often intolerant of poverty. In this tradition, where charity is permissible it must be accorded only to moral worth (to the deserving poor) or as a spiritual investment to enable the poor to join the elect — or, more strictly, to enable them to show evidence of election; their spiritual condition cannot be changed. This attitude finds consistent expression in the moral assumptions, underlying Victorian social Darwinism and self-help. It was a tradition that seemed capable of reconciling an apparently self-interested materialism with an intensely spiritual preoccupation which licensed business zeal. Both Tawney and Weber have argued that it contributed a spiritual and emotional foundation which was necessary to the development of capitaism.

The Leveller movement was probably one of the more important of the politically dissenting minorities to emerge on the Commonwealth side during the Civil War. Its leader, John Lilburne, began as a major in Cromwell's army and, after various periods of exile and imprisonment, ended as a prisoner in Dover Castle in 1657 (more accurately, he died at the end of a ten-day period of parole from Dover). It is difficult to find anything sufficiently radical in their teaching to justify such harassment by a radical regicide government. 'The Levellers were individualists, rather than collectivists, and fought primarily for the rights of the *petite bourgeoisie*' (Gibb 1947 : 15). They asked for reforms that would safeguard civil and personal liberty, and they wanted a bill of rights to guarantee individual freedom.

The reforms that they demanded helped contribute to a political theory that was consistent with, even helpful to, the development of the economic theory that was clearly emerging. In addition to the purely political programme (which a Marxist might interpret as laying down the essential political framework for a completely capitalist society), the Levellers specifically concerned themselves with economic changes. 'Among the rights to be respected and safeguarded ... is the inviolability of property. Already the Leveller notions of reform pretty clearly suggested the programme characteristic of radical democracy: the separation, as complete as may be, of political action from interference with the working of the economic system' (Sabine 1941 : 4).

Political freedom and economic freedom were both essential to the development of an economic society. The Levellers believed that each element had theological sanction. Gerard Winstanley and the Diggers on the other hand represent a more extreme tradition which was to emerge from puritanism, a tradition which would relate less easily to the established order of things. The Diggers got their name when they took possession of common land on St Georges Hill in 1649 and, with dual symbolism, began to dig it on a Sunday, intending to give the produce of cultivating it to the poor. Their beginnings were characteristic. The Levellers had been concerned largely with political reform, the Diggers believed that no political change was of any substance or permanence unless it was accompanied by social changes. The Restoration, as G.M. Trevelyan said, suggested that they were right.

The Diggers were among the more extreme of the factions to emerge after the Civil War. Their leader, Gerard Winstanley, was a mystic whose vague and undoctrinal theism led him to the conviction that life and society must be transformed. He was against churches and clericalism as based on a false learning, 'false in its learned pretensions and, what is worse, pernicious in its social consequences' (Sabine 1947 : 68). He came close to defining the 'divining spiritual doctrine' as the opium of the people. It was, he said, 'a cheat. For while men are gazing up into heaven, imagining after a happiness or fearing a hell after they are dead, their eyes are put out, that they see not what is their birthright, and what is to be done by them here on earth while they are living' (Sabine 1947 : 69).

The birthright certainly did not include the ownership of property or freedom of enterprise and individual initiative; 'initiative and enterprise seemed to him fine names for greed and cunning. It seemed to him impossible that a free and peaceful society could be held together by the impulses that were responsible for aggression and war' (Sabine 1941 : 4). The acquisitive and combative tendencies were set off by a continuous war with co-operative forces in man. Although the conflict was close, the success of co-operation is represented by the success of family life, and it is this which makes human life possible and holds society together. Co-operation and mutual aid, said Winstanley, must be deliberately extended beyond the limited relationships of the family to a wider range of human relationships, so that it can establish a society which is equitable, democratic, and rational.

To achieve this state of affairs poverty had to be abolished because it was contradictory to talk of freedom and poverty co-existing. He went beyond this assertion to argue, as Marx did later, that political and legal oppression could not be eliminated alone by political reforms, they were both, he thought, manifestations of the 'relationships of property that put some men within the economic power of others' (Sabine 1941 : 5). It is an inherent part of his argument 'that English government is controlled by a class in its own interest, even though Parliament legally represents the nation' (Sabine 1941 : 55). His historical explanation for this state of affairs is that it began with the disaster of the Norman conquest when foreign exploitation triumphed over ancient English virtue; Winstanley is perhaps, one of the last English nationalists. The subsequent domination by a number of foreign landowners has been supported by the lawyers and the clergy. Winstanley's solution is the common ownership of the land, the most fundamental liberty for Englishmen is the right to use the land of England.

In *The Law of Freedom* (Sabine 1941) Winstanley presented his case for a communist society. Private property was to be abolished, all crops and manufactured goods were to be held in public store and distributed free on request to anyone who needed them. But this new society was not to be utopian in the sense that it would rely only on the goodwill of its inhabitants for its good order. It was to be regulated by rules and penalties which were to be enforced by officials. There were to be penalties against idleness, waste, and the refusal to practice a useful trade. The first level of enforcement was the father or master of a family, and co-operation, it seemed, was not to be entirely a matter of sweetness and light. The father 'is to command them their work, and see they do it, and not suffer them to live idle; he is either to reprove by words or whip those who offend, for the Rod is prepared to bring the unreasonable ones to experience and moderation' (Sabine 1941 : 545).

The second group of overseers, elected annually, was to concern itself with the regulation of trades. One overseer would supervise every twenty or thirty families in each trade. The overseer's job was 'to see that young people be put to Masters, to be instructed in some labout ... that none be idly brought up in any family within his Circuit' (Sabine 1941 : 548). The overseer was to supervise the learning of crafts within the family, to choose the skilled men, to supervise work, and to supervise the maintenance of tools, stores, and loans.

The criminal code was to be administered by judges who may sentence wrong-doers to lose their freedom. In this case the criminals come under the control of task-masters who make them work at any tasks decided by the task-masters.

'If they do their tasks, he is to allow them sufficient victuals and clothing to preserve the health of their bodies. But if they prove desperate, wanton, or idle ... the task-master is to feed them with short dyet, and to whip them, for a rod is prepared for the fool's back ... And if any of these offenders run away, there shall be hue and cry sent after him, and he shall dye by the sentence of the Judge when taken again.' (Sabine 1941 : 553-4)

The point of this digression into some of the lesser known tributaries of seventeenth-century dissent is not to explore their significance in the development of political or social theory. It is to suggest that from this point onwards, the ideology of work could develop in two directions. The first, the 'respectable' direction, is the development taken by the protestant ethic as it is delineated by Max Weber. This stresses work in relation to business, enterprise, and political freedom. The second, the radical direction, sets the line of development which ends in socialism and communism. The Levellers exemplify the first direction, Winstanley's Diggers the second.

It is worth stressing that despite the radicalism and anti-clericalism of Winstanley there is nothing to suggest that he is outside the new orthodoxy of work and effort. In fact he draws the lines of the new schism in the protestant ethic by taking the importance of work to a pinnacle which it had not reached before. Not only does he emphasize that political forms are meaningless unless they relate to economic foundations, he implies in *The Law of Freedom* that political changes are, in a sense, irrelevant. The proposals for reform which he makes in order to establish his utopian society unlike Lilburne's have nothing to do with the reform of political institutions or the extension of the suffrage. They do not concern politics at all. Winstanley is preoccupied with basing his reconstruction of society entirely on the organization of work. He is as good as saying: 'if work is properly organised, society will look after itself'.

This is the positive side of the argument for establishing Winstanley as one of the founders of the new schism within the protestant ethic, its radical as against its commercial wing. The negative side of the argument is that he did nothing to diminish the puritan emphasis on the moral importance of work. Radical he may have been but not to the extent of questioning the new orthodoxy, that work was important and was to be taken most seriously. While he questioned the temporal and spiritual authority of men, he certainly did not question the authority that the master was to exercise in work. In the world of work, apparently Winstanley thought discipline was not to be questioned.

This is an important point. The Diggers, while not numerically very significant, were among the most radical voices to be heard at a time of radical dissent. But they did not question the new orthodoxy that work mattered. Not only was the new orthodoxy to prevail without question for a very long time, but the zeal for work was to prove most useful to those whose commitment to a work ideology was more immediately self-interested. In this sense, Walzer argues that the transition to a modern society was brought about and made possible by the self-governing industriousness and discipline of the puritans. Taking up Marx's contention that the new discipline of the wage-system was forced upon a brutally recruited and coerced labour force of displaced beggars and peasants, Walzer (1966 : 230) contends that:

> 'Marx's description is true only because the mass of rural labourers and beggars were not yet ready to become the subjects of a systematic self control. But for that very reason they were not taught the "discipline" necessary to the wage system. They were brutally repressed, but they were not yet morally or physically transformed. The making of the English working class came much later, and along with it came ideologies parallel to that of the saints, similarly inculcating self-discipline and teaching a religious or political activism.'

In this sense, the radical Winstanley was to contribute to the ultimate success of the new orthodox ideology. For a final and formal version of his conception of the ultimate importance of work and of economic relationships we have to wait for Saint-Simon and Marx. At this stage we see only the establishment of a schism in which orthodoxy comes to be represented by the business version of the protestant ethic and dissent by radical movements aimed at changing and planning society. But the schism is between those who share a common fundamental belief in work and in economic values.

3. The Division of Labour

If capitalism and industrialization were the consequences of a protestant ethic they made the maintenance of a unified ideology of work impossible; in this sense they negate the concept from which they grew. It would hardly be an exaggeration to suggest that the major problem facing modern industrial and political organization has been the attempt to construct an effective ideology to overcome the results of industrialization. The problem, in particular, presents itself as the necessity of dealing with the division of labour in two senses, the detailed division of labour by function and by task (the consequences of which have come to be represented as the problem of anomy), and the social division of labour by class and by interest (which has come to be represented as the problem of alienation).

Problems, fortunately, do not present themselves in all their fearful complexity on first acquaintance and the great benefits of the principle of the division of labour seemed at first to be unmixed with disadvantage. This was in part because the advantages were presented in persuasive and scholarly terms by Adam Smith before the world had the opportunity to observe the problems which accompanied the factory production process.

Adam Smith, Professor of Moral Philosophy at Glasgow, published the *Wealth of Nations* in 1776. Many people would probably regard him as the inventor of economic man and as the delineator of the complex relationship between economic forces which remains effective only so long as it is uncontrolled. He described in terms of great perception and clarity, the processes of specialization which were at work in factory production. He has become generally identified with the advocacy of capitalist economic theory and of industrial manufacturing and he is often regarded as a founding father of the *laissez-faire* policies, and so is sometimes judged to be guilty by association with the heartless atrocities which those policies produced.

In so far as this description of his popular standing is accurate it does not do him justice. He was described as 'a man of tender feelings and great refinement of character' (Gide and Rist 1948 : 69) and, more to the point, he demonstrates in his work a deep suspicion of the whole class of manufacturers for whom he reserved some of his sharpest and most sardonic comments. The tone of much of his book suggests that he no more approved of much of the phenomena he so brilliantly described than would a clinical pathologist. He developed, before Marx, something like a labour theory of value and he clearly regarded the people who do productive work as the chief foundation of any society.

In terms of its economic fabric, he says, society is very complex and interdependent: 'without the assistance and co-operation of many thousands the very meanest person in a civilized country could not be provided, even according to what we falsely imagine, the easy and simple manner in which he is commonly accommodated' (Smith 1828 : 26). But we do not get this assistance and co-operation from others because of a benevolent regard for each other's welfare, this interdependence rests upon a nice balance of self-interest.

'Man has almost constant occasion for the help of his brethren and it is in vain for him to expect it from their benevolence only. He will be more likely to prevail if he can interest their self-love in his favour, and show them that it is for their own advantage to do for him what he requires of them ... It is not from the benevolence of the butcher, the brewer, or the baker, that we expect our dinner, but from their regard to their own interest.' (Smith 1828 : 27)

The motive force for the economic machine is self-interest. But it requires the introduction of the principle of the division of labour before it can be effectively transmitted to work. In its broadest sense this means, as Plato saw, a general division of tasks among men, but whereas Plato justified this division by reference to differences in talent and ability Adam Smith specifically denies the importance and extent of these differences. He takes a remarkably environmental, even egalitarian line:

'The difference of natural talents in different men is, in reality, much less than we are aware of, and the very different genius which appears to distinguish men of different professions, when grown up to maturity, is not upon many occasions so much the cause as the effect of the division of labour. The difference between the most dissimilar character, between a philosopher and a common street porter, for example, seems to arise not so much from nature as from habit, custom and education.' (Smith 1828 : 28)

This is a remarkable view for the time, or for any other time. It is the antithesis of any sort of justification for the *status quo* in terms of natural selection, and it must lead to the conclusion that things are as they are by chance.

The detailed division of labour is carried to its highest point in industrial production, says Smith. It is a most important principle because it explains and is required by increases in productive capacity, it is most developed in the most advanced countries. The division of labour is effective because it combines three advantages: it leads to an increase in the dexterity of workmen, it leads to the saving of time by avoiding the workers having to move from one place to another, and it leads to the development of machines 'which facilitate and abridge labour'. He illustrates the application and the advantages of the principle of the division of labour by the famous description of pin-making (Smith 1828 : 20).

The direct return for the individual's part in such a process would be small; we would not receive very much for our part in the production of twelve pounds of pinheads. We are generally sustained by other people's labour, a man is 'rich or poor according to the quantity of that labour which he can command, or which he can afford to purchase ... Labour, therefore, is the real measure of the exchangeable value of all commodities' (Smith 1828 : 38). In an ideal state of affairs the wages paid to labour would equal its product: 'In that original state of things which precedes both the appropriation of land and the accumulation of stock, the whole produce of labour belongs to the labourer. He has neither landlord nor master to share with him' (Smith 1828 : 64). But the actual state of affairs is neither original nor ideal: 'As soon as land becomes private property the landlord demands a share of almost all the produce which the labourer can either raise or collect from it' (Smith 1828 : 65). The natural return to labour is reduced by two substantial deductions, rent and profit.

Smith gives a severe account of the considerations that determine the actual extent of a man's wages; they concern the amount to assure the survival not only of the man but of his species of producer. 'A man must always live by his work and his wages must at least be sufficient to maintain him — they must even on most occasions be somewhat more; otherwise it would be impossible for him to bring up a family and the race of such workmen could not last beyond the first generation' (Smith 1828 : 67).

One gets the strong impression in passages like this one, that Smith is using a forbidding and rigorous process of logic to reach more amiable conclusions which are held by him because they are sympathetic to his personality. He ends this particular passage, which sets out from such Athenian premises, by reaching the very humane conclusion that labour should be of moderate duration, carried on by free-men who are well paid. The arguments he uses to get there are of the kind that seem intended to convince a particularly heartless cost accountant. It is as though we argued for the abolition of the death penalty on the ground of the excessive expense of rope. This is how his argument proceeds:

'The wages paid to journeymen and servants of every kind must be such as may enable them one with another, to continue the race of journeymen and servants ... But though the wear and tear of a free servant should be equally at the expense of his master, it generally costs him much less than that of a slave. The fund destined for replacing or repairing, if I may say so, the wear and tear of the slave is commonly managed by a negligent master or careless overseer. That destined for performing the same office with regard to the free man is commonly managed by the free man himself ... the work done by the free man comes cheaper in the end than that performed by slaves.' (Smith 1828 : 77)

The free worker should be paid high wages because just as they result from increasing wealth so they lead to increasing population; to complain about high wages 'is to lament over the necessary effect and cause of the greatest public prosperity' (Smith 1828 : 78).

Smith does not advocate unbridled economic motivation, on the contrary, he argues that wages may be too effective as incentives so that they can have injurious effects on workers. 'Excessive application during four days of the week is frequently the real cause of the idleness of the other three, so much and so loudly complained of. Great labour, either of mind or body, continued for several days together, is in most men naturally followed by great desire of relaxation ... which is almost irresistible' (Smith 1828 : 79).

The conclusions for this last passage are similar to those reached later by Engels, although the tone is more temperate and the style more distinguished. It also shows a degree of psychological perception markedly absent from the work of economists who regarded themselves as following Smith's trail.

He was just as rightminded and well-intentioned in his description of the process by which wages are settled in practice. He has absolutely nothing to do with the theme of common interest which has been so unctuously worked out in more modern times. 'What are the common wages of labour depends everywhere upon the contract usually made between those two parties, whose interests are by no means the same. The workmen desire to get as much, the masters to give as little as possible. The former are disposed to combine in order to raise, the latter in order to lower the wages of labour' (Smith 1828 : 66).

Smith was under no illusions about where the balance of advantage lay in this process and he was free from the cant, to become so popular later, about contracts over wages between free and equal parties:

'It is not difficult to foresee which of the two parties must, upon all ordinary occasions, have the advantage in the dispute, and force the other into a compliance with their terms. The masters being fewer in number can combine much more easily ... In all such disputes the masters can hold out much longer ... In the long run the workman may be as necessary to his master as his master is to him; but the necessity is not so immediate'.

And we should not suppose, he adds, that because we know only of workmen's combinations, because they are so vociferously deplored by the masters, that the masters do not themselves combine: whoever thinks this

'is as ignorant of the world as of the subject. To combine to prevent the raising of wages is the usual, and one may say the natural state of things. Masters, too, sometimes enter into particular combinations to sink the wages of labour ... These are always conducted with the utmost silence and secrecy, till the moment of execution, and when the workmen yield, as they sometimes do, without resistance, though severely felt by them, they are never heard of by other people.' (Smith 1828 : 66)

Adam Smith's perception of motive and behaviour was remarkably clear, his judgements were usually humane and his sympathies often partially concealed behind a cover of irony. But the ingredients of his argument were dangerous. They concern the comparison of costs through (human) wear and tear, the rigorous application of the principle of self-interest to reach the conclusion that a free man is a better investment than a slave because a slave's preservation is managed by someone else, and therefore necessarily less effectively managed than by a free-man looking after himself. His conclusions may have been admirable but the technique by which he reached them was dangerously available for misuse. His sentiments may have been essentially moral but his defence of them can be seen as the triumph of economic measurement which Tawney argued had begun to reach its ascendency in the sixteenth century and which led to the final defeat and collapse of morality in the nineteenth. The deployment of and the dependence on arguments of economic self-interest to reach morally justifiable conclusions are always dangerous; it may lead to purely selfish conclusions which are then unassailable. There is little doubt that Smith helped to establish the primacy of economic rationalism which, once achieved, led to conclusions which seemed morally indefensible because they were based on totally amoral assumptions.

The effects of this process were nowhere more clearly shown that in the systematic exploitation of child labour to which factory production led. Mantoux (1948 : 420-23) says that the employment of children was preferred in spinning because:

'Their weakness made them docile, and they were more easily reduced to a state of passive obedience than grown men. They were also very cheap. Sometimes they were given a trifling wage, which varied between a third and a sixth of an adult wage; and sometimes their only payment was food and lodging. Lastly they were bound to the factory by indentures of apprenticeship, for at least seven years and usually until they were twenty one ... the fate of these parish apprentices in the early spinning mills was particularly miserable. Completely at the mercy of their employees, kept in isolated buildings, far from anyone who might take pity on their sufferings, they endured a cruel servitude. Their working day was limited only by their complete exhaustion and lasted, fourteen, sixteen and even eighteen hours. The foreman, whose wages were dependent on the amount of work done in each workshop, did not permit them to relax their efforts for a minute.'

Mantoux gives Robert Blincoe's account of a Nottingham factory where he was sent with eighty other boys and girls; they were constantly whipped, as a punishment, to make them work harder and to keep them awake. Elsewhere, children who tried to escape were put in irons. One girl who tried unsuccessfully to commit suicide was sent away because her employer 'was afraid the example might be contagious'. The owner of a silk mill in Hertfordshire killed himself in 1801 to escape criminal proceedings in which he was to be accused of literally starving his apprentices to death.

There are few who would now disagree with Thompson's (1968 : 384) judgement that 'the exploitation of little children, on this scale and with this intensity, was one of the most shameful events in our history'. Many of the exploiters took a different view. Manufacturers and their spokesmen took whatever devious and contradictory defence was available: they denied that bad conditions existed, if they did exist then the children enjoyed them, if they did not enjoy them then the conditions could not be improved. Andrew Ure's 'satanic advocacy' is so wholehearted and cheerful that it now reads like a parody of the work of a commited, lying propagandist.

Ure was very clear sighted, at least, about the purpose of machinery: it was 'to supersede human labour altogether, or to diminish its cost by substituting the industry of women and children for that of men; or that of ordinary labourers for trained artisans' (Ure 1861 : 23). The children apparently welcomed this substitution.

> 'I have visited many factories, both in Manchester and the surrounding districts, during a period of several months ... and I never saw a single instance of corporal chastisement inflicted on a child, nor indeed did I ever see children in ill-humour. They seemed to be always cheerful and alert, taking pleasure in the light play of their muscles — enjoying the mobility natural to their age. The scene of industry, so far from exciting sad emotions in my mind was always exhilarating ... The work of these lively elves seemed to resemble a sport in which habit gave them a pleasing dexterity.' (Ure 1861 : 301)

As Ure found existing conditions so admirable he naturally condemned any attempts to improve them. Of the Ten Hours Bill he said: 'It will certainly appear surprising to every dispassionate mind that ninety-three members of the British House of Commons could be found capable of voting that any class of grown-up artisans should not be suffered to labour more than ten hours a day — an interference with the freedom of the subject which no other legislature in Christendom would have countenanced for a moment' (Ure 1861 : 267). The Factories Regulation Act of 1833 forebade the employment in textile mills of children under nine and limited the hours of work of children under eleven to nine per day and of those under eighteen to twelve per day and sixty-nine per week. The Act also sought to ssure children of some hours of education every day. Ure was horrified. The

Act was an absurdity and, like all opponents of reform, he asserted that it flew in the face of fact and reality. It was 'an act of despotism towards the trade and of mock philanthropy towards the work-people who depend on trade for support', it would result in the dismissal of children and 'The children so discharged from their light and profitable labour, instead of receiving the education promised by Parliament, get none at all: they are thrown out of the warm spinning rooms upon the cold world, to exist by beggary and plunder — in idleness and vice'. He went on, 'The Act, under the mask of philanthropy, will aggravate still more the hardships of the poor, and extremely embarrass, if not entirely stop, the conscientious manufacturer in his useful toil' (quoted in Gaskell 1836 : 169-70).

The reference to the 'conscientious manufacturer' was not entirely ridiculous. The manufacturers' advocate, Andrew Ure, urged them to organize their 'moral machinery' on principles of efficiency comparable to those on which they based their mechanical machinery. Ure's description of the advantage of religion cannot be improved upon and it makes commentary unnecessary. The first great lesson of religion is

> 'that man must expect his chief happiness not in the present, but in a future state of existence. He alone who acts on this principle will possess his mind in peace under every sublunary vicissitude ... How speedily would the tumults which now agitate almost every class of society in the several states of Christendom subside, were that sublime doctrine cordially embraced as it ought to be! Without its powerful influence, the political economist may offer the clearest demonstrations of profit and loss ... without furnishing restraints powerful enough to stem the torrents of passion and appetite which roll over the nations.'

Ure is, at this point, recognizing without explicitly describing the distinction between theory and ideology; the most enthusiastic apologist of economic freedom is recognizing the inadequacy of economic theory as a motivator or controller of human behaviour, it is a distinction to which we shall return in the next chapter. What is needed, says Ure, is a motive force which can cause 'self-immolation for the good of others'. 'Where then shall mankind find this transforming power? — in the cross of Christ ... it atones for disobedience; it excites to obedience; it makes obedience practicable; it makes it acceptable; it makes it in a manner unavoidable, for it contrains to it; it is, finally, not only the motive force to obedience,

but the pattern of it' (Ure 1861 : 424-5). In practical down-to-earth
terms: 'Improvident work-people are apt to be reckless, and dissolute
ones to be diseased ... There is, in fact, no case to which the Gospel
truth "Godliness is great gain" is more applicable than to the
administration of an extensive factory' (Ure 1861 : 417).

There is no foreman like God, as we have observed before, and the
organization of the employers' moral machinery became a more and
more urgent requirement as labour appeared to become more clearly
separated from society by industrialization. The organization of the
moral machinery remains to this day a very good description of the
purpose of an ideology of work; the only development in the
twentieth century is that the machinery has been secularized.

The agency of moral organization in the nineteenth century was
religion. E.P. Thompson (1968 : 383) accounts for the role of the
Methodists in order to explain 'why it was their peculiar mission to act
as the apologists of child labour' and their invaluable alliance with the
manufacturers in erecting a moral barrier to discontent. The
explanation is complicated, requiring as it does an understanding of
'the full desolation of the inner history of nineteenth century
Nonconformity' (Thompson 1968 : 385). It seems to suggest a simple,
direct descent from Weber's association between protestant reform
and the spirit of capitalism to Methodism and its defence of factory
exploitation: the business religion becomes the religion of exploitation. The relationship is too neat to be accurate, of course, and it
poses a considerable problem in ideological ancestry, 'a problem to
which neither Weber nor Tawney addressed themselves' (Thompson
1968 : 391). The problem is that Methodism came to serve as the
religion of the industrial bourgeoisie, in direct succession to the
protestant ethic and the spirit of capitalism and, simultaneously as the
religion of the industrial proletariat. 'How was it possible for
Methodism to perform, with such remarkable vigour, this double
service? ... How then should such a religion appeal to the forming
proletariat in a period of exceptional hardship ... whose frugality,
discipline or acquisitive virtues brought profit to their masters rather
than success to themselves?' (Thompson 1968 : 391-2).

The utility of Methodism for the manufacturers, the usefulness of
their own allegiance to it, has often been explained. The utility of
their encouraging Methodism in their employees is also obvious. The
attractiveness of Methodism, on the face of it a contradictory
attractiveness, to the worker is vividly analysed by Thompson in *The*

Transforming Power of the Cross (1968 : Chapter 11). The explanation lies in a compound of indoctrination ('religious terrorism'), the provision of the fellowship of a close community in an otherwise disrupted society, and the appeal of an hysterical emotionalism provided by revivalist preachers.

There may have been other and more practical reasons why master and man should share the same religious doctrine. Religion could become a principle of personnel selection: like chose like, Methodist masters chose Methodist men (the accusation that this is so can still be heard laid against mine managers in south Wales and in the west of England; that the way to promotion lies through the chapel). Is it not also possible that the problem of a religion shared by antagonistic classes emerges, *post hoc*, because we transpose our own apprehension of a divided society in which the interests of master and man are so clearly opposed? The proletariat was, indeed, 'forming' and this was to lead to the development of the labour movement and to continual conflict with the employer. But in the period of formation there may have been no great contradiction in workers sharing their masters' religion. Masters were to be envied and envy could lead to emulation. There is no great contradiction in master and man sharing the same beliefs despite the wealth of the one and the poverty of the other, if those very beliefs are held to lead to success. This was the essential unity of outlook preached in *Self-help*, and it involves no obvious contradiction in an expanding economy as long as diligence and application do appear to be rewarded.

Methodism was an appropriate doctrine, as the inheritor of the protestant ethic, for the industrialist, and as the producer of 'those elements most suited to make up the psychic component of the work-discipline of which the manufacturers stood most in need' (Thompson 1968 : 390).

The inherited association between protestantism and capitalist industrialism emerges almost as clearly if we look at the contemporary opposition to exploitation, at the factory movement for reform. 'The Factory Movement was in many ways a strange agitation. Most of its founders, most of its parliamentary champions and most of its foremost leaders were Tories and Churchmen'. Professor Ward (1970 : 73) goes on to quote Oastler's description of 1835: 'If you chose I will take Yorkshire round, Town by Town; and in each Town, at Public Meetings, we will enquiry the names of 12 of the best masters and 12 of the worst ... and I will engage that, on the average, 9, at least of the

BEST will be Church-goers or Tories, and 9 of the WORST will be dissenting Whigs'. Professor Ward's judgement on this analysis is that 'If "best" and "worst" can be taken as meaning supporting or opposing factory reform, Oastler was undoubtedly right'. He concludes that 'The Factory Movement can only be described as Tory-Radical agitation, with the different components of the alliance varying in influence at different times'.

Professor Ward distinguishes four groups that were active in the demand for industrial reforms. They were the old labour aristocracies who were fighting in self-defence against industrialization; the pioneers of social medicine, northern clergymen who were 'predomin-antly Anglicans', and, lastly, Traditionalists, a group composed of writers, squires, landowners, and Young Englander Tories.

Once again we should be cautious about exaggerating the importance, in terms of the general thesis argued here, of the Anglican church and the gentry in this company. But their presence makes a characteristic and consistent opposition to Methodist support of industrialization. Oastler put the matter simply, opposition to the factories 'was a Soul-question — it was souls against pounds, shillings and pence' and the 'Clergy of the Church of England must either resist the Power of Mammon, or renounce their God'. George Bull believed that the Church of England had to be made the Poor Man's Church, and then the God of the Poor will bless us (Inglis 1971 : 296).

Historians often complain of the inattention to the Tory response to industrialism in the nineteenth century. But it is surely possible to see in those conclusions some evidence of the continuance of an old tradition, not dominated by the transcendent economic ethic and still able to oppose it from the independent basis of spiritual or traditionalistic values. The opposition came in part from Conservatives who could still claim to be speaking on behalf of the people of England before they themselves became totally inundated by industrialism which was to alienate them as thoroughly as it would the proletariat. It is, in fact, a most important question in the development of ideas about society as to whether this critical tradition represents the last protest of a disappearing pre-industrial age or whether it is the lively voice of conscience. The weight of Marxist tradition and scholarship claims that a society dominated by class interests is incapable of ambivalence or confusion, Marx pronounced, as we shall see, that 'the ideas of the ruling class are, in every age, the ruling ideas'. Thereafter, Marxists continue to assert that the ruling class speaks for itself and for the society it rules. The latest version in an increasingly complex process of presentation is the notion of hegemony, 'the predominance obtained by consent rather than force of one class or group over other classes … attained through the myriad ways in which the institutions of civil society operate to shape, directly or indirectly, the cognitive and affective structures whereby men perceive and evaluate problematic social reality' (Femia 1975 : 31). Gramsci said that the capitalist ruling class is represented by two groups of intellectual spokesmen, the organic (or technical and political representatives) and the traditional (whose role is specified in wider cultural and traditional terms), 'all ideas somehow serve the interests of one or another economic class' (Femia 1975). Traditional intellectuals may not begin by sharing the outlook of the ruling class, but they learn to compromise with it if only because compromise pays. The only independence can be found in the ideas of a new group or class rising to challenge the dominance of the ruling group by representing the new emerging productive forces. 'The chief institution for elaborating and discriminating the new proletarian culture is the Communist Party' (Femia 1975 : 39).

These more subtle formulations, although they are presented as transcending the crude materialism of earlier Marxist interpretations, continue to argue a version of cultural consistency or homogeneity. Hegemony means the general acceptance of ideas of the ruling class; it can only be challenged by a class rising to challenge and dominate in its turn. But the evidence of nineteenth century society in Britain suggests cultural dichotomy rather than hegemony. The critics of industrialization were vociferous, disparate in their interests, and often Christian. Were these critics, men like Southey, Wordsworth, Kingsley and Ruskin, simply survivors from a vanishing age? It is certainly difficult to relate them all as representatives of the proletariat, a proletariat which was still forming rather than rising. A great deal of ideological confusion has been caused by a consistent and influential Marxist claim that effective challenge to capitalism can come only from the proletariat or its intellectual champions. The weight of the influence has almost crushed into obscurity a quite distinctive critical tradition unless its representatives can be pressed into the service of the class war. The tradition was strong in the nineteeth century and has continued into the twentieth century. It may be that the only unifying force which binds it is the moral outrage of good men.

Religion was available to both sides but religion was not the only means of achieving a passive understanding among the labour force in the nineteenth century. Next to the 'transforming power of the Cross' was the attraction of the schoolroom, of education as a planned programme of docility and submission. 'The male spinners, even the most rude and uneducated ... always prefer children who have been educated at an infant school, as they are most obedient and docile' (Ure 1861 : 423). Like religion, education could be made to appear both attractive and a duty to the labourer and his family. It was unlikely to be seen as advantageous to the growing number of workers who could regard it as offering some practical improvement, as a means of betterment. Not all industrial workers were slaves or impoverished. The growth of the machine-tool industry created a new 'labour aristocracy', the engineers, well paid, well trained, with the ability and often the ambition to exercise managerial functions. The engineers were also the project of the industrial revolution but they were protected from its savageries and they owed their learning to its processes. Professor Harrison (1971 : 148) quotes a contemporary tribute to the Bradford Mechanics' Institute, given by John V. Godwin in 1859: 'Those who have watched the Bradford Mechanics' Institute are able to state that they have seen year after year an unbroken stream of youths, sons of working men, rising to positions of responsibility, which in all probability they never would have filled without its aid, and in many cases entering upon and pursuing a successful middle class career by the habits, the knowledge and the connections acquired in the Institute'.

We must not forget, in looking for the ideological foundations of discipline and obedience in the factories, that there were also some distinctly practical instruments available for getting workers to do what was wanted of them. Best (1971 : 274), discussing 'the effective agents of social subordination', lists the risk of unemployment and 'the citadel of the law, itself with several batteries aiming straight at the working classes'. Among these he lists the laws restricting trade union activity and, even more important, the law of master and servant: 'The great attraction to employers of the Master and Servant Law was its disciplinary convenience. Under the heading of an action for breach of contract, masters could prosecute men ... for many kinds of unacceptable behaviour, ranging from the real culpable things to disobeying even the most outrageous orders'.

Despite the available apparatus for achieving submission, observers on all sides saw the consequences of mechanization in terms of the emergence of a new class, oppressed and aware of its oppression, and, in a new sense, alienated. But it would be premature for us to pursue, at this point, the reaction which the social problems of industrialization and the division of labour produced; we shall pursue this development in some detail in chapter 7. We have not yet traced the evolution of the official ideology, as we called it, to its developed form. We can hardly credit Adam Smith with the development of an ideology of work that was consistent with factory production. Industrialism had not developed to anything like its full extent when he wrote the *Wealth of Nations* and, in any case, he showed signs of not approving some of its characteristics. Adam Smith gave a theoretical account which explained the machinery of the market and the behaviour of those engaged in. That is not the same thing as constructing an ideology that could comfort and sustain both masters and employees in the factories of the nineteenth and twentieth centuries. The ideologists would, however, not hesitate to seek the authority of his work to support passages in their own which required an appeal to authority to reinforce the weakness of their assertions.

What we have seen so far is the emergence of the problem. The problem consists of the complete change in the nature of industrial tasks, their performance under conditions of rigorous discipline, their concentration in factories and mills, the consequential isolation of the worker from his family and from a 'natural' environment, the extended application of the principle of the specialization of labour. Accompanying these technical and organizational changes in the nature of work were conditions of very severe social dislocation, the exploitation of child and female labour, the concentration of population in urban communities with primitive amenities, and the emergence of a self-conscious class of industrial workers. It is certainly not our purpose to trace the 'solution' to these problems in political terms or in terms of the making of a working class, in the growth of trade unions or the development of town planning. All these and other vast changes followed industrialization. Nothing was the same after factory production was established; we live in a world largely composed of solutions, mostly incomplete, to the problems of industrialization.

As far as we are concerned the problem is more specific. How could the new concepts of respect for work and for economic values survive in the face of conditions, which, as they were the more clearly perceived, must have made those notions appear the more ridiculous? How could an official ideology of work be developed that would comprehend industrialization?

4. The Official Ideology: *Lassez-Faire* and Self-help

We are now going to observe an interesting process of exchange which is essential to the formulation of a modern ideology of work. We have already argued that Adam Smith had constructed a conceptual framework which was capable of debasement by other, less considerable and less humane men. The first stage in the exchange process which followed was the destruction of any remaining ethical element in the new system of economic concepts. Professor Pollard (1965 : 196), describing the limited ethical code of the employers, commented that: 'The human element was merely to be manipulated as if it were an inert piece of machinery. In this sense, by treating human beings as means rather than ends, the essence of Christianity was denied and subverted by the new moralists.' But while a theoretical system may survive or require the abolition of ethics, an ideology which is to influence men's behaviour cannot afford such rigour; morality, or its imitation, is a great motivator. So we then see the construction of a 'moral machine' in which the ethical element is re-introduced. The re-introduction of ethics faced a considerable problem in having to be reconciled with a system which depended for its motive force on self-interest or, more bluntly, on selfishishness.

The resolution of this contradiction was bold; it required self-interest to be seen as a moral principle. Almost every other moral system has emphasized concern for others; Victorian business ideology was distinguished in its promotion of self-regard to a moral duty. Adam Smith begins by recording, often scornfully, that men behave selfishly. We end with the conclusion that men *should* behave selfishly. We have already observed that Smith bore little responsibility for this conversion except to the extent that, as he had defended self-interest on economic grounds, he had contributed to the destruction of an ethical or religious position from which it could be attacked.

Social conditions which accompanied industrialization certainly demanded some sort of practical concern for the welfare of the men and women who were subjected to them but the progress of ideological development largely prevented this concern from emerging. The search for sources of power and of labour required considerable movements of population and the development of large new urban centres with primitive amenities. Small and unimportant villages were required to accommodate city-size populations. The cholera epidemics of the 1830s and 1840s were one result. Those human needs which were able to create a commercial interest for their satisfaction were likely to be met, others were not. Any urban industrial community created in the nineteenth century, in Lancashire or in south Wales, for example, still carries characteristic marks; a large, uniform, and often substandard area of housing, a vast quantity of extant or one time public houses and a very small urban nucleus with a marked absence of civic building (those civic buildings that exist usually reflect the later development of worker influence or latter-day philanthropy: Miners Halls or Carnegie Institutes). The result is that the market centre of a southern English village usually compares well with the centre of large industrial towns like Aberdare of Merthyr.

The country could be seen to contain a large, alienated population. The phenomenon was perceived and described in very different quarters, by Dickens, by Engels, and by Disraeli. Their descriptions reflect, to some extent the concern of some sections of the community, a concern, at least in part, occasioned by fear. But any serious attempt at amelioration of the conditions producing this divided population was thwarted and delayed by the new ideology and by the convergence of political theory and political economy.

Paradoxically, one of the greatest obstacles to improvement was liberal theory. Liberal philosophers, following as behavioural and moral theorists so often do follow the established successes in the physical sciences, had attempted the construction of a mechanism of ethics. The driving force in the mechanism was the hedonistic principle, the pursuit of pleasure or happiness: all people are said to pursue pleasure and avoid pain. The best course was the pursuit of the greatest good of the greatest number. The role of the state was to facilitate a condition in which the greatest good of the greatest number could be achieved.

There are certain well-known philosophical problems which emerge from this position which need not concern us here; after all, no effective ideology has been much hampered by its logical inconsistencies but one of the most worrying of these problems is the difficulty of calculating the greatest good of the greatest number. The principle seems to be one more example of the substitution of accountancy for morality. The analogy with accounting is reasonably accurate. 'The striking feature of the utilitarian view of justice is that it does not matter, except indirectly, how this sum of satisfactions is distributed among individuals ...' Professor Rawls (1972 : 26) continues, 'there is no reason in principle why the greater gains of some should not compensate for the lesser losses of others' and, to bring the analogy with accounting and the market place closer, 'On this conception of society separate individuals are thought of as so many different lines along which rights and duties are to be assigned and scarce means of satisfaction allocated in accordance with rules so as to give the greatest fulfillment of wants. The nature of the decision made by the ideal legislator is not, therefore, materially different from that of an entrepreneur deciding how to maximize his profit by producing this or that commodity ... Utilitarianism does not take seriously the distinction between persons.'

Regardless of its philosophical respectability or otherwise utilitarians and liberals had considerable influence on the reform of society. Jeremy Bentham was responsible for reforms in the law. John Stuart Mill's *Essay on Liberty* is still regarded as a classic statement of democracy and he was largely responsible for the development of a new and more civilized attitude to the position of women in society. Such a movement might have been expected to be sympathetic to the condition of the industrial workers and to have brought about its improvement. If anything, liberalism made it worse and can be said to have resulted in an almost total withdrawal from moral responsibility.

One reason for this paradoxical result was liberal preoccupation with problems which had either changed or disappeared. The major liberal concern was with freedom and the chief liberal hero was the individual man. Early liberal thinking, emerging from Locke's work in the seventeenth century, led to the view that the greatest enemy of individual freedom was the state (as indeed it had been and still frequently is). Liberal philosophy represented a defence against the state; its activities were to be regarded with suspicion, its legislation to be kept to a minimum, its interference in trade to be avoided.

Liberalism failed to meet the demands of new problems because it dogmatized upon principles expounded by Adam Smith. Liberal economists have been described as notable for two characteristics: first, the belief that the principles which guided them were so obvious as to be beyond challenge (as Mac Wickar expressed it in *First Lessons in Political Economy for Elementary Schools*, 'today they are commonplaces of the nursery, and the only real difficulty is their too great simplicity' (Gide and Rist 1948 : 355)) and second, the absolute rigour with which they applied these principles. Gide and Rist (1948 : 354) describe the English economists as pursuing their 'wonted tasks, never once troubled by the thought that they were possibly forging a weapon for their own destruction at the hands of socialists'. The same authors describe Nassau Senior, Professor of Political Economy at Oxford, the first chair of economics established in England, in 1825, as having 'removed from political economy every trace of system, every suggestion of social reform, every connexion with a moral or conscious order, reducing it to a small number of essential unchangeable principles'.

However unpleasant social conditions and however alarmed the reaction to them, liberals were hamstrung by their theory, unable to contemplate any considerable degree of state regulation because the mechanisms of the price system were best left alone. When a public health act was passed in 1848, *The Economist* of the day commented: 'suffering and evil are nature's admonitions; they cannot be got rid of; and the impatient attempts of benevolence to banish them from the world by legislation before benevolence has learnt their object and their end have always been more productive of evil than good.'

The derivation of such references to 'the object and end' of 'suffering and evil' probably lies in the doctrines of Malthus. Malthus propounded the doctrine for which he became famous, that population grows by a geometric progression while the means of its subsistence grows in arithmetical progression, in *An Essay on Population* published in 1798. Malthus was certainly consistent in the gloom of his conclusions and in his view of human nature. The only controls on the inevitable inbalance between population and the means of its subsistence lay in natural or social disasters or in moral control. Poverty could not be avoided although it might be to some extent reduced if the poor could be led to exercise moral restraint by a process of education which it was the duty of the upper classes to provide for them.

Continuing poverty explained the progress that man had made in the world because, without the threat of poverty he would not work. Poverty made man work and was therefore responsible for his welfare;

poverty also caused his unending unhappiness. Attempts to improve his position were bound to fail because while they could not alter the gloomy equation of population and subsistence, they did succeed in obscuring it as a cause of poverty and tended to obstruct the only successful means of amelioration, moral restraint.

Professor Bendix (1956 : 84) draws the conclusion from Malthus's view: No virtue of a poor man could henceforth exempt him from condemnation. The fact of poverty showed that a man had married when he should have stayed single, just as the fact of success demonstrated that a man had exercised proper foresight.

'The implications of this view was convenient and flattering to the rich as they were outrageous to the poor. Landlords and manufacturers could use the principle of population to explain their own inaction, their unending opposition to all proposed reforms, and the inevitability of misery among the poor. All the evils attending the process of industrialisation could be put down to a law of nature and of God and the same law tended to prove that economic success was evidence of foresight and moral restraint.' (Bendix 1956 : 84)

So, there emerges a secular version of the Calvinist doctrine, that success signifies salvation. The amalgam of theory which came to be known as *laissez-faire* had advantages from the point of view of the manufacturer. It protected him from the criticisms of those who might be alarmed at the consequences of his apparently brutal behaviour. It forbade their interference on the ground that their good intentions were certain to harm those they were intended to help. It once again provided an explanation and a defence of relative positions in the new social hierarchy; employers deserved their position and so did the poor. There is no doubt that the economics and the political doctrine of the first half of the nineteenth century were 'capitalists' theory' and that, as Bendix asserts, their final 'justification' was their explanation and support for the enormous commercial and industrial expansion of England. Some such vigorous and self-justifying doctrine had to exist in order to promote and permit expansion on this scale.

However, it is incompatible with morality as it is normally understood. The progressive emptying of economy theory of all moral content brought it into conflict with traditional morality so that a rift opened up between received economic theory on the one hand and ideology as a practical prescription for behaviour on the other.

Professor Bendix (1956 : 68) argues that Sunday school teaching and

charity school education 'did not simply "reflect" the interests of the
entrepreneurs. Evangelical preaching among the poor, as well as the
charity school movement, had developed decades before the accelerated development of industry from 1760 on ... An essential part
of evangelical preaching since the seventeenth century had been the
doctrine that the poor should work hard, obey their superiors and be
satisfied with the station to which God had called them.' Certainly, he
adds, this teaching was used to justify the employers when industry
developed: 'it was also used to explain away all the evils of starvation
and child labour of accidents and ill health.' It also exhorted the better
off members of society to set an example to the poor, 'to reform their
own conduct so that the poor would be able to trust them as guides'
(Bendix 1956 : 72).

Professor Bendix points out one aspect of the conflict: the upper
classes began to reject appeals that they should act with a sense of
responsibility for the conduct of the poor. They began to assert that
the poor were not likely to be reformed by references to their own
conduct and that the poor would have to rely upon their own efforts.
Professor Bendix (1956 : 73) points to a particular ambivalence in this
respect. 'While the intense moralism of evangelical preaching asserted
a tutelage over the poor which the entrepreneurs were eager to deny, it
also inculcated a spirit of discipline and subordination which was
much to their advantage. We might say that while the entrepreneurs
sought to free themselves from moral restraint they saw the practical
advantage in moral responsibility.' This 'ideological break with
tradition', Professor Bendix (1956 : 88) later comes to see as the
rejection of ideology by the manufacturers.

> 'What stands out in this reaction of the early entrepreneurs (and
> many of their followers since them) is their utter unconcern with
> ideas of any kind, and their complete preoccupation with the affairs
> of the moment. If ideology is defined as the attempt to interpret
> the actions of the moment so that they appear to exemplify a more
> or less consistent orientation (if not a larger purpose) then it is clear
> that the most fundamental contrast to ideology is a single minded
> attention to expediency.'

This seems to be very uncertain ground. The assertion that
businessmen are free of ideology has often been made, most recently
by Theo Nicholls in *Ownership, Control and Ideology* (1969). It
remains, as we shall later argue, a contentious assertion. The

definition of ideology as seeking to establish a consistent orientation is very vague and is probably not incompatible with a single-minded devotion to expedience, indeed, a Marxist view of ideology sees it simply as expediency disguised. In any case, expediency in the guise of pragmatism is not merely acceptable as an ideology, it claims to be accepted as a philosophical position. Finally, one's own devotion to expedience is almost certain to be given ideological trappings if one's self-interested actions are to be made acceptable to other people, or to subordinates. Self-interest, when communicated to others, inevitably takes ideological form.

The contradiction in these particular circumstances is not, as Professor Bendix argues, between the ambivalent views of capitalists half-wedded to evangelical tradition and half to moral freedom, it is between an established ideology and a new economic theory. It may be that the economists were giving a clear-sighted account of the businessman's true behaviour and motives but it certainly conflicted with his own traditional view of himself, his relationship to society and to God. But while earlier versions of capitalist theory had merely claimed to describe events in Smith's case, often with sardonic disapproval, later versions claimed also to provide injunctions to conduct and the injunctions were in turn of absolute self-interest. In this sense, economic theory contradicted morality in almost any version known to man.

This might make very acceptable imperatives for conduct as far as the manufacturers were concerned, it gave an authoritative sanction to practically anything they did as long as it was not benevolent; anything was permissible as long as it was not well-meaning. As an explanation to the businessman's subordinates, however, it was not likely to be so successful. There was no shortage of explanations of why the poor should be poor, but the explanations were singularly bleak. There were no longer references to the deferred other-worldly advantages which were certain to follow meekness and acceptance. The explanations given of the existing state of affairs here on earth might make good theory but they entailed a view so gloomy and unalterable that they were hardly likely to win enthusiastic approval from the poor. The views emerging from sources such as the work of Malthus could only add rancour to those whose situation was impossible and, apparently, unimprovable.

Andrew Ure's attempt at the construction of an ideological account at least had the merit, which the economists so obviously lacked, of being deceitful. Professor Bendix (1956 : 97) notes that his 'weakness arose from his failure to make an "untrammelled assertion of moral leadership" and that it was a more or less evasive answer to the accusations of critics. The probability is that any bid for moral leadership arising out of an attempt to defend the nineteenth century entrepreneurs would have to be "more or less evasive".' Ure was a poor ideologist because the evasions were so clearly discernible; it is the work of a second rate hack defending the unforgiveable. In Bendix's (1956 : 99) view it was 'so much concerned with denouncing the infamy of combination among workers that it widened the existing gulf between manufacturers and their employees'. This is the opposite result to what would be achieved by effective ideology.

Theory had destroyed ideology by extracting its moral content. The manufacturers needed a new ideology which could explain existing conditions not only to employers but also to those they employed, which could provide a satisfactory reason for work, which could motivate the employee to carry out his master's instructions with zeal and serve his interests with enthusiasm.

Professor Pollard (1965 : 195) argues that one of the essential preliminaries was a concerted attack on traditional working class habits and outlooks including drinking, week-end leisure, and swearing.

> 'The worker's own ethics were such that he was not normally susceptible to the kind of inducements which his employer could provide within the new working conditions. Ambitions to rise above his own idea of a "subsistence" income by dint of hard work were foreign to him. He had to be made ambitious and "respectable", either by costly provisions of material goods, like the famous gardening plots for miners praised by Arthur Young, or the loan for houses granted by Dowlais to its privileged workers, or by the cheaper means of changing his attitudes, often falsely called his "character". For unless the workmen *wished* to become "respectable" in the current sense, none of the incentives would bite.'

Professor Pollard adds. 'Such opprobrious terms as "idle" or "dissolute" should be taken to mean strictly that the worker was indifferent to the employers' deterents and incentives'.

A tradition of paternalism contributed an ideological element in the relations between employers and workers. The tradition stems from mediaeval society, from the network of obligatory and dependent relations established under the control of God. Many nineteenth century employers saw themselves as inheriting squirarchical authority and responsibility, exercising a religious obligation to control, reward, and punish, to exercise care and responsibility and to expect dutiful obedience. Even an agnostic employer like Robert Owen, unwilling to rest upon the final authority of God, demanded obedience and exercised responsibility for employees whom he regarded as dependent and requiring the moulding influence of a benevolent owner. These employers justified the need for a wise and benevolent concern by reference to the dependence of their workers whom they perceived as illiterate, uneducated, drunken, and wayward. When Owen, with typical modesty, undertook 'the most important experiment for the happiness of the human race that had yet been instituted at any time' (Owen 1920 : 82) at New Lanark in 1800, he found the great majority of the workers 'idle, intemperate and dishonest'.

Professor Genovese, writing of relationships between masters and slaves in the old South, says that

> 'Paternalism defined the involuntary labor of the slaves as a legitimate return to their masters for protection and direction. But the masters' need to see their slaves as acquiescent human beings constituted a moral victory for the slaves themselves. Paternalism's insistence upon mutual obligations — duties, responsibilities and ultimately even rights — implicitly recognized the slaves' humanity.' (Genovese 1975 : 5)

Paternalism protected both masters and slaves from the worst aspects of their relationship, 'it disguised, however imperfectly, the appropriation of one man's labour power by another' (1975 : 6). In this way, Genovese sees paternalism as obscuring the realities of capitalist employment relationships and as an anachronistic survival in a capitalist system of production. The network of personal obligation and relationships cannot survive 'the exigencies of marketplace competition, not to mention the subsequent rise of trade-union opposition [which] reduced these efforts to impediments to the central tendency toward depersonalization' (1975 : 662).

The considerable ideological potential which paternalism offered to an industrializing society was threatened by other internal inconsistencies. To begin with, the employer's benevolent concern is directed at the achievement of the greater maturity of the industrial worker. But this is self-defeating because the worker's dependence provokes a reaction of independent hostility. The justification of paternalism is the development and maturation of the employee but the paternal relationship is doomed by its own logic. Its function is the production of a sober, obedient and able labour force but industrialization promotes requirements for high skill, intelligence, and discretionary judgement from some, at least, of the workers. Advanced industrialization requires labour which is mobile both geographically and socially, which is trained and educated to a level which demands and justifies its independence. Active and voluntary co-operation becomes more important than dependence upon the employer.

Developments in the ideology of the employer also damaged paternalism. We have suggested that *laissez-faire* theory encouraged the pursuit of self-interest and emptied the employment relationship of moral concern and moral responsibility for the employee. Rational bureaucracy introduces processes of control, measurement and a network of rules in place of the arbitrary judgement and concern of the owner. The process is hastened by the intervention of management as distinct from ownership which, as we shall see, seeks a different expression of the legitimacy of its authority and finds it in expertise rather than in benevolence or moral responsibility. The professionalism of the manager comes to replace the paternalism of the owner. These developments are encouraged by the increasingly complex processes of capitalization in joint stock financing, to establish a paternalist relationship the owner must be identified. Paternalism is finally challenged by the growing independence of labour. The first evidence is the growth of the Labour and Trade Union movement. The theoretical expression of this independence is the emergence of social theory which rests upon class conflict. Marx completes the process of developing the independence of labour, a process begun by the employer. Teleological explanations of social change are notoriously dangerous but Marxist theory could be interpreted as providing a necessary impetus to the development of the mature and independent proletariat required by advanced industrialization. Paternalism, like the paternal relationship itself, ends when it achieves the maturity of its children.[3]

The work of reforming the workers to a pattern more suitable for factory production proceeded by the use of a variety of instruments; coercion, the law, poverty, unemployment, incentive, and religion. One of the most successful attempts to follow up such preliminary conditioning with a more or less consistent ideology to bridge the gap between wealthy and poor was made by Samuel Smiles in *Self-help*, published in 1859.

Although the author and his works are regarded as jokes by those who have not read them, Smiles's views probably still supply the foundation for any modern explanation of the success and advantage of capitalism, or at least, for any explanation which does not begin by denying the essential features of a capitalist economy.

Smiles elevated work to a position of absolute importance and made the willingness or ability to undertake it the only proper dividing principle between rich and poor, those who were successful and those who were unsuccessful. Smiles is a radical in the sense that he is not prepared to defend traditional privilege and the advantages of birth and inherited wealth. The potted biographies of successful men which are scattered throughout his books and which compose *Lives of the Engineers*, invariably stress, where they can, the humble origins of the mighty. One suspects Smiles of wishing to invert the normal process in which aristocratic origins are falsely ascribed to the self-made man: Smiles seeks humility in the beginnings of those who began with advantage.

He did not regard poverty as carrying any connotations of wickedness which were irremovable nor as an insuperable obstacle to progress. 'Riches and ease, it is perfectly clear, are not necessary for man's highest culture ... so far from poverty being a misfortune, it may by vigorous self-help, be converted even into a blessing' (Smiles 1908 : 22). In absolute opposition to the more usual view, Smiles believed that the rich may begin with a marked social disadvantage. This was likely to be particularly disabling an obstacle for the rich people of other countries but fortunately, it is a characteristic of the English upper-classes 'that they are not idlers; for they do their fair share of the work of the state', (Smiles 1908 : 27) thus presumably overcoming the natural disadvantage of high birth.

Smiles appeal was thus essentially democratic and egalitarian. Success depends not upon wealth, nor birth, nor inheritance nor even talent — success is open to all who try. 'The greatest results in life are usually attained by simple means and exercise of ordinary qualities ... The road of human welfare lies along the old highway of steadfast well-doing; and they who are the most persistent, and work in the truest spirit, will usually be the most successful.' (Smiles 1908 : 111) The essential quality for success is work. Work and workers, were for Smiles. the foundation of the whole of civilisation. 'The state of civilization in which we live is for the most part the result of past labours. All that is great in morals, in intelligence, in art, or in science, has been advanced towards perfection by the workers who have preceded us. Each generation adds its contribution to the products of the past ...' (Smiles 1907 : 40).

Work was elevated to a position of the greatest importance — both to the individual and to society at large. 'Steady application to work is the healthiest training for every individual, so it is the best discipline of a state. Honourable industry travels the same road with duty; and Providence has closely linked both with happiness ... Labour is not only a necessity and a duty, but a blessing: only the idler feels it to be a curse' (Smiles 1908 : 33).

Work was also self-suficient as a cure-all. Smiles inherited the suspicion of benevolence, particularly when it was directed by agencies of the state. 'Help from without is often enfeebling in its effects, but help from within invariably invigorates. Whatever is done for men or classes, to a certain extent takes away the stimulus and necessity of doing for themselves; and where men are subjected to over-guidance and over-government, the inevitable tendency is to render them comparatively helpless.' Smiles stressed personal responsibility for ones own well-being directed through effort 'great social evils, will, for the most part be found to be but the outgrowth of man's own perverted life; and though we may endeavour to cut them down and extirpate them by means of Law, they will only spring up again with fresh luxuriance in some other form unless the conditions of personal life and character are radically improved' (Smiles 1908 : 3).

Samuel Smiles filled a most serious gap in nineteenth-century ideology. The principle of self-help provided some prospect of hope for the most poverty stricken members of society, as such it provided a motive force for society itself. It had, in this way, a double-edged advantage. It provided the prospect of material success and moral virtue for those who, by hard work, would succeed; and it contributed to the docility and the discipline of those who, by hard work, would fail. It stressed common interests and a common background between employers and workers while encouraging effort as good in itself and as bringing material rewards. If it failed to reward the worker it could contribute to the maintenance of a well-disciplined labour force which it persuaded to accept the same values as those of its masters.

It would be extravagant to argue that self-help alone succeeded in motivating the work force necessary to carry forward industrialization.

To some extent ideology was unnecessary. Workers were attracted by higher wages or recruited by poverty. Engels presented a vivid account of how the factories got and kept their labour. Once workers were recruited, effort was assured by the supervision, the conditions, and the hours under which they worked. Religion, in the form of Methodism, as Thompson argues powerfully, contributed significantly to the maintenance of a work ethic. But an additional exhortation was necessary or was felt to be necessary, which is the same thing. Prevailing economic theory might explain and approve the behaviour of capitalists to each other, but its gloomy rigidity could hardly contribute to the motivation of workers. In any case, it was devoid of any moral appeal and some generally acceptable moral explanation was necessary. Ideology may well be a basic unchanging human requirement in that men have always needed to justify their actions (which are often selfish) to themselves and to others. In the political world there has never been a regime however tyrannical and contemptuous of humanity, which did not seek its own moral justification. In this sense, 'the end of ideology' is merely another utopian dream; men are always likely to be exploited and the exploitation is certain to require justification in a form acceptable to them.

The popularity of Smiles's work demonstrated his success as the ideologist of capitalist industrialization. Its essential features continue to occur in any modern defence of the virtues of capitalism or business enterprise. Such defences of pure capitalism have become rare in Britain where we are used to thinking more in terms of a 'mixed economy'. But in the USA, business ideology is often expressed in terms remarkably similar to those of Smiles. While in England Smiles is remembered with condescending humour, in the USA his sentiments, at least, are taken very seriously. America's exponent, Horatio Alger, has apparently inspired a tradition in which 'the American Schools and Colleges Association polls thousands of "college leaders" to select a few men who have risen from humble origins to great success. When the final tally discloses the names of these fortunate few, they are summoned to New York City to receive the Horatio Alger Award' (Wohl 1967 : 501).

However inconsistent his theory and naive his expression, Smiles was a potent ideologist. Ideological accounts of capitalism and exhortations concerning the importance of work may now take more complex forms, embracing the more recent revelations of sociology and psychology, but they often share the same basic premises.

Part II
The Radical Reaction

5. The Supremacy of Industry

We are now going to return to the dissenting view of society which we last discussed as it was represented by the Diggers in seventeenth-century England. Dissent was then an isolated and eccentric exception to the generally held view in an emergent economic theory. We are now going to discuss the development of a great alternative view of society, a view which has established a tradition which stands opposed, in some senses, to capitalist ideology to which it seems to present itself as an alternative.

We have already seen something of the development of an orthodox view involving the substitution of economic for moral and social values, of accounting for theology, until work becomes established as having paramount importance. The forces underlying the development of industrialization were explained by the economists who urged that the efficiency of the commercial machine depended on its own self-regulation. Their warnings of the dangers of interference were welcomed by entrepreneurs who were grateful for this scholarly defence against intervention in the pursuit of their best interests. The ideological accompaniment to this theme was written by Andrew Ure and by Samuel Smiles, the former, more particularly, an apologist for commercial development who placed the responsibility for improvement upon the individual, however weak, and who made weakness a moral offence. In this philosophy, work and its virtues seemed to be emphasized as never before.

But orthodox ideology gave an incomplete account of the circumstances attending industrialization. Smiles's *Self-help* may have encouraged the worker to better himself but the statistics were against its general acceptance as a view of events. Most people were hopelessly subject to conditions that they could not control.

For most manual workers, perhaps now as then, any ideology of work is an absurdity. Perhaps no one would dare communicate it to the coalbackers whose job was to unload coal from ships into wagons and whose conditions are described by Professor Harrison. They were usually worked out at the age of forty, the strongest among them could not work consistently for more than two or three consecutive days; they usually hired unemployed mates to take their place. Mayhew quotes one of them: 'Sometimes we put a bit of coal in our mouths to prevent our biting our tongues ... but it's almost as bad as if you did bite your tongue, for when the strain comes heavier on you, you keep scrunching the coal to bits, and swallow some of it, and you're half choked' (Harrison 1971 : 44).

Work of this kind has killed an incalculable number of people apart from those whose death it has brought about by industrial accidents. Such conditions and the manifest unreality of orthodox ideology inevitably produced a dissenting explanation of them.

The unavoidable evidence of distress and social dislocation brought about by industrialization inevitably attracted the attention of writers who were more concerned with the effects than with their economic causes. What followed was an attempt to develop theory which would not only try to account for social dislocation but which would try to change the framework within which industrialization took place so as to remove or improve its worst consequences.

This reaction was not simple or unified and it contained many contradictory elements. But the prime cause of dissent both from existing circumstances and from the orthodox account of them must have been the massive and indigestible fact of industrialization. Professor Bowle (1963 : 101), arguing that the dominant economic fact of the early nineteenth century was the development of new industrial techniques, wrote that: 'Hitherto no political theory had fully taken account of them. Adam Smith and his followers had attempted to explain the working of economic laws, and Bentham to adjust political institutions to them, but no one had advocated a way to bring the process under fuller control and even enhance the new possibilities of production.

The attempt was to be made but it took several different forms. We shall begin this observation of the radical reaction by briefly examining the views of two Frenchmen, Sismondi and Saint-Simon. Sismondi described the causes of industrialization and its excesses, but his prescriptions were ameliorative rather than radical. Saint-Simon has variously been described as the founder of socialism and as an 'authoritarian revolutionary'. Other branches of the reaction were to lead to communism or to anarchism. But few anywhere, apart from some representatives of the old conservative tradition, disapproved of industrialism as such. Later, Durkheim was to regard the division of labour, which was inseparable from industrialization, as a factor leading to social solidarity. Saint-Simon regarded industry as the most important social function, so important that it was, he thought, to provide the framework of government. The savagery with which Engels or Marx attacked the effects of industrialization was not directed against industry itself so much as against the economic fabric within which it operated: as Gouldner puts it, Marx 'did not regard modern society as an adolescent industrialism but as a senile capitalism'.

In the radical theorists we are never very far from the paradox of a similarity to the classical economists with those work they are so often contrasted. So much is this the case that Durkheim has specifically to refute the 'misunderstanding' which would have Saint-Simon as 'the apostle of industrialism' or as having 'completed Adam Smith'.

This puzzling similarity between some early socialists and classical economists comes about because both share an admiration for industrial processes and a belief in the benefits they can bring; they are both, in a sense, slaves of 'steam-age intellect' although the socialist believes that a considerable change in economic relationships is necessary before the potential good created by industrialization can be released.

There is no consistent alignment, however, of those who advocate and those who oppose industrialization. Some, like Gaskell in England and Sismondi in France, were more concerned with the immediate and obvious effects of industrialization than with its long-term benefits. Sismondi in particular was consistently preoccupied with subordinating notions of economic progress to the ultimate test of whether it improved or worsened the condition of men. His absolute concern with the paramouncy of human as against economic values was rare in the nineteenth century, unknown among economists and has probably not been expressed with such confidence and clarity until recently. Economists regarded their study as the science of wealth and saw national activity as primarily concerned with its accumulation which it was the duty of governments to facilitate, certainly not to impede. Sismondi took a different view, that

> 'the accumulation of wealth in abstract is not the aim of government, but the participation by all its citizens in the pleasures of life which the wealth represents. Wealth and population in the abstract are no indication of a country's prosperity: they must in some way be related to one another before being employed as the basis of comparison.' 'Political economy at its widest, is a theory of charity, and any theory that upon the last analysis has not the result

of increasing the happiness of mankind does not belong to the the science at all.' (Gide and Rist 1948 : 191)

He attacked the classical economists' enthusiasm for machinery because although he agreed that new products will give rise to new consumption in the long run, in the short run the machines would put people out of work. He was most concerned with the social consequences which the economists blandly ignored in their preoccupation with long-run advantages. Perhaps he was one of the first observers to point out that in the long run we shall all be dead.

He was concerned about mechanization because he believed that workers did not share, except as consumers, in the benefits of mechanization. He was sceptical about the view that mechanization was a response to an increase in demand preferring a more cannibalistic explanation, that mechanization and increased production resulted quite simply from one producer trying to increase his profits at the expense of other producers. In an analysis similar to Marx's, he argued that producers in their competitive pursuit of cheapness force each other to economize in men and materials, to reduce wages, to lengthen the working day, to require greater labour effort, and to employ women and children as the cheapest forms of labour available.

'The earnings of an *entrepreneur* sometimes represent nothing but the spoliation of the workman. A profit is made not because the industry produces more than it costs, but because it fails to give the workman sufficient compensation for his toil. Such an industry is a social evil.' In a phrase which was to anticipate Marx even more clearly he added: 'We might almost say that modern society lives at the expense of the proletariat, seeing that it curtails the reward of his toil' (Gide and Rist 1948 : 197).

Anticipating Marx still further, Sismondi argued that society tended, as the result of competition, to split into two classes, those who own and those who work, the rich and the poor. The separation is encouraged because the weakest producers and trades are eliminated by competition; the intermediaries between rich and poor, the yeomen farmers, village traders, master craftsmen, and small manufacturers are all removed, resulting, as we would put it, in a polarization of society. 'Society no longer has any room save for the great capitalist and his hireling, and we are witnessing the frightfully rapid growth of a hitherto unknown class — of men who have absolutely no property' (Gide and Rist 1948 : 200).

Gide and Rist, commenting on the significance of Sismondi's work, suggest that he illuminated the other side of the coin presented by the classical economist, so that it would no longer be possible to speak of a spontaneous harmony of interest. Sismondi attacked *laissez-faire* theory and advocated social intervention in economic affairs, he was 'the first of the interventionists'.

But there was something partial and half-hearted about the kind of intervention he recommended. He advocated the reunion of property and labour (by peasant proprietorship and by small-scale manufacture), the right of combination, the abolition of child labour, a reduction in hours of work, the payment of a guaranteed wage in sickness and in old age (by the employer, not the state). These are ameliorative solutions which are all familiar to us in a twentieth-century welfare state but there is nothing thorough-going or radical about them. Sismondi apparently apologized for his failure to produce cohesive programmes of reform, he hoped it would be judged sufficient to have exposed what was wrong.

It is ironic that these half-hearted attempts at improving and, therefore, maintaining the existing situation are based on an attitude much more hostile and antipathetic to the system than is the theory underlying many more apparently total programmes of reform or revolution. Unlike Sismondi, Saint-Simon would have overturned the system, but his proposed reforms grew out of an absolute admiration for its operation.

Saint-Simon held an evolutionary theory of society: its characteristic institutions and relationships grew out of tendencies emerging in its predecessors. There were three important periods in world history: 'The first had a polytheist ideology and a societal order based on slavery; the second an ideology called "theological" and a feudal system; the ideology of the third which had not yet attained fullness was scientific or positive and its social system was industrial' (Manuel 1956 : 220). Just as in Marx's later dialectical process of change, the process was to be ended in a final phase of development or fulfillment which, for Saint-Simon, was to produce the new society of science and industry. Saint-Simon seemed to regard the unfolding of the new society as inevitable but, again like Marx, his certainty did not prevent his constant exhortation of others to assist in its arrival, nor his exasperation at their apparent apathy.

Saint-Simon not only observed the water-shed which we have mentioned, in a sense he constituted it. Theoretically we could, he says, decide to revert to a feudal and theological society; practically we are forced to go on, to take the only course of development open to us. Industry is now the main force in society. 'Modern societies will be definitely in equilibrium only when organised on a purely industrial basis ... The production of useful things is the only reasonable and positive end that political societies set themselves.' The only interests serving as objectives for the ordinary concern of men are economic interests. 'This group of interests is the only one which all men understand ... All societies rest on industry. Industry is the only guarantee of society's existence ... The most favourable state of affairs for industry is for this reason the most favourable to society' (Durkheim 1959 : 134).

It is hardly possible to exaggerate the importance with which Saint-Simon regarded industry and economic concepts.

'The whole art of government in civil society would become the application on a universal scale of the truths of political economy. Economics was more than a compilation of precepts for the accumulation of private wealth or the enrichment of individual nations; it was the morality of the temporal order in civil society.'

'The doctrines of work and progress were the driving ethical concepts of the new society ... Production was the one positive end of society and the maxim "Respect for property and for property owners" had to be superseded by "Respect for production and for producers" ...' Producers of useful objects were the sole legitimate directors of society.

'Man progressed ethically, to the degree that industry became perfected. It was therefore moral to spread and inculcate ideas which tended to increase the productive activity of one's own nation and fostered respect for the production of others.' (Manuel 1956 : 240)

So far, Saint-Simon seems to share the entire view of economists emphasizing the primacy of economic interest. But Saint-Simon does not see their primacy reflected in the dominant institutions of society as it exists. This is because the dominant institutions are survivals of a bygone age of military power and theological mysticism. He contrasted the real and the apparent importance of things in the famous 'parable' of 1819. 'Let France suddenly lose the leaders of productive industry ... its creative scientists, artisans and writers, and it would become an inferior among nations, deprived of its genius and most vital forces. Should, however, the royal family and thousands of unproductive churchmen, functionaries and military men die, their loss would not appear disastrous' (Manuel, 1956 : 210).

Saint-Simon advises us to get rid of all these archaic survivals of past feudal and theological societies. Our whole conception of government would also have to change. In a sense, the need for government would disappear, the government of a country would be replaced by the planning and administration of its trade and industry, the economic structure would come to replace the traditional governmental apparatus. 'There was no need for a government expert or a man trained in administration. Before the triumph of the industrial society men had been governed, in the order of the future they would be administered.' Saint-Simon drew up comparisons between the old traditional order and the new industrial society. 'Under the old the people were regimented by superiors; under the new they were related to one another by occupational ties' (Manuel 1956 : 308).

The whole new system of management which would replace government would be composed by different principles of representation and would take decisions by scientific processes of thought, the government of people would be replaced by the administration of things. In his proposals for a new administrative Chamber 'Men were not to be selected as representatives of a body of voters but were to be chosen solely for their professional competence. These experts would assemble in the chambers to plan and direct public works, rather than to deliberate about abstract principles' (Manuel 1956 : 312).

The whole fabric of social life is composed essentially of industrial relationships so it follows that the only men competent to direct it are men of industry taking impersonal decisions, experts interpreting the problems imposed by things and understanding the solutions which are demanded by circumstances. These 'industrials', as he came to call them, constituted the elite which was to dominate his new society. Other classes would be subordinated to the industrials who would, by nature of their jobs, become responsible for the administration of society. The distinction which we have become used to, between political authority and 'workshop leadership' was artificial, it was natural for those who organized work to organize social life because work was social life.

Saint-Simon's attitude to workers, as opposed to those who organize it, changed over the years. In his earlier work he seemed to have regarded the workers with some contempt, as being ignorant and irresponsible. After 1820, Manuel argues that he developed a much more humanitarian outlook towards them, wishing to improve their situation and at the same time regarding them as sufficiently able and responsible to take their part in the new society. He next came to recognize that they were both numerous and powerful and he therefore began to appeal to them as likely agents of change.

But his appeals were of a different kind and had a different intention from those that were later to be launched by Marx. Saint-Simon turned to the workers as Robert Owen turned to whoever he could persuade to listen, as a possible ally who might be persuaded to implement his blue-print for society. It would be in the workers' interest to bring these changes about, they would then become more prosperous, they would be liberated from exploitation and particularly from the necessity of dying in wars which were not their concern. He could certainly offer them improvement as a reward for their assistance, but their situation was not to be transformed in the new society. In a model address which he urged them to direct at their employers, they were to accept certain unavoidable realities in their situation: 'You are rich and we are poor. You work with your heads and we with our hands. From these two facts there result fundamental differences between us, so that we are and should be your subordinates.' Manuel (1956 : 255) therefore concludes that Saint-Simon 'was clearly not the herald of a proletarian revolution, whatever else he was'. His workers were not to occupy the apex of the new society although they might be removed from its base.

But even if their advance was to be a limited one, at least they were to occupy a place in the ruling group. They were important because they made things and their relationship to each other, to their organizers, and to the rest of society was to be determined entirely by functional considerations. Their condition would also be improved because the decisions which affected it were to be based, in the new order, in accordance with the modern recommendations of social-scientists, on impersonal and scientific considerations — 'decisions can only be the result of scientific demonstrations, absolutely independent of any human will' (Manuel 1956 : 311). It was to be not the boss who would give his subordinates instructions; 'the law of the situation' would tell them what was to be done.

That phrase, 'the law of the situation', is, of course, Mary Parker Follett's and it illustrates the proximity of Saint-Simon's outlook to a much more contemporary view. One should be careful about making such comparisons. Saint-Simon has suffered more than most from distorting interpretation by other writers and from the claim to have legitimately sired many strange intellectual offsprings. This is partly because of the fecundity and appropriateness of his thinking to the economic circumstances of his time and partly because of the cult of Saint-Simonism which he deliberately cultivated but over which even he was incapable of exercising posthumous control. Thus there are debates over the extent to which he has 'anticipated' Marxism, anarchism, collectivism, fascism, and socialism. We are now going to add an additional claim that he anticipated managerialism. The simplest explanation for these contradicting arguments is that all these movements, and others, are intellectual accompaniments to a world of intense industrialization; Saint-Simon was one of the first to identify this world and to explain its new forces; therefore Saint-Simon truly did foreshadow movements which are inseparable from industrialization, self-contradictory though some of these may at first sight appear to be.

Durkheim (1959 : 21), grinding his own axe, regards Saint-Simon as the founder of socialism, if 'one calls socialist these theories which demand a more or less complete connection of all economic functions or certain of them, though diffused, with the directing and knowing organs of society'. This particular ascription of paternity depends both upon a suitable interpretation of Saint-Simon and a suitable definition of socialism (as concerned with central economic planning rather than with the ownership of property and the distribution of wealth). Durkheim then goes further in order to help establish his own argument that the division of labour is an essential principle of social co-operation.

A rather less tenuous connection can be traced from Saint-Simon to the corporate State. The advocacy of the displacement of political government by scientific administration of the planning and discretion of public works by suitably qualified experts clearly leads to some modern forms of totalitarian government. Manuel (1956 : 313) concludes that 'the similarity of the chamber organisation with recent fascist corporate practice as well as technocratic proposals is patent'. Durkheim's association between the emphasis given to work and economic production on the one hand and socialism on the other should demonstrate the fallacy in assuming that a work or worker based political philosophy has any necessary connection with democracy or with freedom. Nothing could be more dictatorial than the absolute supremacy which Saint-Simon gives to things and the scientific principles which can be elucidated in their administration. There is no room for alternate views because, for any problem there is a right solution. There is no room for a clash of interests because everyone will get out of society what he puts into it (thus, incidentally, reducing the undeserving poor and the indigent to a worse position than they would enjoy under Victorian capitalism). There is no room for arguments based on values because values themselves (other than those so thinly concealed by this total respect for science, technology, and industry) have disappeared with the last vestiges of theocratic society. There is, in short, no room for arguments at all.

This is managerialism inflated to a level at which even the most overweening managers in our own 'new society' would hardly dare voice their amibition to arrive. Saint-Simon is strangely representative in this other sense, that he exhibits the potential for absolute authoritarianism in what is apparently the most radical of outlooks. The new technical order of things points to a world in which communist or syndicalist alternatives to capitalism will differ in every respect except their common complete subjection of man to the economic and technical machine which he has constructed.

In this sense, it is Saint-Simon, rather than Adam Smith or Ricardo or Andrew Ure or Samuel Smiles, who represents the apotheosis of the spirit of capitalism. Leaving aside comparatively unimportant considerations such as the ownership of property (which Saint-Simon, again with uncanny appropriateness, dismissed as of trivial significance), his view of the new world is of a logical and natural extension of capitalism to its completed state, removed of those inhibitions to its progress which Saint-Simon correctly identified as traditional. All these ingredients identified in the protestant ethic: work, measurement, rationalism, materialism, are present not as confused alternatives to other and more widely accepted notions, but as dominant themes which demand that others must be removed. Saint-Simon's new society would not be a perfect world, but it would be a perfect world for manufacturers and businessmen.

The apotheosis is achieved by an attack on morality which matches the practical onslaught by liberal economists on the same objective. The economists argued that traditionally accepted moral values were a threat to the functioning of the economic system. Saint-Simon argued that there was no other system and no other values. The appearance of alternative systems of thought and belief were, he argued, throwbacks to survivals of previous patterns of social organization. Saint-Simon, and his later followers who propounded the 'new religion' as an appropriate faith for the 'new society', insisted that obstacles and alternatives to the industrial society were the result of traditional mystifications and that they were essentially irrational. Auguste Comte, outlining a similar demise of theocratic society and its replacement by the new social system representative of the dominance of science and industry, proposed that 'scientific men ought in our day to elevate politics to the rank of a science of observation' (Comte : 130). [4] The application of the science was to be a matter for the informed elite; just as it was absurd to require liberty of conscience in physics or chemistry so it would be ridiculous to let every Tom, Dick, or Harry have his say in politics. Comte granted a difference between the science of politics and the natural sciences in that, for politics, established principles had not yet been formulated but this was merely a 'transitory fact'. The confidence of the social scientists in announcing the imminent arrival of the established principles of their science has not diminished in the 150 years since Comte wrote. Social physics, or sociology, was needed, he said, in order 'to complete the natural sciences' and then mankind will have 'entirely completed its intellectual education, and can directly pursue its final destination' (Comte : 237).

The confidence of the sociologist in the march towards this final destination has not greatly diminished either. Professor Fletcher believes that 'it is essential that we should now mount a deliberate, sustained, constructive effort — certainly on a European, preferably on a world-wide scale — to establish both theoretically and practicably, the outline of the New Social System' (Fletcher 1974 : 11). Everywhere, he says, traditional societies are slowly adapting themselves to 'the New Social System as best we can — and to move increasingly from the more negative and destructive criticism of the old, towards the constructive realization of the new. It is a massive task' (Fletcher 1974 : 73). It must indeed be massive in that it still seems necessary to tell us to start on it after 150 years.

Saint-Simon said 'politics is the science of production'. This slogan and the conceptions it rests upon has, whatever myths it has destroyed, contributed to the most potent myth of our own industrial society, that scientists, managers, social scientists, and administrators are peculiarly exempt from criticism because they are value-free. Paradoxically, while the 'pure scientists', upon whose work Comte's confident analogy was based, have become less certain of their own objective certainty, engaged in a speculative range from the statistical variables of the uncertainty principle to the almost metaphysical speculations of quantum physics, the social scientists remain impatient for the established principles which will provide the outline of the new social system. The invigorating, if brash, self-confidence of this outlook was shared, once upon a time, by socialists who believed, with Saint-Simon, that the new society was a matter of the rational application of the principles of sound administration. The problems of politics would disappear when science, industry, and reason would combine to provide abundance and health. This is the clean, clinical and inhuman socialism of Aldous Huxley's *Brave New World*. It is the confidence of the American reporter returning from the USSR and saying, 'I have seen the future and it works'. Those of us who survived the future have lost our confidence. Socialism has reverted to the politics of the possible rather than the science of production.

The myth still haunts us, however, so that the objectivity of science is a model for social theory and social planning. There is still an ideal of rationality and freedom from values. The work of scientists and, hopefully, of social scientists may be subjected to technical criticism but because its techniques are said to be its ends, its ends and the purpose to which they are put, cannot be criticized. Scientists may make mistakes and can then be criticized (always and only by other scientists) because they have to that extent ceased to be scientific, but when they are correctly scientific they can do no wrong because the concept of wrong is inappropriate in application to their work: they uncover correct solutions to problems. The only criteria which can be applied to the activity of our 'industrials' are technical criteria, any other reference is to some traditionalistic mystification.

We have come to believe this nonsense because Saint-Simon and his numerous followers have convinced us that it is so. Or, to put it another way, we have come to believe it because we have changed the world so that it *is* so. Objectively speaking, if we could imagine ourselves detached from the world in which we live, scientists have values. They have values in at least two senses. The first is as ordinary citizens of the world, deprived for the moment of any special rights, qualifications, and privileges. In this sense they are as likely as the next man to punish their children for telling lies or for being cruel to animals. In the second and more special sense, they have values as scientists. In this, specific sense, their values are embedded in and can be revealed in their work. The work in itself is usually highly valued, to the extent that opportunity to pursue it is regarded as compensation in itself. The way in which the work is carried out also has all sorts of value connotations. There are quite scrupulous standards concerning verification and methodology, fraud is discouraged, original work is acknowledged, and so on. Many of these 'special' values are not simply imported into the work of the scientist from, for example, the Christian ethic. Many, probably most, are necessary to the pursuit of scientific work. Most overriding in this respect is the absolute conviction that scientific enquiry is important. Scientists or their representatives may defend this conviction with arguments about the advance in the standard of living, the subsistence level in underdeveloped countries and so on, but ultimately their argument rests upon the absolute rightness of scientific work, they are morally convinced that what they are doing is right.

This conviction is not confined to scientists. It is probably shared by all workers in the respected professions. Managers are not so certain. But they give us an interesting example of the way in which the world still has to be changed a little to fulfil Saint-Simon's prophecies (or his exhortations). Managers, we are told, do not yet enjoy the status that they should, there is still some uncertainty about the moral value of their work. We are earnestly requested to conclude this particular debate by agreeing to accord them greater respect, greater respect than, for example, doctors, teachers or politicians. In other words, our new society is still incomplete; we should change so as to allow managers a place in the patheon of 'industrials' which we have already agreed, contains the scientists.

When the process of change is completed (it has aparently been completed some time ago in the USA and the USSR) we will all agree that the manager, like the scientist, is completely value-free. Some of us, like Theo Nicholls, are apparently already convinced of it. What we will mean, of course, is that our conception of the world has so changed and our acceptance of the managers' values is now so total that we can no longer identify them, just like the scientists', as values at all. A simpler way of putting it is that the managers and the scientists will have simply succeeded in superimposing their values on the whole of society, ourselves included. They will look at the world and at each other just as we will do.

There may be a few isolated eccentrics of course, some whose archaic values will give them an independent platform from which the industrials seem to be pursuing highly questionable values. But these will be dismissed as survivals of a long-gone-theocratic age. They will be left to complain, like Oastler, that a preoccupation with capitalist or economic ends is incompatible with a Christian ethic. But by that time no one will care, least of all most of the Christians. Other critics will be treated like dissidents or deviants, as they have been treated in the United States. The best evidence of the triumph of these values comes, of course, when the critics can be confined for psychiatric care, as in the Soviet Union.

6. Anarchists and Syndicalists

Anarchism is peculiarly difficult to relate to this or to any other general argument. It is a word which embraces a number of very different theories about the relationship of man to society, often asserting that he has been brutalized by government but will be liberated or cleansed when government is overthrown. Anarchist theories are usually concerned with politics and society but they are always occupied with the problem of authority and they have often been driven to propose solutions to the economic problems which their general theories illustrate, so they often concern themselves with work. Anarchist theory also provides a foundation for a great deal of the contemporary reaction to the official ideology of work, to what has come to be known as the counter-culture.

Anarchist views are often expressed in extreme forms, either in slogans or in interminable works of nineteenth-century prose, often untranslated. They are therefore particularly suitable for interpretation by a wide variety of commentators with an axe to grind. Proudhon, for example, has been variously associated with the development of anarchism, socialism, and fascism. Some of these interpretations have been distortions; *The Times Literary Supplement* (19 February, 1970) reviewing a book on Proudhon by Alan Ritter said that it contained 'a hilarious survey of Proudhon's various interpretors'. Finally, anarchists are always concerned with human freedom so that it may be difficult to discern a coherent movement among writers who were as concerned to distinguish their individuality from each other as much as from their opponents.

Woodcock defines anarchism as a 'system of social thought, aiming at fundamental changes in the structure of society and particularly ... at the replacement of the authoritarian state by some form of non-governmental co-operation between free individuals' (Woodcock 1963 : 11). He distinguishes five main anarchist 'schools':
1. Individualist anarchism — represented by Max Stirner (memorable as the victim of a bitter attack by Marx) who envisaged a union of egotists drawn together by respect for each other's ruthlessness.

2. Proudhon, advocating a rebuilding of society based on mutualism, on the free association of co-operative and interdependent interests.
3. Collectivism — in which Bakunin replaces individual possession with control of the means of production by voluntary associations which continue to allow the individual to enjoy the product of his work.
4. Anarcho-communism, in which Kropotkin proposes that local communes should control production, wages are abolished, and goods are taken from the community's stores as they are needed — 'from each according to his means, to each according to his needs'.
5. Anarcho-syndicalism — essentially a French movement which was influential in Western Europe and North America, in which the revolutionary trade union is regarded as an essential instrument of change by using the general strike to bring about a free society founded on industrial associations.

We are not going to follow the labyrinthine development of these ideas and movements. We shall examine some strands in anarchist thinking which seem to be particularly closely associated with the development of syndicalism because that movement is especially concerned with the organization of work.

Anarchist theories are often concerned to find in the interplay of economic activity a basis for voluntary association which will replace the need for authority. Proudhon argued along lines very similar to Saint-Simon that:

> 'Division of labour, collective force, competition, exchange, credit, property, and even liberty — these are the true economic forces, the raw materials of all wealth, which without actually making men the slaves of one another, give entire freedom to the producer, ease his toil, arouse his enthusiasm, and double his production by creating a real solidarity which is not based upon personal conditions, but which binds men together with ties stronger than any which sympathetic combination or voluntary contracts can supply.' (Gide and Rist 1948 : 304f).

Proudhon agreed essentially with Saint-Simon, 'we would substitute organization for government'. The essential co-operative spirit would be provided by labour and by mutual need. Like Saint-Simon he was convinced of the irrelevance of political action, of the dominance of economic relationships in society, and of the need to reflect these relationships in society. But there is an essential difference in emphasis between them. There is an inescapably authoritarian end to Saint-Simon's government by industrialists and intellectuals and the authoritarianism is made no less burdensome in prospect because it is based on the dictates of scientific method or on the unarguable requirements for the most efficient administration of 'things'. Proudhon could not tolerate any such rigidity because at the centre of any system of which he could approve, is man. Proudhon, too, advocated a network of co-operating associations but he emphasized that 'association, considered as an end in itself, is dangerous to freedom, but considered as a means to a greater end, the liberation of individual men, it can be beneficial' (Woodcock 1963 : 123).

Proudhon also differed from Saint-Simon in that he was a moralist and a puritan, despite his total opposition to religion. His friend Herzen (1968 : II, 817) found him in some respects, peculiarly bigotted — in certain matters

> 'he was incorrigible; thus the limit of his character was reached and, as is always the case, beyond it he was a conservative and a follower of tradition ... his conception of family relationships were coarse and reactionary, but they expressed not the bourgeois element of a townsman, but rather the stubborn feeling of the rustic *pater familias*, haughtily regarding women as a subordinate worker and himself as the autocratic head of the family.'

Herzen quotes him as commenting on a friend's good fortune: 'his wife is not so stupid that she can't make a good *pot au feu* and not clever enough to discuss his articles. That's all that is necessary for domestic happiness'.

His attitude to work was certainly puritan. 'Work is the first attribute, the essential characteristic of man'. Bowle (1963 : 66) says that in Proudhon's view 'work was the characteristic of man's nature; not to work was not to be a true man leading a full life ... labour was both a social necessity and a moral virtue'. Honest work protected those who did it from moral corruption, its victims were normally the intellectuals, writers, artists, and priests, moral perversion resulted from satiety, boredom, and from over-sophistication. In the long established tradition of claiming work as a panacea he argued that 'one of the virtues of hard work ... was that it would diminish sexual desire and provide a natural means of controlling the population' (Joll 1964 : 69).

Apart from its moral characteristics, the chief advantage accompanying hard work was the sense of social communion and human solidarity which it conferred on the worker. These benefits result 'from the workers' sense that he is making full use of his faculties — the strength of his body, the skill of his hands and the agility of his mind; it comes from his sense of pride at overcoming difficulties, at taming nature, at acquiring knowledge and at guaranteeing his independence' (Edwards and Fraser 1970 : 81).

In this passage Proudhon goes on to stress the natural element in labour and contrasts it with the unnatural entertainments and occupations of leisure which have accompanied what he sees as the impoverishment of work. If labour is properly organized with the necessary conditions of variety, health, intelligence, art, dignity, passion, and legitimate gain, then it can 'even as far as pleasure is concerned, become preferable to games and dancing, fencing, gymnastics, entertainments and all the other distractions which man in his poverty has invented as a means of recovering from the mental and physical fatigue caused by being a slave to labor' (Edwards and Fraser 1970 : 82).

No stronger claim could be made for its beneficent influence, work has never had a more ardent apologist than Proudhon. But he recognizes that its ideal or its natural advantages are frequently not provided by the reality of work as it exists. Marx was to explain its shortcomings by the facts of its organization which stemmed from the private ownership of the means of production, from capitalist exploitation. Proudhon believed that the moderate enjoyment of property was an essential element in social cohesion. He was also realistic enough to see that, although workers could be robbed by calculating the value of their work on an individual basis while the employer enjoyed the much greater product of their collective labour, the essential explanation for the degradation of work was not ownership but technology and organization.

Proudhon recognized that the real problem was that of large-scale industry, factory production, and the detailed division of labour. In these conditions, he said, 'manual skills have been replaced by perfected equipment and the role of men and machines have been reversed. It is no longer the worker who uses his intelligence; this has been passed on to the machine. What ought to constitute the workers' pride has become a means of stultifying his mind. Spiritualism demonstrates in this way that souls and body are separate' (Edwards and Fraser 1970 : 84).

His solution to what was to be identified as the problem of alienation was as realistic (and, incidentally, as modern) as his recognition of the special problems posed by factory production. He advocated programmes of complete job rotation during the workers' apprenticeship in industry, followed by partnership in management and profit sharing. Workers, before they become thoroughly specialized in one manufacturing process, should also, he argued, gain experience in a variety of other industries and they should be presented with open career structures which he summed up in the progression: apprentice, journeyman, master. Modern techniques of personnel management have not, so far, caught up with Proudhon just as, in England, they have not yet gone beyond Robert Owen.

This passage (in *Justice in the Revolution and the Church* (Edwards and Fraser 1970 : 82-5)) suggests that Bowle (1963 : 156) is less than fair to Proudhon when he argues that his 'self governing federal society was, of course, incompatible with industrial capitalism. Like Godwin and Cobbett, Proudhon's agrarian mind never fully understood the problems of great industry.' Proudhon showed a sympathy with the proletariat and the artisan which Bakunin was to discount in favour of the peasantry which, he regarded as a much more likely instrument of revolution. Proudhon's distinction between the beneficent qualities of work and the disabling characteristics of factory production was later to be echoed by William Morris, Durkheim, and most contemporary commentators.

Yet there is something in the contention that Proudhon, along with many anarchist thinkers, is antipathetic to industrial organization.

'The anarchist's cult of the natural, the spontaneous, the individual, sets him against the whole highly organized structure of modern industrial and statist society, which the Marxist sees as the prelude to his own Utopia. Even efforts to encompass the industrial world by such doctrines as anarcho-syndicalism have been mingled with a revulsion against that world, leading to a mystic vision of the workers as moral regeneraters; even the syndicalist could not foresee with equanimity the perpetuation of anything resembling industrial society as it exists at present.' (Woodcock 1963 : 23)

Anarchism is a protest against the extension of authority and centralized control, as such it is bound, in the end, to be incompatible with integrated industrial society. It is a protest against authority and, in answer to the inevitable question with which anarchists are always plagued, 'how will society work without it?' they latch on to the co-operative economic elements in Saint-Simonism. This makes it virtually impossible for them to advocate the overthrow of an industrial structure on which they have had to rely in substitution for traditional political authority. They then solve the problem of industrial production (which, in reality, they have succeeded in exaggerating) by ignoring it.

Bakunin and Kropotkin came much nearer to rejecting industrial society than Proudhon. Bakunin despised the proletariat as 'a privileged class of workers who, thanks to their considerable wages, pride themselves on the literary education they have acquired; they are dominated by the principles of the bourgeois, by their ambition and vanity, to such an extent that they are only different from the bourgeois by their situation and not in their way of thinking' (Joll 1964: 90).

Marxists regard industrialism with approval, as a means of creating a revolutionary, self-conscious, and strong proletariat, they see no evil in its survival as long as the economic context is changed. Anarchists seek to strengthen co-operative relationships at the expense of external authority, for this purpose the institutions of work seem valuable to them. They do not always recognize that authority is more closely present to the worker in his work than is political authority outside it. The concept of political liberty is, as Marx held, a bourgeois conception and the anarchist preoccupation with it is also to some extent, bourgeois.

But there is more than a theoretical foundation for Proudhon's veneration for work. Work and the family, for Proudhon, together assured independence and dignity. If work had to be undertaken in factories then Proudhon wished to guarantee as much independence and dignity as possible by programmes of education and career development, programmes essentially designed to secure the worker's freedom from reliance on one highly specialized operation. But these were desperate measures, perhaps advocated to make factory work resemble as closely as possible the 'real' work of the peasant, craftsmen or small proprietor, who were partly freed by their labour, from the necessity of subordination to others.

Proudhon seemed not to realize that factory work entailed subordination. More surprisingly, he seemed not to recognize the fundamental authority implied in all work and the subjection of the individual to necessity or routine which it nearly always involves. It is strange that this French peasant was reminded of this reality by a Russian gentleman. Herzen (1968 : II, 817) admonished him as follows:

'... nothing is left but the dull, exhausting, inescapable toil of the proletariat of today, the toil from which at least the aristocratic family of ancient Rome, based on slavery was free ...'
'Man is doomed to toil: he must labour till his hands drop and the son takes from the cold fingers of the father the plane or the hammer and carries on the everlasting work. But what if, among the sons, there happens to be one with a little more sense, who lays down the chisel and asks:
"But what are we wearing ourselves out for?"
"For the triumph of Justice", Proudhon tells him.
And the new Cain answers:
"But who charges me with the triumph of justice? ... Who set up the objects? ... It is too stale; there is no God but the commandments remain. Justice is not my vocation; work is not a duty but a necessity; for me the family is not lifelong fetters but the setting for my life, for my development. You want to keep me in slavery, but I rebel against you, against your yardstick, just as you have been revolting all your life against bayonets, capital and Church."'

These are difficult questions which are directed at an examination of the mystifications involved in an ideology of work and which it has taken one hundred and fifty years to formally place on the agenda for scrutiny. The anarchists probably came nearer than most to being able to examine them. They were prevented from doing so because their scepticism about society's assumptions was not total. In part they were trapped in an emotional veneration of workers as the sturdy independent peasantry which most embodied a spirit of co-operative freedom and independence. In part they had to construct a theoretical basis of economic co-operation to replace the political structure of authority which they sought to destroy. Their thinking and their analysis also emerged from a process of theoretical development which was rooted in economic concepts and values which had been developed most consistently by Saint-Simon. The anarchists were economic men as surely as the intellectual descendents of Adam Smith, the point we have previously attempted to argue is that their presence in the radical wing of the schism in that development

is of minor significance and gives a misleading impression of the depth
of their opposition to it.

Yet there was more ambivalence and less consistency in the way in
which the economic arguments were deployed by anarchists. Their
'failure' to take account of industrial conditions is a mark of this
ambivalence. It is as if the logic of their argument was determined by
the premisses on which it rested while the drift of the argument was
conditioned by their temperament. The anarchists were largely radical,
economic reformers whose major concern was not economic reform but
human dignity and freedom.

Although it is beyond the scope of the ideology of work this noble
inconsistency is best illustrated by Proudhon's magnificent reply to
Marx's letter, asking for his co-operation in organizing correspondence
between international socialists. Proudhon agrees, although he cannot
promise to write 'either at length or often since my various occupations
as well as my natural laziness do not allow me to make these epistolary
efforts'. He goes on to make some reservations.

> 'for God's sake when we have demolished all *a priori* dogmas,
> do not let us think of indoctrinating the people in our turn.
> Do not let us fall into your compatriot Martin Luther's incon-
> sistency. As soon as he had overthrown Catholic theology he
> immediately, with constant recourse to excommunications and
> anathemas, set about founding a Protestant theology. For three
> hundred years Germany's whole concern has been to destroy
> Luther's hodgepodge. Let us not make further work for humanity
> by creating another shambles. I wholeheartedly applaud your idea
> of bringing all shades of opinion to light. Let us have a good
> and honest polemic. Let us set the world an example of wise
> and farsighted tolerance, but simply because we are leaders of a
> movement let us not instigate a new intolerance. Let us not set
> ourselves up as the apostles of a new religion, even if it be the
> religion of logic or of reason.'

Even more characteristically, if on a less elevated scale, his letter
goes on to reply to a rancorous attack by Marx on one 'M. Crün in
Paris'. Proudhon appeals: 'M. Marx, to your well-balanced judgement, Crün is in exile with no fortune, with a wife and two children
and with no source of income but his pen.' Proudhon understands
Marx's philosophic wrath and realizes that we should all be saints and
angels, but we must live and, good heavens, 'a man who sells ideas

about society is no less meritorious than one who sells a sermon' (Edward and Fraser 1970: 149-51). This passage well illustrates the old anarchist preoccupation with the individual rather than with the achievement of a dogmatic consistency.

Syndicalists shared and developed the preoccupation with economic relationships and regarded the ties which bound man as a worker to his society as the only significant associations which he formed. Because men 'in society are interested above everything else in the satisfaction of their economic needs' this simple self-interest becomes the vehicle for man's assertion of power (Laidler 1949: 295). Industrial unions would recognize the reality of the workers' interests and the ties which bound them to their comrades while widening their horizons and developing their sense of class consciousness.

Once organized, industrial unions would engage in hostile and violent conflict with employers and with the still extant remnants of political society in strikes which were always to have revolutionary significance. Any means, short of the destruction of human life, were recognized as appropriate. The dedication to revolutionary objectives obviously associates the syndicalist with a communist position but the syndicalist is distinguished by his contempt for political means and political institutions. Syndicalists are also as devoted to the means as to the end, and the means for them, are trade unions. This also distinguishes them from communists and socialists who are sometimes ambivalent about trade unions and sometimes openly hostile. Sturmthal (1964: 1968), for example, argues that

'Classical Socialist Theory has been at a loss to determine the place of unions in a collectivized economy. Presented in conventional Marxian terms the problem was simply that unions were instruments of the workers' resistance to capitalist exploitation: with the transfer of the ownership of the means of production to the community, exploitation was bound to disappear and with it the main *raison d'etre* of the unions ... as long as exploitation was by definition excluded from a Socialist society, Socialist theory found no easy solution for the problem of union functions beyond the decline of capitalism.'

Syndicalists are not so sanguine and, in any case, they differ from socialists in their rooted objection to the State as an instrument of class rule. Workers cannot succeed, they believe, unless they overthrow the State by their own direct action. Political action, even by workers' parties, is likely to produce only the illusion of success because political activity is particularly suitable, indeed it demands, a process of bargaining, compromise and collaboration and, as such it is likely to corrupt the workers' objectives. As Laidler (1949: 296) puts it, 'an analysis of democratic reforms, the syndicalists assert, will show that those of value have been wrested by force. Too many reforms granted by legislations are devised to weaken the revolutionary movement by developing class harmony.' Syndicalists are therefore suspicious, not only of politics, but of reformers and reform which they see as aimed at making conditions tolerable which ought to be destroyed.

Syndicalists believe that work, and the economic relationships which it involves transcends class, country, and patriotism. Patriotism, as it is reflected in armies, is merely a device to ensure the subjugation of workers, so syndicalists have often been preoccupied with the subversion of the armed forces because they are composed of misguided workers who ought to recognize their friends instead of shooting them.

The new classless, stateless society will be created by a general strike. Even if a general strike fails it is to be welcomed as a necessary rehearsal for the success of the next general strike. When the general strike ultimately succeeds and the new society is established then unions, or syndicates, composed of workers in the same industry or trade-groups will control production. These groups will not regard themselves as owning the means of production so much as managing it on behalf of and 'with the consent of society'. This consent, however, is regarded as having been expressed through the medium of the 'syndicates'. The planning and co-ordination of these activities on a regional and inter-regional scale would be achieved by institutions resembling local trades and labour councils and ultimately by a kind of managing TUC, if such a thing can be imagined.

Syndicalists argue that the kind of relationships established in such a society would be so based on reality that they would make coercion unnecessary: 'the discipline they exact is that from within, decided upon by those whose duty it is to carry on the process in question ... the rules they would impose would follow from a knowledge of the conditions of their social functions and would be, so to speak, a "natural" discipline made inevitable by the conditions themselves' (Laidler 1949: 299).

The influence of Saint-Simon is obvious and once again we can suggest that there is likely to be no discipline more absolute than a 'natural' discipline imposed by the 'conditions themselves'. After all, even the most complete tyranny may be overthrown by a revolution, or by a general strike, but presumably, not even a syndicalist can object to rules imposed by 'conditions themselves'. The syndicalists' version of the new society is, then, not only likely to be oppressive but it seems certain to be permanent because, as in Marxist theory, the process of continual conflict seems to come to an end once the millenium has arrived. Not only is the end questionable but syndicalists seem to have rid the process of construction of some of the normal safeguards which are commonly believed to require some degree of popular approval for the changes in contemplation. Syndicalists have no respect for democratic processes of decision-making based on universal suffrage and majority rule. Majorities, they say, are usually controlled and exploited by powerful minorities pursuing their own interest. Majorities are usually misled, wrong and a cumbersome impediment to progress and to progressive minorities.

Syndicalists, therefore, stress the importance of the conscious militant minority, the activists who are intelligent, sensitive and vigourous, but who must look to support from the mass of the workers. The influence of syndicalist thinking in terms of revolutionary tactics has been considerable. Any self-respecting contemporary university student, concerned to win the revolutionary struggle for control of the refectory committee, knows of the importance of the conscious minority as a detonator of the mass. The extent of the influence of this argument does nothing to conceal the poverty of its content. The whole process of the 'proctor' mentality at work has been attacked by Arnold Beichmann (in *Encounter*, August 1970), as characteristic of members of an intellectual elite of the left who insist on advising the working class as to its own best interest and who are constantly aghast at the working class's lack of gratitude when it does not pay the slightest attention to the advice so generously given it. The position of the conscious minority comes dangerously close to patronizing the very class that syndicalists put at the centre of social and economic life. What is to distinguish this particular conscious minority from any other exploiting group which may (despite its bourgeois origins) be more successful than the syndicalists in establishing its influence over the masses? Are the only safeguards to be class origins and goodwill? But goodwill is surely a dangerous guarantee among the powerful, it is the syndicalists who tell us, after all, that minorities rule in their own interest. Or is the test to be more pragmatic, concerning success in winning the solid active support of the working class? In this case it seems to be a long time coming. To this the syndicalists say that that is because the working class has been corrupted by other powerful minorities. This reveals the essential paradox of the argument. Majorities cannot be trusted because they are easily corrupted. The syndicalist minority must win the support of the mass. If they fail it is because majorities cannot be trusted. If they succeed it is because the majority has approved.

But ideologies should not be taken too seriously, their statements are never intended as doctoral theses or to pass examinations. Messianic doctrines such as this can never be attacked because they have not delivered the goods, their success as ideological statements and exhortations in fact depends upon the inclusion of uncertain delivery dates. Some day it will happen.

George Sorel, perhaps the leading theoretician of syndicalism, recognized the importance of a belief in the general strike as a social myth. It did not matter whether the general strike succeeded, or even whether it ever took place, what mattered was the belief in it. Sorel held the view that a governing class was influenced by a particular reigning mythology or set of beliefs and expectations, the objective reality of which was irrelevant. Myths were indispensable to every revolutionary movement and the myth of the general strike was necessary to the working class in order to encourage it in its intermediary battles. The myth also ensured that the revolutionary struggle was likely to be waged continually because it meant that the conflict between bourgeois and worker was never likely to be healed. Sorel was sufficiently realistic to see that people whose lives are influenced by such myths are likely to be particularly difficult to convert because they are secure from all refutation, particularly if they steadfastly refuse to advance any positive programme of what is to take the place of the structures when they have successfully assaulted and destroyed them. Syndicalists and their associates seem particularly grateful for this advice.

Syndicalism is a significant doctrine because, apart from its practical influence, it reveals two problems which are important in any discussion of left-wing, or worker-orientated theory. The first concerns the role of the intellectual — the worker by brain as the Guild Socialist was to call him. The second, 'the central issue of the labour movement in the twentieth century: its relation to the state' (Lichteim 1966 : 26).

The importance with which syndicalists regard the conscious minority or the revolutionary elite is bound to lead to a discussion of the role of intellectuals and their relationship to the workers. Hannah Arendt (1970 : 73) puts the matter very forcefully: 'For better or worse — and I think there is every reason to be fearful as well as hopeful — the really new and potential revolutionary class in society will consist of intellectuals, and their potential power, as yet unrealised, is very great, perhaps too great for the good of mankind.' She bases this argument on the fact that the growth in productivity results from the scientists' development of technology rather than from increases in productivity brought about by the contribution of workers, the intellectuals have 'ceased to be a marginal social group and have emerged as a new élite' (Arendt 1970 : 72) who are essential to society's functioning. But, she continues, 'they have no drive to organise themselves and lack experience in all matters pertaining to power. Also, being much more closely bound to cultural traditions ... they cling with greater tenacity to categories of the past that prevent them from understanding the present and their own role in it.' As a result, 'it is often touching to watch with what nostalgic sentiments the most rebellious of our students expect the "true" revolutionary impetus to come from those groups in society that denounce them the more vehemently the more they have anything to lose by anything that could disturb the smooth functioning of the consumer society' (1970 : 73).

This is to suggest that revolutionary theorists after Marx have continued to think of the proletariat as the revolutionary agent when changes following industrialization which Marx may not have predicted have made it unlikely that the proletariat will fill this role and more likely that the intellectuals will. If this is so, the efforts of syndicalists and others, to build a bridge from the intellectuals to the workers, seem to be not only unsuccessful but unnecessary.

It is ironic, in terms of these speculations that Sorel regarded the intellectuals as one of the main targets to be attacked by syndicalists. The working class was to be the agent of change and it was the syndicalists' role to develop the workers' capacities by training them to take over the 'workshop created by capitalism'. Sorel saw the danger of domination by intellectuals and believed that it had to be resisted; he regarded socialist intellectuals as 'bourgeois intellectuals in search of a proletarian clientele' (Lichteim 1966 : 25).

The real difficulty in this position is whether the domination of the intellectuals can be resisted simply by identifying it. Lichteim says that

Marx, commenting on 'the functional division in modern industry between (intellectual) overseers and (manual) executants ...' was anticipating the key issue of the future. Later Lichteim (1966 : 28) adds that Sorel would probably 'have scented in the Communist authoritarianism the gem of a new hierarchy subordinating the toilers once more to a directing stratum'.

This last comment suggests an argument which is now frequently conducted, that analysis of class conflict within a capitalist environment misses the point of current problems and is not likely to be fruitful in terms of their solution. Every analysis that we have examined since Adam Smith has been set firmly within an economic context, its discussion bounded by parameters of economic value. However rigorous and thorough-going the attack on capitalist society, both its analysis and any proposed alternative have been set in economic terms and have been built on the same foundations as the institutions which are to be replaced. The criticisms, however, revolutionary, in fact entrench the values of the situation they seek to overthrow.

Thus syndicalism, amongst the most extreme of the criticisms of capitalism, emphasizes the supreme importance of economic relationships and the paramount importance of the place of work. Syndicalists create for themselves the impossible dilemma of trying to solve the problem of authority by emphasizing the importance of work, which is, in the present day, inseparable from the presence of authority. It is as though the syndicalists themselves were trapped in the myths of the previous century's economic understanding, just as Sorel accuses the bourgeois of being trapped in the enlightenment. It may be that the essential problems of the twentieth-century worker cannot be usefuly presented in terms of the economic relationship in which he operates but that they exist, rather, in terms of his role as an industrial employee, whoever owns the capital of his factory.

Explanations and promises of improvement which rest upon his importance as worker or as producer seem likely to enlarge rather than to diminish his difficulties as his position as worker becomes more tedious, less important to society and to himself and as he becomes more thoroughly subordinated, not to an economic oppressor but to an industrial authority. Syndicalists compound the fallacy still further when they argue, along with Saint-Simon, that the new industrial authority will be more expert; there is no authority less challengeable than that which is legitimated by its own absolute rationality.

Not only the syndicalists seem unable to escape from the horns of the dilemma which they have constructed but also the intellectuals seem not to be as easily dismissed from consideration as Sorel believed. For, unless the syndicalists are to manage society by some quite other principles than those they elucidate in its analysis, the intellectuals, the professionals, and the experts will be recruited for the directing role in the new society. Not only does authority refuse to be displaced but it is manned by the very personnel of whom the syndicalists seem most suspicious.

There are signs, recently, of considerable criticism of 'the system' beginning to emerge from outside it. The other principles which the syndicalists failed to discover are beginning to be constructed. We shall be examining proposals for the alternative rather than the new society later but it is worth considering, at this point, the kind of perceptive criticism that is now being directed at the syndicalists' new world. The following passage sets out to contrast the old radicalism with the new in terms of their attitudes to science and technology but, in doing so, it illustrates the more general point, that the economic myth in which we have been locked is most visible and can best be attacked from outside it.

'Centralized bigness breeds the regime of expertise, whether the big system is based on private or socialized economies. Even within the democratic socialist tradition with its stubborn emphasis on workers' control, it is far from apparent how the democratically governed units of an industrial economy will automatically produce a general system which is not dominated by co-ordinating experts. It is both ironic and ominous to hear the French Gaullists and the Wilson Labourites in Great Britain — governments that are heavily committed to an elitist managerialism — now talking seriously about increased workers' participation in industry. It would surely be a mistake to believe that the technocracy cannot find ways to placate and integrate the shop floor without compromising the continuation of super scale processes. ''Participation'' could easily become the god-word of our official politics within the next decade; but its reference will be to the sort of ''responsible'' collaboration that keeps the technocracy growing. We do well to remember that one of the great secrets of successful concentration camp administration was to enlist the ''participation'' of inmates.'

Roszak cites Cohn-Bendit as an instance of the failure of some radicals to analyse the cultural consensus which, he says, underlies the technocracy. 'What results from ignoring this level of analysis shows up in Cohn-Bendit's treatment of "communist bureaucracy", which he seems to blame on the sheer opportunistic bastardliness of Bolshevik leadership. The relationship of the technocracy — whether Stalinist, Gaullist, or American capitalist — to these universally honored myths of high industrial society eludes him' (1970 : 206).

We can take it that Cohn-Bendit's is a position not too far distant from the syndicalism we have been discussing. Its influence on him and on the events of Paris in May 1968 proves its continuing potency. Its continued failure to meet its own requirement of winning widespread worker support is not, in itself, too serious — the myth can, after all, continue indefinitely to claim that they will join next time and, if they do not, that this is proof of their subjugation to 'power élites'. Success may come, one day, failure illustrates the beastliness of bourgeois institutions. The real tragedy of syndicalism would be demonstrated only in the event of its triumph; that it is totally enclosed within the framework of the same ideology that produced the spirit of capitalism.

7. Marx and Alienation

I *Marxism, The General Theory*

We have delayed too long an examination of Marx's theory; its influence on outlooks that we have already discussed has been apparent.

Marx dominates the subsequent development of labour ideology and a great deal else besides. His account of labour and of its 'alienation' cannot be separated from his world view, from the general explanation he˙gives of history, of society, and of the economic relationships on which it is founded. For that reason it would seem to be wise to give a general account of the theory, however inadequate and superficial it is, and however unnecessary as far as the average reader is concerned. This account will be given, as far as possible, in his own (translated) terms because one of the major problems concerning his meaning lies in his interpretation by various ideologists intending to construct quite different buildings with stone from the same extensive quarry.

Men are distinguished from the animals, says Marx, 'as soon as they begin to produce their means of subsistence', in this way they 'are indirectly producing their actual material life' (Marx & Engels 1965 : 33). The nature of individuals depends on the material conditions which determine their production; production and exchange determine our behaviour and our outlook and it is an illusion to think that our thoughts are independent of the material conditions of our lives. 'They [that is morality, religion, ideas] have no history, no development; but men developing their material production and their material intercourse, alter, along with them their real existence, their thinking and the products of their thinking. Life is not determined by consciousness but consciousness by life' (1965 : 38). 'The phantasms formed in the human brain are necessarily sublimates of their material life process, which is empirically verifiable and bound to material premises' (Marx & Engels 1965 : 37).

Just as the nature of the individual depends upon productive forces so do the relationships between states and their internal structures. In particular, successive developments of the division of labour which, in its simplest form is found within the family, represent 'just so many different forms of ownership the first of which is tribal, the second of which is the communal state or city which is threatened by the gradual extension of private property and in which slavery is the basis of production. The third form is feudalism' (Marx & Engels 1965 : 33).

The continued development of the division of labour leads to contradictions and to inequalities in distribution. An estrangement is set up between what the individual contributes and the society to which he contributes. A man's work becomes alien, he must do it or starve, he has no choice in what he does.

'This fixation of social activity, this consolidation of what we ourselves produce into an objective power above us, growing out of our control, thwarting our expectations, bringing to nought our calculations, is one of the chief factors in historical development up to now'. The interests of the individual and of the community are in conflict and the community's interest becomes independently established in the state, divorced from the real interests of individual and community but always based on real interests 'especially ... on the classes, which in every such mass of men separate out and of which one dominates all the others' (Marx & Engels 1965 : 45).

Struggles within the state between democracy, aristocracy, and monarchy, or struggles over the franchise, are merely illusory forms of the real struggle fought out between the different classes, 'it follows that every class which is struggling for mastery even when its domination, as is the case with the proletariat, postulates the abolition of the old form of society in its entirety and of demarcation itself, must first conquer for itself political power in order to represent [itself] in turn as the general interest' (Marx & Engels 1965 : 45).

Marx's prediction of the inevitability of proletarian revolution depends first upon the establishment of his theory of surplus value and of the accumulation of capital. These are essential cornerstones in the construction (or, perhaps, the destruction) that follows because they relate to certain preconditions of a revolutionary situation; the working class must be extensive in numbers and must have been the victim of expropriation, at the same time the contradiction must have been established 'of an existing world of wealth and culture', which presupposes advanced productive development.

The value of any commodity is determined by the amount of labour necessary to produce it. The value of labour is similarly determined, like any other commodity, by the number of hours of labour necessary for its production. The value of labour is determined by the cost of keeping it in a state of productive efficiency. Labour, however, normally produces more that the cost of its own keep. Gide and Riste (1948 : 455f) point out that although Marx does not prove this assertion, it is unexceptionable because, if it were not true, in general terms, then there would have been no saving, no accumulation of capital, and no civilization.

The worker receives that proportion of what he produces which is necessary to his own efficient maintenance, the rest goes to the capitalist. In the first part of his period at work, the worker produces his own wages, after this, he works for nothing, or, more accurately, he works without charge for someone else. The proportions between the parts of the productive period vary, according to Nassau Senior, entrepreneurs in nineteenth-century British manufacturing derived their profit entirely from the last hour of work in the day.

The difference that goes to the capitalist is surplus value. The capitalist naturally tries to increase surplus value while reducing labour value. 'The object of all development of the productiveness of labour, within the limits of capitalist production is to shorten that part of the working day during which the workman must labour for his own benefit, and by that very shortening, to lengthen the other part of the day during which he is at liberty to work gratis for the capitalist' (Marx 1901 : 311). He does this by various means, by, for example, lengthening the working day but he goes so far that he is likely to be limited by a reaction which enforces legal limitations on the hours of work (there is still no such limitation for adult males in the UK), by reducing the cost of living, by more efficient industrial organization, by philanthropy, by employing women and children.

In his discussion of capital, Marx distinguishes between variable capital, needed to maintain labour, and constant capital, which assists labour's productive capacity by equipping it with machinery. Constant capital is unproductive of surplus value, it produces its own equivalent value so it is in the interest of the capitalist to employ more variable capital. This is one of several parts of Marx's analysis where he appears to be flying in the face not only of subsequent developments but also of the behaviour of people; capitalists normally appear to do the opposite, they try to reduce variable and increase fixed capital. Cole came to his rescue on this issue by arguing that he was not giving an account of the behaviour or the profit of any particular capitalist but that rather he was dealing with the return to the capitalist class as a whole, with the 'general class-reationship between possessing classes and workers'. Marx, he claimed, distinguished between 'the amount of surplus value that accrued to a capitalist in the first instance and the amount which the working of the capitalist system allowed him to keep for himself. The former ... was derived solely from the "variable" part of the capital' (Cole 1954 : II, 282). The latter, for each individual capitalist would be reduced to equality by competition. The profits of a particular business depended on competitive conditions.

In *The German Ideology* (1965 : 85), Marx and Engels set out the whole historical process of which this accumulation of surplus value represents the penultimate stage:

1. 'In the development of productive forces there comes a stage when productive forces and means of intercourse are brought into being, which, under the existing relationships, only cause mischief and are no longer productive but destructive forces (machinery and money), and connected with this a class is called forth, which has to bear all the burdens of society without enjoying its advantages, which, ousted from society, is forced into the most decided antagonism to all other classes; a class which forms the majority of all members of society, and from which emanates the consciousness of the necessity of a fundamental revolution ...'

2. 'The condition under which definite productive forces can be applied, are the conditions of the rule of a definite class of society, whose social power, deriving from its property, has its *practical* — idealistic expression in each case in the form of the state; and, therefore, every revolutionary struggle is directed against a class, which till then has been in power.'

3. 'In all revolutions up till now the mode of activity always remained unscathed and it was only a question of a different distribution of this activity ... whilst the communist revolution is directed against the preceding *mode* of activity, does away with *labour*, and abolishes the rule of all classes with the classes themselves ...'

4. For the communist consciousness to be created and to be successful 'an alteration ... can only take place on a mass scale ... in a practical movement, a *revolution*.'

The inevitability of revolution, says Marx, rests upon the theory of surplus value and on the accumulation of capital. The bourgeois continues to expropriate the proletariat while the progress of capitalist production swells its ranks; thus the same forces make it both more impoverished and more powerful and, therefore, a potent revolutionary force.

Marx's most succinct statement of the revolutionary character of communism is in *The Communist Manifesto*: 'A spectre is haunting Europe — the spectre of communism'. Bowle points out that this was not true but that its predictive value was greatly enhanced by its quality as propaganda. 'The history of all hitherto existing society is the history of class struggles'. Bourgeois society has not replaced class conflict in society, it has simply 'established new classes, new conditions of oppression, new forms of struggle in place of the old ones' (Cole 1948 : 120). The bourgeoisie, having successfully struggled against the domination of feudal nobility, has now established itself and parallel to the establishment of its own production patterns and economic relationships, the institutions of government also represent its domination: 'The executive of the modern state is but a committee for managing the common affairs of the whole bourgeoisie' (Cole 1948 : 122). Just as law is a reflection of bourgeoisie economic domination, so, Marx tells an imaginary member of the class, 'Your very ideas are but the outgrowth of the conditions of your bourgeois production and bourgeois property, just as your jurisprudence is but the will of your class made into a law for all' (Cole 1948 : 140).

The triumph of capitalism has removed the necessity for any comforting illusions, it 'has left no other nexus between man and man than naked self-interest, than callous "cash payment" ... It has resolved personal worth into exchange value ... The bourgeoisie has stripped of its halo every occupation hitherto honoured and looked up to with revered awe. It has converted the physician, the lawyer, the priest, the poet, the man of science, into its paid wage labourers.' (Cole 1948 : 123).

While the bourgeoisie is establishing its own supremacy it is also producing changes in the proletariat which make the workers' conditions more desperate.

'In proportion as the bourgeoisie, i.e., capital, is developed, in the same proportion in the proletariat, the modern working class developed a class of labourers who live only so long as they find work, and who find work only so long as their labour increases capital ... the cost of production of a workman is restricted, almost entirely, to the means of subsistence that he requires for his maintenance, and for the propagation of his race. But the price of a commodity, and therefore also of labour, is equal to its cost of production. In proportion therefore, as the repulsiveness of the work increases, the wage decreases.' (Cole 1948 : 128)

The bourgeoisie, in the course of its own conflicts with its enemies, is also forced to recruit the proletariat to help it and in this way it contributes to the organization of the proletariat, the bourgeoisie 'supplies the proletariat with its own elements of political and general education, in other words, it furnishes the proletariat with weapons for fighting the bourgeoisie' (Cole 1948 : 132).

While the proletariat is in this way both impoverished and organized, its ranks are swollen. 'All previous historical movements were movements of minorities, or in the interests of minorities. The proletarian movement is the self-conscious, independent movement of the immense majority in the interest of the immense majority' (Cole 1948 : 133).

The bourgeoisie finally goes too far in its oppression, 'in order to oppress a class, certain conditions must be assured to it under which it can, at least, continue its slavish existence'. But the modern labourer sinks as industry progresses. 'He becomes a pauper, and pauperism develops more rapidly than population and wealth. And here it becomes evident that the bourgeoisie is unfit any longer to be the ruling class in society ... It is unfit to rule because it is incompetent to assure an existence to its slave within his slavery, because it cannot help letting him sink into such a state, that it has to feed him, instead of being fed by him' (Cole 1948 : 134).

Modern industry promotes the co-operative association of workers. 'The development of modern industry, therefore, cuts from under its feet the very foundation on which the bourgeoisie produces and appropriates products. What the bourgeoisie therefore produces, above all, are its own grave-diggers' (Cole 1948 : 135).

The revolution and the victory of the proletariat are inevitable. The proletariat will take all capital from the bourgeoisie and will capture the means of production which will be organized and controlled by the state. The state will be the 'proletariat organised as the ruling class'. This is the penultimate stage of social conflict which has characterized, says Marx, all historical development. The feudal nobility fought the new, emergent middle class. Out of that conflict, the bourgeoisie emerged as the ruling class and superimposed its own characteristic forms of law and government upon a capitalist society. But the very progress of its domination provoked the hostility of the growing proletariat. The consequence of this conflict is the domination of the proletariat. The proletariat then has to fight class enemies and reactionary forces and, finally, the negation will be negated when the pre-conditions of class conflict will have been destroyed by the complete victory of the working class. Class-conflict will disappear with the final disappearance of classes. The proletariat will finally succeed when it abolishes its own supremacy. At this point we will see the withering away of the state and also, in a sense, the end of history; as class-conflict has provided the dynamic force which has caused all historical development, the end of class-conflict will, presumably, see the end of historical development.

Marx's general theory claimed, at one and the same time to be analytic, predictive, and exhortative; it revealed the inevitable while requiring us to assist in its arrival. It provided a large section of society with an explanation of its situation and of its importance, it developed a sense of class loyalty and a sense of social purpose over and above the immediate aim of survival.

Marx's economic theory has provoked a great deal of criticism, directed primarily at the theory of labour value, and the accuracy of his predictive statements has been widely questioned. In industrialized countries the proletariat has not grown larger, it has been reduced and it has not grown poorer, it has been enriched. Peasantries seem to have proved more effective revolutionary instruments than proletariats and neither has the revolutionary potential of the military. The bourgeoisie is entrenched and its ranks have been swollen. Alternative and ameliorative economic theories such as those of Keynes, the new deal and the welfare state, seem to have worked, at least, so far.

Some other predictions about communism have been more accurate. Bakunin said of it that

'power corrupts those who wield it as much as those who are forced to obey it ... all who put science before life, defend the idea of the state and its authority ... the difference between such revolutionary dictatorship and the modern state is only one of external trappings. In substance both are a tyranny of the minority over the majority —

in the name of the many and the supreme wisdom of the few — and so they are equally reactionary, devising to secure political and economic privilege to the ruling minority and the enslavement of the masses, to destroy the present order, only to erect their own rigid dictatorship on its ruins.' (Bowles 1963 : 321)

Marx may also, paradoxically, have succeeded in freeing the economic force of industrialism by seeking to change the environment which contained it. If industrialism was indefensible in its current, capitalist setting, the modification of the setting might be necessary to secure its permanent establishment. To this contention, a Marxist would probably reply that the current nature of industrialism and capitalism are inseparable co-variables.

It is time now to look in more detail at Marx's attitude to industrialization and to the division of labour.

II *Labour Co-operation and the Division of Labour*

Marx argues that the purpose of all capitalist development of labour productivity is 'to shorten that part of the working day, during which the workman must labour for his own benefit and, by that very shortening, to lengthen the other part of the day during which he is at liberty to work gratis for the capitalist' (Marx 1901 : 311).

In chapters 13 and 14 of *Capital*, in particular, Marx outlines and explains the great productive advantage which social or mass labour in co-operation enjoys over individual labour. It can be applied in large numbers at a concentrated and critical time, as in harvesting, or its application can be extended over a great space, as in dam building. It can be employed in the simultaneous performance of many operations, it has the advantage of economizing in the use of the means of production and it tends to average out differences between the abilities and the performance of individual workers. In addition to the more obvious advantages Marx sees subtler advantages in co-operative labour: 'Apart from the new power that arises from the fusion of many forces into one single force, mere social contact begets in most industries an emulation and a stimulation of the animal spirits that heighten the efficiency of each individual workman ... The reason of this is that man is, if not as Aristotle contends, a political, at all events a social animal' (Marx 1901 : 316). Or, as a modern management consultant might put it: 'the problem for management is to capture the naturally co-operative forces residing within the primary groups'.

Marx argues that this enhanced power of co-operation is not only natural to man but that it contributes to a higher level of activity than he would be capable of achieving solely as an individual. 'This power is due to co-operation itself. When the labourer co-operates systematically with others, he strips off the fetters of his individuality, and develops the capabilities of his species' (Marx 1901 : 319).

But labour co-operation requires organization to bring together a number of labourers and this in turn requires capital, the capitalist must be able to pay at least for their food and shelter for a limited period, it depends 'in other words, on the extent to which a single capitalist has command over the means of subsistence of a number of labourers' (Marx 1901 : 320), a minimum amount of capital is necessary in order to convert isolated processes into one, combined social process.

The achievement of co-operative production is a necessary function of capitalism; Marx argues that, at a given stage of development, co-operative labour cannot be achieved without capital. But the sheer necessity for capitalist control and organization inevitably leads to antagonism between capital and labour. He explains this process clearly in the last two chapters of the first volume of *Capital*.

'By the co-operation of numerous wage-labourers, the sway of capital develops into a requisite for carrying on the labour process itself, into a real requisite of production. That a capitalist should command on the field of production is now as indispensable as a general should command on the field of battle.

All combined labour on a large scale requires, more or less, a directing authority, in order to secure the harmonious working of the individual activities ... A single violin player is his own conductor; an orchestra requires a separate one. The work of directing, superintending, and adjusting becomes one of the functions of capital, from the moment that the labourer under the control of capital, becomes co-operative.' (Marx 1901 : 321)

But, the purpose of capitalist production, we must remember, is to extract the greatest possible amount of surplus value for the capitalist,

'to exploit labour-power to the greatest possible extent. As the number of the co-operating labourers increases, so too does their resistance to the domination of capital, and with it, the necessity for capital to overcome this resistance by counter-pressure. The control exercised by the capitalist is not only a special function, due to the nature of the social-labour process, and peculiar to that process, but it is, at the same time, a function of the exploitation of a social labour process, and is consequently rooted in the unavoidable antagonism between the exploiter and the living and labouring raw material he exploits'. (Marx 1901 : 321)

Labour co-operates, not as the result of voluntary associations or activities on its own behalf (although these come later), the co-operation of labour is brought about by the capitalist. The capitalist organizes labour and promotes its co-operative activity in order to increase its productive efficiency, in order to exploit it more thoroughly. But the co-operative activity of labour, once brought about by the capitalist, brings about a reaction by labour against its exploitation: the capitalist has created the conditions which make this reaction possible while, at the same time imposing conditions which make reaction inevitable.

Even the nature of the co-operation between workers, a co-operation essential to their ultimate advantage, is not spontaneous or rational to them, it is imposed on them;

'the co-operation of wage labourers is entirely brought about by the capital that employs them. Their union into one single productive body and the establishment of a connexion between their individual functions, are matters foreign and external to them, are not their own act, but the act of the capital that brings them and keeps them together. Hence the connexion existing between their various labours appears to them, ideally, in the shape of the powerful will of another, who subjects their activity to his aims.' (Marx 1901 : 322)

Capitalist control is, however, essentially despotic and as it extends the range of labour co-operation, the control begins to assume specialist forms. First, the capitalist is relieved of the burdensome necessity of working himself. Next,

'he hands over the work of direct and constant supervision of the individual workman, and groups of workmen, to a special kind of wage labourer. An industrial army of workmen, under the command of a capitalist, requires, like a real army, officers (managers), and sergeants (foreman, overlookers), who, while the work is being done, command in the name of the capitalist. The work of supervision becomes their established and exclusive function.' (Marx 1901 : 322)

The extension of this class in terms of its numbers and possibly also in terms of its power and influence in society is one of the most characteristic features of industrial development in the twentieth century, a development which took place largely after Marx's death. It is also one of the most contentious developments in terms of his analysis for, while Marx saw the group as exercising control and authority on behalf of the much more important class of owners and employers, the group has developed almost independently of ownership to become, apparently, a class in its own right, to the point at which some observers would say that it is now a self-governing élite in whose interest society at large tends to be organized. This is certainly the position of writers like James Burnham who emphasize the emergence of a managerial class and of an ideology of managerialism.

Marx emphasizes the inevitable and unavoidable relationship between the capitalist's ownership of the means of production and the function of control in industry. 'It is not because he is a leader of industry that a man is a capitalist. The leadership of industry is an attribute of capital, just as in feudal times the functions of general and judge were attributes of landed property' (Marx 1901 : 323).

In co-operative work, labourers 'enter into relations with the capitalist, but not with one another', they are incorporated in capitalism and they co-operate with it as members of a working organism, 'the productive power developed by the labourer when working in co-operation is the productive power of capitalism.'

So capitalism is necessary in order to facilitate the large-scale co-operation of labour but it also entails the more complete exploitation of labour.

Marx goes on, in chapter 14 to give a detailed examination of the causes and consequences of the divisions of labour in large-scale manufacturing. He regards the division of labour as representing a particular form of labour co-operation and he distinguishes between the division of labour in manufacturing, which was characteristic of capitalist development from the sixteenth century to the end of the eighteenth, and in modern machine industry. The former he deals with in the last chapter of Volume I, the latter in the first chapter of Volume II.

Manufacture involves the gathering together in a workshop, under the control of a capitalist, of labourers from different independent handicrafts through whose hands an article must pass before it is completed. Manufacture can also involve the opposite process, the employment by a capitalist in one workshop of a number of workers all doing the same kind of work. An example of the first kind of manufacturing process is the production of carriages, of the second, the making of paper.

The great advantage of manufacture is that more is produced in a given time because of the increase in the productive power of labour. Marx's explanation of the means by which this increase is brought about is very similar to the explanation given by Adam Smith. The result of the practical application of these advantages is an intricate arrangement of distinct operations which must be carried out in strict sequence; Marx clearly saw that the maintenance of the sequence or, as we might now describe it, the pursuit of the critical path, is a matter of great importance to management. 'Each labourer or each group of labourers prepares the raw material for another labourer or group. The result of the labour of the one is the starting point for the labour of the other' (Marx 1901 : 337). He might have added, at this point, that a process in which labour effectively controls the essential supply of raw materials of another group of labourers, is bound considerably to increase the power of the workers, a truth which has been grasped in modern strike strategy.

'Manufacture not only finds the conditions for co-operation ready to hand, it also, to some extent, creates them by the sub-division of handicraft labour. On the other hand, it accomplishes this social organization of the labour-process only by riveting each labourer to a single fractional task' (Marx 1901 : 337). This is one of several ways in which the manufacturing process influences the way in which labour is treated, the manner in which it is employed, and the tasks which it is required to perform. 'After manufacture has once separated, made independent and isolated the various operations, the labourers are divided, classified, and grouped according to their predominating qualities' (Marx 1901 : 341). Marx adds that if natural abilities are the foundation on which the division of labour is built, it develops these powers and develops new ones which are highly and unnaturally specialized. 'The habit of doing only one thing converts him into a never-failing instrument, while his connexion with the whole mechanism compels him to work with the regularity of the parts of a machine' (Marx 1901 : 342).

This process, as it develops, also entails the development of a hierarchy, a development of which Marx observed only the beginning. It has constantly evolved since then, accompanied by systematic training, the application of job-evaluation, and wage-structure differentiation on a rational basis, all related to an extended hierarchy of jobs and of control. Marx described the beginnings of this process:

'...individual labour powers, require different degrees of training and must have different values. Manufacture, therefore, develops a hierarchy of labour-powers, to which there corresponds a scale of wages ... Every process of production, however, requires certain simple manipulations, which ever man is capable of doing. They too are now severed from their connexion with the more pregnant moments of activity, and ossified into exclusive functions of specially appointed labourers. Hence, manufacture begets, in every handicraft that it seizes upon, a class of so-called unskilled labourers, a class which handicraft industry strictly excluded. Alongside of the hierarchy there steps the simple separation of the labourers into skilled and unskilled. For the latter the cost of apprenticeship vanishes; for the former it diminishes, compared with artificers, in consequence of the functions being simplified.' (Marx 1901 : 343)

This, of course, results in a fall in the value of labour, the reduced cost of training increases the amount of surplus value available to the capitalist.

Marx admits an exception to this process, an exception which 'holds good whenever the decomposition of the labour process begets new and comprehensive functions, that either had no place at all, or only a very modest one hin handicrafts' (Marx 1901 : 343). The exception has since assumed great proportions. Much of the argument over the relevance of Marx's analysis to the process of industrialization in the twentieth century concerns precisely the size and significance of the exceptions to his general account of continual de-skilling. The specific form of the question is whether industrialization has led to an increase in the relative proportion of unskilled labour, which is what Marx predicted for capitalism, or whether it has led to a general extension of skill and to an increase in the numbers of managerial, technical, and professional workers. On the face of it, it seems that the second proposition is the more accurate, i.e. industrial development increases the demand for skills. But the choice between these views is likely to be complicated by whether we chose a particular industry or industrial society as the environment within which comparisons over a period of time are to be made. The development of sections of relatively highly skilled labour in a particular industry may not be so apparent or important if the labour has to transfer to another industry in which its acquired skill is so specialized as now to be worthless. The appearance of increasing skill may in fact be simply a symptom of labour being rivetted to a part division of the productive process.

The same subject comes up in another form when Marx extends the division of labour to the distribution of intelligence and skill. Manufacture means that knowledge, judgement, and intelligence are now required

> 'for the factory as a whole. Intelligence in production expands in one direction because it vanishes in many others. What is lost by the detailed labourers, is concentrated in the capital that employs them. It is a result of the division of labour in manufacturers, that the labourer is brought face to face with the intellectual potencies of the material process of production, as the property of another, and as a ruling power. This separation begins in simple co-operation, where the capitalist represents to the single workman, the oneness and the will of the associated labour. It is developed in manufacture which cuts down the labourer into a detailed labourer. It is completed in modern industry, which makes science a productive force distinct from labour and presses it into the service of capital.' (Marx 1901 : 355)

Marx thus gives a comprehensive account of the development of co-operative labour and of its division into special tasks. The development is inflicted by the capitalist upon workers, he says, to the advantage of the former and to the disadvantage of the latter. But there are, as it were, unplanned consequences in the process which is forced along by capitalists. Workers are organized where they were before disunited and their strength and number increase in proportion to their misery. The process goes further as higher levels of industrial development and of productive complexity are reached. It reaches its limit in machine production and in the detailed division of labour. The consequences of this last stage of development lead us on to a discussion of one of the most controversial concepts in Marx's analysis.

The result of the development of machine production is that 'capital is constantly compelled to wrestle with the insubordination of the workmen' and Marx quotes the testimony of an enemy, Andrew Ure, as a witness in his case, 'the more skilful the workman, the more self-willed and intractable he is apt to become, and of course, the less fit a component of a mechanical system in which ... he may do great damage to the whole' (Marx 1901 : 362). This is why, says Marx, capitalists are constantly complaining about the difficulty of achieving labour discipline.

The use of machinery lengthens the working day until a public outcry demands its effective limitation, after that point the capitalist is forced to pursue the progressive intensification of labour because its continued extension has been prevented. This 'closer filling up of the pores of the working day' is pursued by various devices, by piece-work payment, by demands for more energetic work, by the increase of machine speed, and by the introduction of more machines. The result is that 'the denser hour of the ten hours working day contains more labour, i.e. expended labour-power, than the more porous hour of the twelve hours working day' (Marx 1901 : 408).

The effect of the extension of the division of labour on the worker is to aggravate his condition, even the reduction of the effort which it requires of him is not the blessing that it is so often made out to be.

'At the same time that factory work exhausts the nervous system to the uttermost, it does away with the many-sided play of the muscles and confiscates every atom of freedom both in bodily and intellectual activity. The lightening of the labour even becomes a sort of torture, since the machine does not free the labourer from work but deprives the work of all interest. Every kind of capitalist production, in so far as it is not only a labour process, but also a process of creating surplus value has this in common, that it is not the workman that employs the instruments of labour, but the instruments of labour that employ the workman.' (Marx 1901 : 422)

Marx argued that in earlier societies, the developing separation of labour had been frozen and made permanent by law and custom. The social division of labour was, in any case, not so harmful as the detailed division of labour in the factory, but even on the plane of society as a whole the division of labour entails 'some crippling of body and mind', but 'manufacture carries the social separation of branches of labour much further, and also, by its peculiar division, attacks the individual at the very roots of his life, it is the first to afford the materials for, and to give a start to industrial pathology'. Manufacture 'converts the labourer into a crippled monstrosity by forcing his detail dexterity at the expense of a world of productive capabilities and interests' (Marx 1901 : 357).

Engels (1969 : 149) was, if anything, more violent in his descriptions of the effects of this process. The compulsion to work is bad enough in itself, he says, because compulsory toil is a degrading punishment, but the division of labour has made the punishment much worse, it has 'multiplied the brutalizing influences of forced work ... It is still the same thing since the introduction of steam. The workers' activity is made unmeaning and monotonous to the last degree ... And a sentence to such work, to work which takes his whole time for itself ... how can such a sentence help degrading a human being to the level of a brute?'

These conditions, says Engels, confront the worker with a choice, to conform or to fight. He also suggests that the employer has accompanied his demand for labour control and for discipline with a moral apparatus which incorporates the notion of work as a duty. 'The worker must choose, must either surrender himself to his fate, become a "good" workman, heed "faithfully" the interest of the bourgeoisie in which case he most certainly becomes a brute, or else he must rebel, fight for his manhood to the last, and this he can only do in the fight against the bourgeoisie.'

III *Alienation*

A considerable controversy rages amongst students of Marx, over his commitment to the concept of alienation as well as over its meaning. The controversy, which is sufficiently complicated in itself, is further confused by the entrenched ideological position of some of the protagonists. Very roughly, these are those who have detected in his early writings a more humanist and less doctrinaire Marx and they have chosen to set the young Marx up as the theoretical champion of 'communism with a human face'. The inference from this position is that a misleading concentration upon the later works gives a false justification (as though in holy scripture) for Stalinist rigidity and the communist state as it is represented in the example of the Soviet Union.

Marx's treatment of the concept of alienation has become a part of this controversy. One view is that Marx developed his case about alienation in the *Economic and Philosophical Manuscripts* (1844) but that in his later works, *The German Ideology* (1845), the *Communist Manifesto* (1848), and *Capital* (1867) he stopped making references to alienation unless it was in a very critical context. Robert Tucker (1964), on the other hand, argues that whether the concept is referred to by name or not (and complications of translation intrude here, for there are at least three German terms which can be taken to connote our understanding of the term 'alienation'), it virtually underlies the whole of his analysis. Meszaros argues that there is no break in the development of theory between a young and idealistic Marx and the later mature and more scientific analyst. Meszaros refutes the interpretations which have been put upon the later 'critical' references to alienation and proceeds to give numerous examples of the appearance of the term in later works. The most decisive argument seems to lie in the recently discovered Draft of the Outlines of the Critique of Political Economy, which we shall refer to here, following McLellan, as the *Grundrisse*. This incomplete sketch of Marx's whole analytic system has been called by Meszaros (1970 : 240) 'probably the greatest single theoretical monument of Marx's life'. The work was completed in 1857 and 1858. McLellan (197 : 13) comments that the term alienation 'is central to most of the more important passages of the *Grundrisse*'. Meszaros (1970 : 233) says that the concept has become the 'structural common denominator ... the centre of reference of his entire conception'.

The pedantry which seems to surround some parts of this controversy may obscure what appears obvious to the less learned reader of Marx: that his whole conception of historical development and of its underlying economic relationships depends upon two processes, alienation and its subsequent transcendence. In more practical terms nearer to our immediate purpose, the whole of the exposition of Marx's attitude to machine production and to co-operative labour has been concerned with his explanation of the causes and effects of alienated labour. In this sense, Marx is never *not* concerned with alienation, but his clearest reference to the term as such seems to lie in the Manuscripts of 1844 and the *Grundrisse* of 1857-8.

It is soon apparent that Marx (McLellan 1971a : 135-8) uses the term to denote several different sorts of relationship, or rather, of broken relationships. The first of these is that labour is necessarily alienated from what it produces, its product

'confronts it as an alien being, as a power, independently of the producer ... In political economy the realization of labour appears as a loss of reality for the worker, objectification as a loss of the object or slavery to it, and appropriation as alienation, as externalization.

The appropriation of the object appears as alienation to such an extent that the more objects the worker produces, the less he can possess and the more he falls under the domination of his product, capital.

All these consequences follow from the fact that the worker relates to the product of his labour as to an alien object. For it is evident from this presupposition that the more the worker externalises himself in his work the more powerful becomes the alien objective world that he creates opposite himself, the poorer he becomes himself in his inner life and the less he can call his own.

According to the laws of political economy the alienation of the worker is expressed as follows: the more the worker produces the less he has to consume, the more values he creates, the more valueless and worthless he becomes, the more formed the product the more deformed the worker, the more powerful the work the more powerless becomes the worker, the more cultured the work the more philistine the worker becomes and more of a slave to nature.'

Marx goes on then to assert that the worker is alienated in two senses, first, from his product, second, from the process of producing it 'to his own activity as something that is alien and does not belong to him'. He has also by now explained that as man 'makes' the world, his alienation from what he makes is, at the same time, alienation from the sensuous and natural world. Marx then further extends the completeness of alienation, man is (1) alienated from nature; (2) from himself, from his own vital activity; (3) from his human essence; and (4) from other men.

Marx (McLellan 1971a : 142) proceeds to a still further extension of the term. If the product of my work opposes me it must belong to someone else, to another man. If the object of the worker's labour is 'an object that is alien, hostile, powerful and independent of him, this relationship implies that another man is the alien, hostile, powerful and independent master of this object. If he relates to his own activity as to something unfree it is a relationship to an activity that is under the domination, oppression and yoke of another man.' In alienated labour man 'creates the domination of the man who does not produce over the production and the product. As he alienates his activity from himself so he hands over to an alien person an activity that does not belong to him'.

Schacht (1971 : 91) regards this use of the term of alienation as equivalent to subordinated labour, as a weakness, a concept which would be better dropped. As an instance of its inconsistency, Schacht argues that labour under the direction of another man need not be alien activity (that is, the labour may not be dissociated from the worker's own interest *because* it is dictated by another man) and he gives the example of the orchestral player. There are several objections to this criticism. First, orchestral players volunteer to work under the direction of another in a sense that an assembly-line worker does not. Orchestral players are in no way conscripted, they do not have to be orchestral players, they spend years of training in order to take part in an activity which, for the most part, is not possible unless it is directed by another man. Labour under another man's direction does not normally connote the degree of choice left to an orchestral player. Second, orchestral playing is more game-like than most examples of subordinated labour; game players have to seek out other players and submit themselves to the authority of a set of rules and of a captain who will give them orders, but it would be absurd to assert that they are therefore alienated from the game or from the captain, and the absurdity lies in the fact that neither orchestral playing nor game playing can be compared to subordinated work.

Schacht also cites the examples of small hill-farmers and shop-owners whose work is alienating but who are free from subordination. But many others would see these people as un-alienated simply because they are free in a sense in which subordinated employees are not. They are, to an extent, free to be poor in that they have some measure of control over the degree to which they will exchange effort for leisure and money for freedom. The whole point of the extensive comparison of the factory system to domestic manufacture, which is largely to the former's disadvantage, is not that the domestic worker was richer but that he was more free, and in several senses, which are well-known and easily recognized, not alienated.

Marx's association of subordination with alienation was certainly intended by him, it was no accidental lapse. And it relates to a long tradition in which subordination in work has been regarded as un-free, restricting, and likely to produce consequences harmful to the worker. It is not only the Greeks who believed that it was subordination rather than the nature of the task performed, which was debasing to a human being. There is some research evidence to suggest that the authority imposed by the task, the system or the technology is less harmful or, at least, less resisted in its effect on the worker than the authority of another man. Schacht (1971 : 92) accepts that: 'It might of course turn out to be the case that this alienation very frequently does involve the surrender of labor to the direction of another man; but this would be a factual correlation rather than a matter of definition.' But it would become a matter of definition if the correlation were sufficiently complete. It also becomes a matter of definition if we assert that only the worker who is free from external control is free to ensure that his work is not alienated. One form of external control, but not the only one, is subordination to another man. Another form would be the external control imposed by a market economy and Marx certainly recognized that 'civil society' produced alienated labour; in this sense the small farmer or shopkeeper is also alienated, to an extent, because they are subordinated to market forces if not to other men. Subordination to other men may not then be a sufficient cause of alienated labour, but Marx could certainly continue to argue that market forces increased the number of subordinated labourers, gradually eliminated the number of independent peasant farmers and finally resulted in the employment of a subordinated proletariat by a bourgeoisie. 'Agriculture comes to be more and more merely a branch of industry and is completely dominated by capital' (McLellan 1971b : 41).

When everyone works for himself the worker must exchange his product

'in order to transform his own production into means of subsistence for himself. Exchange negotiated through exchange value and money, implies a universal interdependence between the producers, but at the same time the complete isolation of their private interest and a division of social labour, whose unity and mutual fulfillment exists as an external, natural relationship, independent of the individuals. The tension between universal supply and demand constitutes the social network that binds the indifferent individuals together.' (McLelland 1971b : 67)

In this sense, Marx sees capitalist society as producing alienation from other men. Capitalism exaggerates competitive relationships between men and encourages them to pursue their own self-interest, regarding their fellows as means to this end. Capitalism, in a word, develops egoism and egoism leads to the alienation of man from other men.

Schacht (1971 : 88) summarizes Marx's use of the term as always connoting separation involving the surrender of the worker's control over his labour and its product, 'Marx terms the product "alienated" from its producer when it comes under the sway of an alien hostile power, human or inhuman'. Schacht (1971 : 112) concludes that in the course of Marx's treatment he uses alienation in connection with labour, its product, the senses, communal life, other men, and man himself and that 'the use of the term "alienation" to designate all of them severely limits its descriptive content'. The term has acquired even more general usage after Marx until it has come 'to refer to virtually anything which is not as it should be as an instance of "alienation" '. Blauner (1964 : 2) takes this view: 'The alienation thesis has become the intellectual's shorthand interpretation of the impact of the industrial revolution on the manual worker. Non-Marxists and even anti-Marxists have followed Marx in this view that factory technology, increasing division of labour and capitalist property institutions brought about the estrangement of the industrial worker from his work.'

The point of this quite justifiable comment is that it surely reveals the importance of the contribution of Marx's concept of alienation to all subsequent ideological exchange on the subject of work in industrial conditions. There is no doubt that the use of the concept produces serious problems in any programme of research concerning employee attitudes. But we are not concerned with research or with the utility of the concept in social theory. The potency of 'alienation' in the vocabulary of ideology has been demonstrated by the very criticisms that are made of it. 'Alienation', perhaps because of its vagueness and its multi-reference, has become an inescapable concept of the ideology of work; it may have become an even more important element in capitalist or management literature than in post-Marxist doctrine. There is, after all, some natural reluctance to recognize the possibility of the phenomenon's extent in a state which is advancing to socialism; for capitalist economies, on the other hand, it remains a constant obstacle (and therefore a major preoccupation) in the way of the achievement of improved productivity and higher profits.

This brings us to an attempt at assessing its contemporary ideological status and significance. One aspect of the question concerns the predictive value of Marx's analysis. Marx has often been accused of having advanced a self-fulfilling prophecy; because he predicted revolution he made it certain that it would take place. Marx pleaded guilty to this accusation, the point he said is not to understand the world but to change it. It seems equally possible, however, that he advanced a self-falsifying prophecy: because he predicted revolution he made it certain that it would not occur. In this sense, capitalists and their managers have, after Marx, been constantly aware of the characteristics of the employment relationship which he so vividly presented and have therefore consistently attempted to reduce their effects. Modern management theory, at least those aspects of it concerned with employment, is almost entirely concerned to overcome alienation. In this sense Marx may have supported the capitalist system, postponing its decay by so clearly diagnosing the maladies from which it would 'inevitably' die.

A serious criticism of Marx's discussion of alienation asks how far it is correctly associated with the effects of the division of labour in a purely capitalist society. A Marxist will no doubt argue that this is an absurd question because the division of labour and alienation are inseparable characteristics of capitalist production, if capitalist society is destroyed it characteristics disappear. Marx (1901 : 44), indeed, says something very like this himself. In what he calls 'natural' society, man's work becomes alien, enslaving him instead of being controlled by him, but in communist society, on the other hand, 'society regulates the general production and thus makes it possible for one to do one thing today and another tomorrow, to hunt in the morning, fish in the afternoon, rear cattle in the evening, criticise after dinner ...' But this idyllic situation is almost certainly a description of the final stage of the evolutionary process, the negation of the negation, when classes have disappeared with the end of class hostility. In the meantime, what is to be the situation during the dictatorship of the proletariat? More particularly, who is going to work the night shift and who to work in the slaughterhouse?

Marx is, in any case, almost ambiguous about the division of labour. It represents, along with machine production, a necessary stage of development and a higher stage of development than that which preceded it; 'co-operative labour' not only raises the productive capacity of man but makes him more truly himself. Engels writes of 'man's silent vegetation' before the industrial revolution as a state not 'worthy of human beings'. It may be necessary to distinguish between Marx's hostility to capitalism and his attitude to machine production, about which at times he could become quite lyrical and, over the steam-hammer, almost poetic. There certainly seems little concern in Lenin and subsequent Soviet Marxists, as we shall see, over the de-humanizing results of machine production.

The argument about the contemporary status of alienation seems to fall into two patterns. On the one hand, there seems to be a measure of agreement that Marx's analysis did not take into account subsequent developments in capitalist production, 'the progressive pauperization of the proletariat and its necessary evolution to the realisation of its revolutionary role, has been rendered obsolete ... far from aiding a proletarian revolution the economic infrastructure of society has made for the progressive integration of the working classes into the existing social order.' In this sense, Marx was wrong. But McLellan (1971a : XLI) goes on to suggest that 'the second of Marx's major analyses, which aimed at showing that in a commodity society the products of men's labour acquired an independent, anti-human power, has become far more relevant than he could have imagined'.

The conclusion of this second form of analysis is illustrated in a passage from the *Grundrisse*.

'The historical vocation of capital is fulfilled as soon as, on the one hand, demand has developed to the point where there is a general need for surplus labour beyond what is necessary, and surplus labour itself arises from individual needs, and on the other hand, general industriousness has developed (under the strict discipline of capital) and has been passed on to succeeding generations, and finally when the productive forces of labour, which capital spurs on in its unrestricted desire for wealth and the conditions on which alone capital can achieve this have developed to the point where the possession and maintenance of general wealth requires, on the one hand shorter working hours for the whole and working society conducts itself scientifically towards the progressive reproduction of wealth, its reproduction in even greater profusion, so that the sort of labour in which the activities of men can be replaced by those of machines will have ceased ... capital, with its restless striving after the general form of wealth, drives labour out beyond the limits of its natural needs.' (McLellan 1971b : 85-6)

In the sense that this and similar passages suggests the advance of capitalism to what is now fashionably called the consumer society, Marx certainly predicted a future in which man seems to be enslaved by demands which he is forced to create. But there are references, here and elsewhere, which suggest both that Marx imagined a future for labour (or for the proletariat) which has more accuracy than is often conceded to him and that it contained elements which contradicted what is often understood as his major prediction. In a passage entitled 'The Labour Process and Alienation in Machinery and Science', Marx appears to predict a future for capitalism in which the last phase 'is the *machine*, or rather an *automatic system of machinery*'. In this phase, 'the production process has ceased to be a labour process in the sense that labour is no longer the unity demanding and transcending it', the unity of the system now seems to be imposed by the machinery itself. Social labour and productivity become represented not in labour but in capital in the form of machinery, 'the worker appears to be superfluous in so far as his action is not determined by the needs of capital ...' the production process 'has become a technological application of science' (McLellan 1971b : 135).

The contradiction inherent in the capitalist system now emerges in a different form, it lies in the fact that value is determined simply by the quantity of labour engaged in production while labour, in fact, becomes less and less important in the production process. Labour is reduced quantitatively and qualitatively to a 'subordinate role as compared with scientific labour in general, the technological application of the natural sciences, and the general productive forces arising from the social organisation of production'. In this process 'labour does not seem any more to be an essential part of the process of production. The human factor is restricted to watching and supervising the production process. (This applies not only to machinery, but also to the combination of human activities and the development of human commerce)' (McLellan 1971b : 136).

Marx returns to the paradox that labour time is the basis of value but no longer the basis of production.

'The theft of other's labour time upon which wealth depends today seems to be a miserable basis compared with this newly developed foundation that has been created by heavy industry itself.... The surplus labour of the masses has ceased to be a condition for the development of wealth in general ... Production based on exchange value therefore falls apart, and the immediate process of material production finds itself stripped of its impoverished, antagonistic form. Individuals are then in a position to develop freely. It is no longer a question of reducing the necessary labour time in order to create surplus labour, but of reducing the necessary labour of society to a minimum. The counterpart of this reduction is that all members of society can develop their education in the arts, sciences, etc., thanks to the free time and means available to all.' (McLellan 1917b : 142)

The implications of these astonishing passages in the *Grundrisse* are considerable. As they stand they suggest that Marx may have concluded that the development of capitalist machine production would not lead to an extension of the size of the proletariat, that the intensification of production would be achieved by machinery, that is by capital itself (albeit itself a crystalization of past labour), that labour would cease to be the measure of production and of value. Now these interpretations are enough in themselves to stand Marx's general analysis of historical development, as it is normally understood, on its head. It is not at all clear, in fact, whether he is arguing that these conditions are brought about in the last phase of capitalist production (the 'automatic system of machinery' as he called it) or in the phase of communist society which is to supercede it. In either case he seems here to be substituting the contradiction that capitalism 'reduces labour time to the minimum while at the same time establishing labour hire as the sole measurement and source of wealth' (McLellan 1971b : 143) for the whole principle of class antagonism resting on the exploitation and expropriation of labour. Not only does this new concept flatly contradict what is normally understood to be a Marxist analysis but it makes for a far less dramatic and exciting principle of revolutionary change than does the notion of class war: capitalism is to go out with a technological squeak rather than a revolutionary bang.

There is, finally, the equally disturbing possibility that Marx is here promoting the forces of technical production to a place of greater analytic importance than the economic relationship which he has elsewhere emphasized as dominant 'Productive forces and social relationships — the two different sides of the development of the social individual — appear to be, and are, only a *means* for capital to enable it to produce from its own cramped base. But in fact they are the material conditions that will shatter this foundation' (McLellan 1971b : 143). In this way, apparently, the technical production system which is the highest development of capitalism finally serves to destroy it.

IV *Conclusion*

The interpretation of these passages becomes important in determining the progress of the class war. The commonly understood version of Marxism is that an enlarged and enraged proletariat is finally driven to take over the means of production from its exploiters. The Marxist answer to the charge that this prediction had been falsified by events was that events had not yet unfolded. Communism was then furnished with the infallable defence of untestability, it could not be refuted until tomorrow which, of course, never comes. But communist theory has several other tricks up its sleeve. Like other 'autocracies tempered by insurrection' it is always capable of denouncing past errors by claiming that they are purged by current revelation. In this sense, there is an ever changing pantheon of new representatives of the truth of Marxism, the current ideological contender is probably Gramsci. There are also constant reformulations of doctrine. The determinism of the Second International is now dismissed as crude, it has given way to more subtle notions of *praxis*, of the need to apply theory to a particular and changing historical context.

The class war and the identity and importance of the proletariat have all come up for revision. As the manual work force of the advanced industrial societies declined in both numbers and revolutionary zeal, account began to be taken of that class which seemed to be replacing it. There was much talk of the significance of the white collar workers and an emphasis on the essential similarity of their relationship to the employers — that manual worker and office worker were both exploited. If the office worker did not behave with revolutionary propriety this was, it seems, because the 'objective' reality of his class position had not been revealed to him. 'False consciousness', which had been so useful in explaining the strange behaviour of the proletariat, was also available to explain the reluctance of the white collar workers to join the class struggle. The evidence of the growth of white collar unionization has put some life into the case for 'proletarianization' but it takes a truly committed imagination to see the National Union of Bank Employees in the forefront of the revolutionary struggle.

Professor Giddens suggests that the naivety of these arguments has led to a new shift in focus on the class struggle. The new emphasis is on

> 'the crucial importance of scientific and technical ideas to neo-capitalism: the production and dissemination of scientific knowledge becomes the primary "force of production" in neo-capitalist society. Engineers, scientists, technicians of all sorts thus occupy a pivotal place in the socio-economic order. But rather than affiliating themselves with other groupings in the "middle class" these worker constitute a new vanguard of the working class — not because they are "proletarian" in the conventional sense of the term as regards income and economic rewards, but because they experience, in acute form, a "contradiction" between their need for autonomous control over their work (the production of knowledge) and the bureaucratic exigencies of the organization to which they are subject.' (Giddens 1973 : 195)

The class struggle goes on but the actors in the drama change and the plot thickens. The process is held up as an example of the way in which Marx's analysis is consistently and constantly applied to the unfolding process of historical reality. While we cannot predict the precise nature of historical change, Marxist theory, we are told, is capable of providing an understanding of the current realities. There is enough in the passages which have been quoted from the *Grundrisse* to substantiate this claim. If this particular development was not foreseen by Marx, his analysis makes sense of it. The process illustrates both the strength and the weakness of Marx's theory. Theory at such a level of generalization succeeds because it can explain all phenomena, but its universal potential means that it is irrefutable. It can never be ovethrown by contrary evidence. When contrary evidence does appear this cannot serve to challenge the theory because history has moved on, new 'realities' have appeared, the very fluidity of the theory is evidence of its extraordinary adaptability. It can never be wrong. The proletariat gives way to the white collar workers who are displaced by the scientists and technologists. When the evidence of proletarian stability appears, social and economic relationships are said to have changed so that the test of proletarian revolt is no longer relevant. When our scientists will demonstrate no awareness of a contradiction between the need to control their work and the bureaucracies which control them they too will have been removed from the stage of history. Who is next? The process of rescuing Marx from erring is the theoretical equivalent of the older practical process of predicting the day for the revolution, or for the end of the world.

It all makes poor theory, but admirable ideology. It is aided by the massive extent and the considerable obscurity of Marx's writing. The interpretation of the word is hedged about by formidable scholarship. A priesthood intervenes to explain the doctrine, contrary explanations are pronounced anathema and, above all, the laiety is told to mind its own business and get on with its work. The *Grundrisse*, we are told, 'is a demanding text to read and a hazardous one to quote, since the context, the grammar and the very vocaburlarly (sic) raise doubts as to what Marx 'really' meant in a given passage. Let the quoter, the excerptor beware. Beneath these choppy waters are reefs to sink many a hasty cargo of interpretation' (Nicolaus 1973 : 25).

Such a reprimand should be followed by a respectful silence. Perhaps we might be permitted to return to more orthodox versions of what Marx might have meant in order to attempt, with humility, a summary of his theory of alienation and of his significance in the development of the ideology of work.

The first position which Marx established concerns the unprecedented importance to be attached to the worker. Marx was more than merely sentimentally predisposed to regard the worker as hero, philosophically he asserted that man created his world, and therefore himself, through work. Work has never before and may never again be elevated to a position of such absolute importance. As a corollary of this elevation, the worker was given an unusual dignity. Man's essential being comes to be seen in man as worker and his essential activity in his work.

The second position emerging from the analysis concerns the misery of his existence. However ambiguous and imprecise the term, we know what Marx means when he says man is alienated. The very importance of work demands that the actual conditions in which it is carried out should fracture his relationship to the world.

The third position concerns the special conditions of his existence. Capitalism entails that man in work is exploited. The worker has produced his surroundings but they have been stolen from him.

The general conclusion from Marx must be, in accordance with his general veneration for contradiction, that the worker is in a state of inevitable tension, within himself and in relation to his surroundings. He is important because of his work and yet his work robs and impoverishes him. The descendents of this view can be seen in those writers who have concerned themselves with the socio-psychological aspects of alienation including Fromm, Marcuse, and, representing a considerable managerial concern, Chris Argyris.

The emphasis on the workers' position extends well beyond the relationship of employment. Production is the fundamental foundation of society, its relationships, its developments, its ideas, laws, and institutions; the worker is the fundamental agent in production so the worker assumes a position of transcendental importance in the world and in history. The final development of the whole historical process is in fact, simply a recognition of this position, the worker is established in a position of supreme importance at last.

In this sense, Marx continues and completes a tradition, which we have seen grow and develop from Gerard Winstanley, Saint-Simon and the syndicalists; economic relationships and the institutions of work came to replace established society. Marx represents the final stage in the development of that schism which we observed developing between the orthodox and the radical ideologies of work, both emerging directly as different manifestations of the protestant ethic, both marked out in revolutionary opposition to the traditionalistic values which they overthrow (as a matter of fact, Marx frequently commented on the revolutionary nature of capitalism). One of the many paradoxes in this situation is that the fundamental similarity of the two ideologies emerges most clearly in the extreme statements of their mutual opposition. But the strongest paradox embedded in the Marxist theoretical system is that it is, in a sense, a managerial conception.

For Marx, alienation represents an imperfection in the purity of the ideal of work, which is the only activity that gives man his identity. The essential paradox of alienation is that it is a pathological state of affairs produced in work as the result of an over-emphasis on a work ethic and on work-based values. It becomes possible to speak of man alienated by his work only when he is asked to take work very seriously.

We shall see that, following recent studies by Lockwood and Goldthorpe, (Goldthorpe et al. 1968) the concept of the alienated industrial worker has been held in serious question because of evidence which points to his instrumental attachment to his work; he works, in short, for money. This astonishing disclosure[5] leads to the question as to how far anyone calculatively involved in work can be alienated by it or, how can the worker be alienated if work has ceased to be a 'central life interest' for him. The evidence can just as easily be interpreted as supporting Marx; an extrinsic instrumental relationship to work is precisely what he meant by alienation. These questions raise several further problems of an ideological rather than of a sociological kind.

The first is that a worker who *is* instrumentally attached to his work is attached to it in a manner which is perfectly appropriate to a 'business-like' relationship. An economic explanation of work and of the relationships of dependence which surround it entails that they are instrumental or self-interested. It is not out of regard for our welfare, as Adam Smith tells us, that the baker bakes our bread. Marx sees this fundamental impersonality of market relationships equally clearly but, unlike Adam Smith, he deplores it. It is just such cold-blooded and calculated attachments which rob work of its meaning and which alienate the worker. Now the proposition that this represents a fundamental change from a situation which once existed is, of course, unprovable and irrefutable. But Marx is as capable of being sentimental about a warm and vanished past as any pre-Raphaelite dreamer. There is nothing to suggest that a worker on the track is any more 'instrumentally' attached to his work than a medieval labourer but the suggestion that things were better once is suspiciously familiar in the description of any vanished golden age.

Marx argues that the worker has become alienated because capitalism has de-humanized his relationship to work. The implication of a process of historical change which has reduced him to an alienated state is, to say the least, contentious. But the assertion that a de-humanized relationship to work is implied in business theory or in capitalism is unarguable. Marx clearly understood the implication of capitalism in ideological terms and the consequential problems of motivation which it involved. Capitalism is virtually a closed conceptual system and it hardly permits the accompaniment of exhortations to behaviour which are based on ethical statements. Commercial imperatives and moral imperatives do not mix.

There are many possible illustrations of this contradiction. We have already noticed one in passing; the extraordinary difficulties and convolutions in the nineteenth century attempt to produce and promote an ideology of work which was compatible with *laissez-faire* and liberal economic doctrines. The task was a formidable one and we concluded that the solution entailed the promotion of selfishness to a moral principle. We suggested that this was a process, literally, of demoralization which might be without precedent in history. We also suggested that the attempts to close the gap between economic theory and a necessary and effective ideology of work, were none too successful. We are now arguing that the attempt cannot succeed, that the historical failure to succeed in this task in the nineteenth century was inevitable because capitalism's pretensions are universal and its premises are singular. Capitalism depends upon the motive force of self-interest, on the 'invisible hand' which will guide the intricate machinery of calculation. Capitalism, as Oastler saw, is incompatible with any alternative system resting on different values, it represents and it requires the triumph of material, calculable, self-interest.

We can see a sociologist's illustration of this incompatability in Professor Etzioni's study of organizations. He contends that there are three possible bases for achieving the compliance of subordinates in organizations; bases in coercion, in shared norms, or in remuneration. Business organizations are predominantly based upon remunerative sources for the achievement of compliance and, he adds, organizations suffer losses in efficiency to the extent that they rely on mixed sources of compliance; incentives and moral appeals do not mix.

There are innumerable contemporary and practical examples of the way in which economic values refuse to co-exist with alternative value systems. The confrontation is never direct, and for that reason it goes unnoticed as it may have been unnoticed when, in the sixteenth century, a change took place which 'set a naturalistic political arithmetic in the place of theology [and] substituted the categories of mechanism for those of theology' (Tawney 1925 : 106). But the confrontation is to be observed whenever a cost benefit analysis is proposed to study the amenity value of un-polluted countryside or to estimate the social cost of noise. Even when the results of such calculations apparently favour the non-commercial choice between two alternatives, the process by which the decision has been made illustrates the complete ascendancy of a process of calculation based upon economic values.

Capitalism makes absolute claims and it is more than feasible that these claims have to be met in order to permit capitalism's survival and growth. But one of the inherent contradictions within it is that it can permit appeals and imperatives only when they are couched in its own terms and these terms can seem ineffective, even repellent, when they are directed at subordinates. Capitalism requires a degree of commitment to work which it is incapable of commanding. Capitalists can require merely that their employees will work 'for the money', at least, that is the limit that consistency imposes on them. Capitalists can be, in practice, as inconsistent as the next man but when they appeal for co-operation out of a sense of duty (to the firm, to the community, or to the nation) there is a palpable effect of their having reached beyond a rule book which they claim to be universal and which so obviously directs their own affairs. Capitalist theory will explain why men work but the explanation will not encourage work, at the lower levels, of sufficient energy and intensity to meet the capitalists' own interests. It provides a motive which is insufficient to overcome bounds set by reality (insatiable economic needs in a dustman can only lead to lunacy or despair), by fatigue, or by boredom. And in many categories of employment, particularly in crafts and professions, simple economic motivation may be positively dysfunctional. In this sense, it is not so much that capitalism has actively alienated labour, it is rather, that capitalism has never succeeded in synthesizing labour. The capitalist, however, needs synthesized labour so he is driven to break out of his own conceptual system.

The agent for the pursuit of productivity and profit, the manager, probably sees this contradiction more clearly than the entrepreneur. In any case, as his function concerns the control and co-ordination of subordinates, it appears to the manager as a special problem in his own work. What Marx called alienated labour and what we have called un-synthesized labour is a major obstacle in the way of achieving management objectives. The problem, as modern management theorists so often identify it, is how to release the worker's potential for co-operative effort. Obstacles to this release constitute management problems in the employment of labour, which Marx identified as the problem of alienation. In this sense, alienation is a managerial problem. It is managerial not only in that it represents a problem of special concern to the manager but also in that it emerges as a concept in the same process of development which leads to industrialization.

Industrialization exposes, as Marx argued, the impersonality of economic and employment relationships. The exposure and the other grim characteristics which accompanied industrialization made the construction of an ideology of work necessary. But an ideology of work is almost inseparable from the notion of alienation which is both entailed by it and which contradicts it. Alienation is almost literally a mirror image of a work ethic, it reflects what is projected into it but it reverses it. The concept of alienation emerges from a work ethic because of an inevitable recognition that men are not as totally involved in their work as the ethic demands that they should be, there is always a managerial problem of imperfect commitment to be overcome. Alienation is a constant problem which demands a more effective ideology of work, but refinements in the ideology will only re-emphasize the problem of alienation.

The paradox of alienation, like all the best paradoxes, is therefore inescapable, because it resembles a logical loop. It illuminates the unreality and the unreasonableness of regarding work as *the* essential and characteristic human activity. The consequence of exaggerating the importance of work is that it magnifies, in the process, the de-humanizing characteristics which have always accompanied it and the magnification requires a further exaggeration of the importance of work which leads to still greater emphasis on its alienating features.

Capitalism, in its pure and doctrinaire form is less susceptible to these difficulties because of its straightforward advocacy of economic doctrine. But its honesty is a motivational weakness and, for that reason, capitalism comes more and more frequently to be overlaid by ideological disguises. Capitalism, even in its more advanced formulations, is never capable of mounting the ideological exhortation to work which is embodied in communism. This is why communism, in terms of its foundation of economic values, its veneration of work, and its emphasis on alienation, can be presented as, in effect, capitalism set free of its imperfections. To put the matter the other way around, and with an emphasis not too different from Marx's, we might say that capitalism represents an imperfect stage in develop-ment towards the absolute transcendency of economic values and an associated ideology of work, the fullest development of which is represented in Marxism.

This complicated theoretical diversion explains more fully, perhaps, the earlier contention which we have asserted rather than argued, that the radical and the orthodox ideologies are merely schisms within the same dogma. Communism is not so much opposed to capitalism, it is the refinement of capitalism.

8. Division and Demoralization

Marx believed that the division of labour in machine production turned the worker into a 'crippled monstrosity', 'riveted to a single, fractional task', 'working with the regularity of parts of a machine', and that these unfortunate consequences alienated the worker from his environment.

Durkheim argued a different but equally pathological consequence of the disordered state which he considered to exist in economic affairs, a consequence also related in some measure to the division of labour. Durkheim believed that a state of anomy existed in the economic relationships of society. The actual reflection of this state of moral disorder is to be found in the constant conflicts and disorders which characterize economic affairs. Arguing, with Saint-Simon, that economic activity and relationships had now achieved paramount importance, displacing administrative, military, and religious functions, Durkheim asserted that we now live in an essentially economic and industrial society. The character of contemporary life is economic, but Durkheim noted that character was insufficiently respected. Saint-Simon, from the basis of the same contradiction, had concluded that industrial management was to be made the principle of social organization; Durkheim concluded that economic relations should become the basis of public morality. Economic affairs and occupational relationships are, in fact, in a 'state of juridical and moral anomy' (1960 : 1). Apart from the limited influence of professional ethics, there are no precise ideas on what ought to be the relationships between employers and workers, between competing tradesmen, or between tradesmen and consumers. Those vague notions that exist are sanctioned only by opinion, not law, so that 'the boundary between what is permitted and what is prohibited ... seems susceptible to almost arbitrary change by individuals'. The very basis of our collective life is, therefore, exempt from any moral regulation and this must be 'a notable source of demoralization' because most of those who live in industrial society live outside any moral environment (Durkheim 1960 : 2).

One would expect Durkheim to develop an attack on the moral

disorders of a commercialized, industrial society and on the dire consequences of the divisions of labour, the kind of attack that has become totally familiar to everyone. However, this is not Durkheim's intention. He means to recreate the conditions in which morality can develop and, as morality must be related to the essentially economic character of society and, as the division of labour is inseparable from economic society, the moral system cannot contradict the principle of the division of labour. The division of labour, far from being the villain of the piece, appears as hero, as the foundation of social and moral order.

The division of labour has been misinterpreted by economists, says Durkheim, who wrongly regarded it as a purely economic phenomenon whereas it is essentially the source of social solidarity: 'great political societies can maintain themselves in equilibrium only thanks to the specialization of tasks, that the division of labour is the source, if not unique, at least principal, of social solidarity' (1960 : 62). It is also the foundation of contract and of contract law. 'The involvement of one party results either from involvement assumed by the other, or from some service already rendered by the latter. But this reciprocity is possible only where there is co-operation, and that in its turn does not come about without the division of labour' (1960 : 124). The division of labour has progressed, he says, because it follows the increasing density and condensation of society. It does not precede collective life, it follows from it. Increased density means that the pressure exercized by social units upon one another become stronger and so they are obliged to develop in different societies.

But if the division of labour is to be the prime cause of the development of social solidarity then there are obvious and awkward facts to be explained. Durkheim is aware of them, or of some of them, at least. The progressive extension of the division of labour has *not* always been accompanied by a progressive extension of social solidarity, if that had been the case, then the moral disorder which Durkheim says has developed in economic affairs might be a development for which it would be difficult to account. Many observers have, indeed, argued that the disorder results from the division. There are also more obvious phenomena like economic depressions, disorders in industrial relations, class conflicts, even civil wars, not to mention suicide, to the study of which Durkheim had made a major contribution.

Attacks on the division of labour as the cause of these misfortunes are misplaced than they are the result of the economists's narrow preoccupation with its economic aspect. How then are we to account for all these disorders? Durkheim proceeds like a mediaeval logician defending a vulnerable syllogism. The division of labour is a positive force, but we must distinguish: the 'natural' development of the division of labour produces social solidarity, an awareness of the interdependence of man in society. There are also unnatural or pathological forms and these are of two kinds, the anomic and the forced division of labour.

The anomic division of labour results, often, in conflict between capital and labour which became a typical feature of society after the introduction of large-scale industry in the seventeenth century. Specialization of tasks thereafter developed much more rapidly and, because the workers found conditions imposed upon them which they were unable to change, their resistance to them became a chronic condition in society. Durkheim concedes that the division of labour has led to the increasing isolation of the individual in specialized activity which seems no longer to involve him in any sense of making a common contribution in his work. He agrees that this aspect of the division of labour threatens to decompose society. He agrees with Auguste Comte, that the division of labour can be carried too far and that it can prove a threat to social progress. Comte believed that the continued extension of the division of labour must be controlled and that its control must be exercized by the state.

Durkheim thought this an impractical solution because the proliferation of tasks and functions is so vast and the activities of government so general that effective control was impossible. He seems to rely, as an alternative process of control, on some natural tendency to restore stability and co-operation. Each individual should feel that 'he is not self-sufficient, but is a part of a whole on which he depends' (1960 : 361). He acknowledges that this is a vague notion to set against the very concrete and often divisive impressions that are attached to the performance of certain jobs but, he says, this feeling of interdependence is likely to be established by habit. Collective feelings become more and more important in resisting the centrifugal tendencies in which the division of labour may encourage, the 'patterns of mutual reactions' between functions establish habits which are changed by constant practice into rules of conduct: there is a 'sorting of rights and duties which is established by usage and becomes obligatory' (Durkheim 1960 : 366).

The appearance of negative characteristics, of decomposition, which seems to surround some particular aspects of the division of labour, follows from concentrating on isolated instances which ignore the slow process of development in which a network of links is established which is finally consolidated into permanent, organic solidarity.

The absence of solidarity follows when there is no harmony of functions. The division of labour fails to produce solidarity because of a state of anomy and a state of anomy could not arise where functions or tasks are in sufficient contact with each other for sufficient time; given sufficient time, spontaneous relationships develop into a body of rules. If the relationship between tasks is constantly interrupted only the strongest stimuli can be communicated between them so the formation of habits or rules governing the relationship is impeded: 'relations being rare are not repeated enough to be determined' (Durkheim 1960 : 368). At a stage when markets and industries are developing, industrial processes are subjected to considerable change and this may mean that adjustment and regulation is difficult.

The consequences can be serious. If the individual

> 'does not know whether the operations he performs are leading, if he relates them to no end, he can only continue to work through routine. Every day he repeats the same movements with monotonous regularity, but without being interested in them, and without understanding them ... He is no longer anything but an inert piece of machinery, only an external force set going which always moves in the same direction and in the same way. Surely ... one cannot remain indifferent to such debasement of human nature. If morality has individual perfection as its goal it cannot thus permit the ruin of the individual, and if it has society as its goal, it cannot let the very source of social life be drained.' (Durkheim 1960 : 371)

The second 'unnatural' form of the division of labour is forced. The division of labour is forced when it no longer corresponds to differences between talents, capacities, and skills but is the result of constraint. 'Labour is divided spontaneously only if society is constituted in such a way that social inequalities exactly express natural inequalities' (1960 : 377). Inequalities result in class war when 'the distribution of social functions on which it rests does not respond — to the distribution of natural talents' (1960 : 375). Lower classes become dissatisfied with their customary or legally sanctioned roles, they 'aspire to functions which are closed to them and seek to dispossess those who are exercising these functions' (1960 : 374). The division of labour in a spontaneous form requires the possibility of combat and competition so that he who can best perform a task can displace the less able. But this traffic requires contiguity and the elimination of great differences between classes which acts as constraints on competition; 'for needs to flow from one class to another, differences which originally separated these classes must have disappeared or grown less' (1960 : 375).

The anomic and the forced forms of the division of labour are, however, 'unnatural' manifestations and they cannot detract from the importance of the principle itself: 'not only does the division of labour present the character by which we have defined morality; it more and more tends to become the essential condition of social solidarity' (Durkheim 1960 : 400). In a phase that clearly emerges from the foundations of Saint-Simon and points to its elaboration in Elton Mayo, Durkheim adds that all other social relationships other than those found in work are decaying and cannot, therefore, be the basis of moral order; 'As we advance in the evolutionary scale, the ties which bind the individual to his family, to his native soil, to traditions, ... to collective group usages, become loose ... since the division of labour becomes the chief source of social solidarity, it becomes at the same time the foundation of the moral order' (1960 : 400).

Durkheim's enthusiasm for the division of labour, apart from his qualifications concerning its 'unnatural' forms, is boundless. He urges us to shrink ourselves. Our duty in the higher societies is to concentrate and specialize. 'We must contract our horizon, choose a definite task and immerse ourselves in it completely ... this specialization ought to be pushed as far as the elevation of the social type, without assigning any other limit to it' (1960 : 401). In a revealing footnote, Durkheim considers the objection that the extreme division of labour can be damaging on grounds of hygiene and health. He reassures us:

'the extreme specialization at which biological functions have arrived does not seem favourable to this hypothesis. Moreover ... has not the division of labour, in its historical development, been carried to the last stage in the relations of man and woman? Have not there been faculties completely lost by both? Why cannot the same phenomenon occur between individuals of the same sex? Of course, it takes time for the organism to adapt itself to these changes, but we do not see why a day should come when this adaptation would become impossible.' (Durkheim 1960 : 401f)

Apparently, we are to look forward to the 'crippling of mind and body' not with anger or resignation, but with impatient enthusiasm.

Durkheim's work has been described as one of the most penetrating pieces of analysis of the division of labour and he stands high among the founding fathers of sociology, but there is undoubtedly something scholastic about his approach to industrial work and something impractical about his conclusion. The distinctions between natural and pathological forms of the division of labour are drawn at great length but they leave none too clear an impression in the mind. It is difficult to recall, when all is said, how it is that a cause giving rise to solidarity should have produced anomic conditions by the intervention of abnormal states of the division of labour and how, precisely, these abnormal conditions came about from such a beneficent source. At one stage, Durkheim argues that it is all the fault of the economists for reducing the division of labour to 'being merely a means of increasing the produce of social forces' (1960 : 373) and for not seeing that it is above all a source of solidarity. This seems very hard on the economists; they may have misinterpreted the facts but they did not create them. And one of them, Adam Smith, made what is essentially the same point with more lucidity, wit, and a great deal more human sympathy.

We are not only none too sure about the circumstances that produce anomy but we are also rather unclear as to how it can be avoided or removed. We should not tamper with the natural, organic development of the division of labour, but presumably we can only discover the unnatural and distinguish it from the natural when we observe its consequences, by which time the distortion has already taken place. Durkheim suggests that anomy may be a temporary state, that with a certain degree of stability, repeated relationships will form moral bonds and mutual dependencies. Anomy may thus be a transitory characteristic in an evolutionary development. In this sense we have only to wait for it to go away but there is a depressing pessimism about the promise of evolutionary adaptation that is to accompany the process.

Durkheim tells us that we must take care to provide equal opportunities, we must arrange a careful match between tasks and talents, between the allocation of functions and the abilities to carry them out. This requires a very precise piece of social engineering. Friedmann points out that, in order to achieve positive results from the division of labour, each worker would have to be free to choose his own functions, but this is a rare privilege (and, in any case, some of us would occasionally make mistakes). If this match of tasks and talents is not achieved, however, a very 'dangerous atmosphere of discontent' is likely to be produced. It is all very well for Durkheim to say that it is constraints upon the 'natural' forms of the division of labour which produce anomy and conflict, but constraints seem to be inseparable from industrialized social life and many of the most irksome seem to flow from its promotion of the intense division of labour. In short, perhaps anomy is a necessary condition of the division of labour in society.

There is some support for this view, indeed, its general popularity may explain the reputation which Durkheim enjoys as an analyst of industrial processes in that it is based upon this single concept rather than on an understanding of his general analysis. Many of the accompanying characteristics are present in modern production processes. Nothing could be more interdependent than the various tasks carried out in a car assembly plant. The workers work in close proximity in a fixed relationship, the dependence of one upon the finished work of another is obvious to all, they are well aware of their mutual dependence but solidarity, in Durkheim's sense, is hardly the result. Marx drew attention to this very characteristic or production processes in which the finished work of one man becomes the raw material for another as an example of the way in which even the instinct for co-operation had been captured by the capitalist and is used to control the worker more effectively. Friedmann (1961 : 77) introduces a number of careful qualifications before he recognizes any relationship between technical and moral interdependence: 'mechanical interdependence does not necessarily cause moral solidarity. Many other factors must be taken into account, the chief one being the structure and quality of the technical organisation itself. If this is faulty ... the close dependence of one job upon another will often cause irritability and a state of nerves and may set one worker against another.'

There is no doubt that, to some extent and at some level, the division of labour implies co-operation and interdependence and implies also the consciousness of this co-operation and produces, therefore, moral solidarity. But the principle cannot be infinitely extended so as to produce solidarity with society at large. Marx, once again, reached a very different conclusion, that the solidarity which resulted contributes to the alienation of a whole section of society from the rest. Friedmann (1961 : 77) makes this distinction very clear:

> 'we must distinguish between two kinds of solidarity, both found in real life to-day. There is the firm's unity, which brings together all the personnel of a business or a factory, of a big store, a workshop or a mine, and so causes a group solidarity *within* the firm. And there is the solidarity of the workers as wage-earners, linking them to other wage-earners outside the firm, to the employees ... of other firms. The latter is what Marxism, with its theory of social "classes", calls class solidarity, making of it, through the 'class struggle', the chief cause of all political and social movements and the main instrument of its revolutionary dynamic. This too is the form of solidarity which constitutes a common denominator underlying different types of trade union activity.'[6]

It certainly seems to be the case that the more extreme forms of the division of labour in highly integrated production processes have given trade unionists a bargaining power which would be denied them in less inter-related activities, power which they can use as an effective weapon; in these circumstances the division of labour appears to enhance the power to disrupt rather than to solidify.[7]

A Frenchman, Bouglé, writing in 1903, said that 'from Durkheim's defence of the division of labour one gains almost as pessimistic an impression as that given by its socialist critics'. Durkheim is often pessimistic: 'In the present state of our societies work is not only useful, it is necessary; everyone feels this and this necessity has been felt for a long time. Nevertheless, those who find pleasure in regular and persistent work are still few and far between. For most men, it is still an insupportable servitude ... work is for most men a punishment and a scourge' (quoted in Friedmann 1961 : 79).

In order to make it tolerable and to bind those in servitude to it into a network of rules and moral obligations, Durkheim tries to legitimate the principle upon which it has been extended into the manufacturing process, the principle of the division of labour. But the pathologies which he tried to account for and explain loom larger than the theory that purported to make them aberrations from a norm. When all is considered, it is Durkheim's concept of anomy which is memorable and significant, not the theory of the division of labour of which anomy was an intractable constituent.

The unavoidable paradox seems to be that, while Durkheim sought to make work the basis of morality, characteristics of modern work seem to lead to demoralization and anomy. The paradox is well illustrated by his rejection of the familiar argument that industrial workers should be given a broad, liberal education in order to widen their horizons and to compensate them for the effects of cramped and limiting work. Durkheim sees this as a dangerous course: 'if a person has grown accustomed to vast horizons, total views, broad generalities, he cannot be confined, without impatience, within the strict limits of a special task. Such a remedy would make specialization inoffensive by making it intolerable and consequently, more or less impossible' (1960 : 372).

There is no doubt that Durkheim takes a sensible view. A liberal education would make work unsupportable or, at least, it would reveal as farcical the moral appeal for it to be taken seriously. Durkheim's morality thus demands that, in order to prevent the farce from being exposed, liberal education should be suppressed. The dangers of demoralization demand that education should be subordinated to the demands of work.

The debate concerning education and the demands of work continues to this day. The two points of view are clearly described by Michael Carter. In the first:

'A country may look upon its educational system as a means of ensuring a direct supply of appropriately qualified workers for industry, commerce and administration. This is the rationale underlying the educational system in Soviet Russia, for example, where the "polytechnic" principle relates instruction in the schools to "socially productive" work. At all levels of the educational system, the constant aim is "to prepare young people psychologically ... for taking a future part in socially useful work, in labour, in creating the values necessary for the development of the Socialist State".' (N. Kruschev *Memorandum on School Reorganization*, (1958), quoted in Carter 1966 : 25)

The second view is one in which public education is regarded

'as a rescue operation ... Adam Smith, indeed, saw education as Vaizey has put it, as "a counterbalance to the inhuman results of

the division of labour". Smith declared that "some attention is necessary in order to prevent the almost entire corruption and degeneracy of the great body of the people". He considered that this is particularly so because the division of labour alienates the worker from society and reduces him to a remarkable degree of stupidity in which he is not able to exercise his civic duties".'
(Carter 1966 : 27)

Carter (1966 : 167) later suggests that it is surely 'an affront to the human being that work thus finishes off the process of deadening the curiosity and inauguration that is often begun in an adverse home environment and continued in school'. But it may be an even greater affront if we regard the process as reversed so that, instead of work completing a process begun in school, education lays the foundations for a process completed in work. This is certainly one strand of the outlook that would subordinate education to the demands of work. The process of preparation is, in part, said to be 'vocational', education is regarded as 'a preparation for real life' and, ideally as incorporating some practical matters which involve training for work. The other ingredient is more subtle and it involves 'psychological' preparation: since divided labour cannot accommodate complete men, education must begin the process of fracturing them at school so that they will be ready to play their part in adult manufacturing processes.

The results of *not* pursuing a policy of educational conditioning can certainly be pathetic. In a Harlech Television production called 'The Murder of Enthusiasm', produced by Aled Vaughan, a number of young 'C' and 'D' stream school-leavers were followed into their first jobs in factories and shops. One of their most bitter complaints was that, while at school, they had been encouraged to appreciate and to write poetry and that the world of imaginative possibility that had been opened to them was obscured when they began doing the jobs that they knew they would have to do for the next forty years. Surely then, Durkheim was right: it would be inhuman to open windows on horizons which can never be reached and which simply serve to illuminate the tiny confines of industrial life.

For one reason or the other, and it is the vocational preparation argument which is most often publicly expressed, education in this country seems to be increasingly regarded as a preparation for work. We have been told to admire the disciplined production of an administrative élite by such means as the *École Polytechnique* (the intellectual patron of which must surely have been Saint-Simon). A brochure published by the University of Warwick in 1967 said that British universities 'have traditionally provided training which, whilst excellent in itself,' [isn't that enough?] 'has not developed the type of mental discipline in its graduates needed for the problems which they subsequently face in industry and commerce'. It was clearly the intention at Warwick that the unfortunate tendency should be corrected.

There has been considerable development of the 'applied' fields in British universities and, more recently, of business and management studies. There have been signs that these attempts by the unversities to adapt themselves more rapidly to urgent vocational requirements have not been sufficient to save them from a preference for public investment in the relatively new and much more vocationally directed polytechnics. In the *Guardian*, February 6 1973, Professor Asa Briggs (who, as Vice Chancellor of Sussex University is an interested party) commented that: 'With a bleak quinquennial settlement universities will be preoccupied with making ends meet while polytechnics will be left to chart out their new opportunities'. This follows the government's decision to expand polytechnic education and it is associated with policy statements which will impose important qualifications on the traditional role of universities.[8]

The subordination of education to a process of psychological preparation for work extends to the schools as well as to the universities, not least by the encouragement being given to headmasters and teachers to regard themselves as managers of educational resources rather than simply as teachers. In this way the independent, professional defence of educational standards and purposes is gradually eroded; if headmasters are managers, like every other salaried bureaucrat, then the standards and concepts of management must be acceptable within the school or, at least, they are not likely to be subjected to critical review. Just as in medicine and nursing, managerial posts in large comprehensive schools begin to form a hierarchy (heads of years, heads of school, deputy heads, headmaster) which, salaries, prospects and the general climate of opinion begin to make more attractive than teaching. Managerial notions do not have to be introduced by the back door, they are the baggage carried in through the front by the tenant.

There is a persuasive attractiveness in the conception of education as a preparation for work. Not only does it favour the acquisition of skill and the improvement of productivity, it seems to increase pleasure and avoid pain because it closes the gap between expectation and reality. It limits expectation to the dimensions of reality and, in this way, it produces workers who are more happy or, at least, less discontented. It meets the demands of education in an industrial democracy because it is practical, popular, and contributes to a stable and orderly society.

It might seem a more offensive notion in the context of university education because the view has long been held that universities exist to establish a basis of *critical* thought, that the university exists 'to set our affairs within the wider context, to distinguish and defend ideals and standards that easily suffer from the pressures of everyday life, to maintain an informed, perceptive and independent criticism of the life our society makes possible for us', and again, 'one of the university's most characteristic functions in a democratic society is to help make public opinion more self-critical and more circumspect' (Pratt 1973). This critical role is expected of, or has been tolerated in universities,[9] but its extension to other levels of education has always been regarded as much more dubious. The division in society's expectations of its educational process may be based on the dilettante associations of universities in earlier times, gentlemen were expected and could afford to be detached, objective, and critical. The only occupational associations stemming from a university education were the learned professions and, in that particular context, a critical detachment *was* a vocational advantage. In the natural sciences, a spirit of objective enquiry, unclouded by undue respect for authority, was a necessary part of a scientific outlook.

In schools and institutes, however, this tradition of scepticism has never enjoyed the same vocational advantage. Clerks, apprentices, and operatives need, above all else, to be submissive and respectful. There is a long tradition in which Mr Gradgrind's 'little pitchers' have to be prepared for Mr Bounderby's use. The curriculum has changed, in some respects it may have a more liberal appearance, but in recent years the direction of education in the schools at preparation for work has been more openly acknowledged. The Schools Council on Education Reform recently set out the objectives of education as the self-development and self-realization of the child, 'the general adaption of students to the world of work and life beyond school and the development of an awareness of social environment'. It proposed the development of flexibility 'to enable students to accept new life styles', 'the formation of facilities for vocational training for those not suited to two years academic study at sixth form level' (IPM Memorandum January 11, 1973). The Institute of Personnel Management has raised some questions concerning the adequacies of preparation for work which take place in the schools. 'Are the highly specialised requirements of industry met by the more limited degree of specialisation attained in schools? With levels of technology advancing at an even faster rate, can the skills learnt in schools be specific enough for the needs of industry? Could they even be a hindrance in the learning of new skills and the adaptation to new ideas? The Institute notes that the Schools Council 'considers that a broad education is more attractive to industry because of its emphasis on flexibility, effective learning techniques and thought processes'. But, the Institute wonders whether receptiveness to new skills and ideas are 'more important than ready learnt skills'. So we see that the pathetic readiness of educationalists to subordinate their goals to the requirements of industry may not produce adaptation quickly enough to satisfy the managers.

The alternative view is rarely well stated because it is usually made to rest only upon the value of university education where the defence of objectivity and the maintenance of critical standards appears to be élitist and allows the case for the independence of educational values in the school to go by default. There *is* a case to be defended at all educational levels. It is not simply a question of compensating for the limited dimensions of the world of work, the critical quality of education could be directed at exposing the banalities on which the moral appeal of work is made to rest.

Carter (1966) argues that the gap between the expectations of youth and the realities of work should be closed by bringing about a change in the content of work. Many other contemporary writers make the same case, that work must be changed. It is very doubtful if this can be done within a framework of social values which are essentially economic in character and which have produced the work-world that we know. It is certain that it cannot be done unless those same social values are subjected to critical review, not only by a privileged minority of university students, but by the general attention of education. Within the existing framework, the case for changing work will surreptitiously be transformed so that it continues to support the environment within which it has developed. Just as William Morris dismissed the notion that machines could be developed in order to save and dignify labour in a society in which machines were made to produce goods and profits, so work, as we shall argue later, is only changed so as to serve more effectively the interests of those who control it, unless society is changed.

The naive mistake of so many critics of contemporary society is their belief that it can be changed only by a revolution. But, we have argued, the intention of the revolutionaries is, for the most part, to produce a 'new society' where our domination by work would be more total. A much more significant change in society could be produced almost imperceptibly and education could become a most effective agent of such a change. Far from requiring any positive or deliberate shift in the aims and objectives of educational programmes, it seems that education need only be occupied with its traditional concerns for it to be, in effect, a revolutionary force. It is surely the perception of this very fact that explains the constant pressure that has been directed at education to make it more exoteric, to make it more concerned to inculcate the values and skills of work. The independent, professional, and traditional direction of education is almost bound to produce dissonance and dissatisfaction with the world of work and that is why the work-world is so concerned about the control of education. It is not that industry and commerce really require the schools to produce ready-made machine minders or computer operators, they can do it themselves in a week. What industry and commerce require is docile raw material. And unless education is subordinated to their purpose it creates workers who will remain dissatisfied with their moribund routines and the ridiculous hierarchies of authority which are necessary to maintain them. The problem was clearly seen by Ruskin who, outlining a programme of comprehensive and compulsory education, acknowledged that 'sensible people' would ask 'Is this man mad, or laughing at us, to propose educating the working classes this way?' when education would only make them wretched (Ruskin 1905 : XVII, 402). To take this view, said Ruskin,

> 'was to admit that a certain portion of mankind must be employed in degrading work: and that to fit them for this work, it is necessary to limit their knowledge, their active powers and their enjoyments, from childhood upwards, so they may not be able to conceive of any state better than the one they were born in, nor possess any knowledge or acquirements inconsistent with the coarseness, or

disturbing the monotony of their vulgar occupation.' (Ruskin 1905 : XVII, 403)

Ruskin thought it was a profound state of slavery to be kept 'low in the forehead, that I may not dislike my work'.

Workers who have emerged from an education which was not directed at 'the general adaptation to the world of work' will be intractable, likely to regard their work as instrumental to the attainment of other ends which, perhaps, they were taught in school to value more highly. They will also be likely to demand high compensation for the limitations of work. These are characteristics which their managers will deplore and, in an attempt to remove them, the managers will try to extend their control to the educational process which has produced such evidence of 'alienation'. The managers may even attempt to convince us that education should not result in the 'demoralization' of the worker, that education should make men happy in work. But it is surely better that men should see that their work confines them than that they should find the confines comfortable. In a contemporary industrial world education cannot but be revolutionary unless it is banausic. Is it because a classical education in the humanities still produces a 'contempt for the useful' that classical education has been suppressed? Scott-King explains to his headmaster. "I think it would be very wicked indeed to do anything to fit a boy for the modern world". "It's a shortsighted view, Scott-King". "There, headmaster, with all respect, I differ from you profoundly. I think it the most long-sighted view it is possible to take'" (Waugh 1947 : 88).

We have extended the discussion of work to the field of education because it illustrates the dire consequences of subjecting all other considerations to the test of whether they meet the demands of work. Divided work requires severely limited education; an extended education will expose the limitations of work. An investigation into the effects on young workers of character development courses such as those provided in Outward Bound Schools reported that

'those who had been on the courses appeared generally less settled at work. They were less likely to be completely satisfied with their jobs, less likely to feel able to use their abilities fully at work, less likely to enjoy harmonious relationships with their supervisors, more prone to regard labour-management relations in terms of conflict rather than teamwork, and more likely to be definitely intending to change both their occupation and employer ... If the courses do result in personality changes making young people more lively, critical and independent, this in itself may interfere with their adjustment to the work situation.' (White and Roberts 1972)

Durkheim was right. Business may claim to acknowledge 'that freedom for self-development is the finest value in life' and that 'a basic principle of personnel management concerns the "sacredness" of individual personality' (Calhoon 1967 : 19), but educational programmes that develop the individual and thereby threaten business are not likely to receive its support. Some of the latest techniques developed by business reveal a very different preoccupation than the promotion of self-development: 'Now, managers receive a quarterly human resource report on employees for whom they are responsible. It shows investments made in additional personnel, replacement personnel, training and development, as well as write-offs incurred through turnover and obsolescence of prior investments ... By estimating the expected life of each human investment, long-term manpower planning becomes more feasible' (Lawrence 1971).

Work and the techniques for its control have contributed a great deal to the brutalization of the worker, not least by the inhuman language in which the techniques have been described. The effects of brutalization are infinitely extended when work is set up as a mould which must determine the dimensions of education. Durkheim did no service to human welfare in his analysis of the division of labour because, sharing a socialist view of its importance to social co-operation, he maintained an unreal optimism about its consequence.

The description of reality from which he set out was more accurate than his predictive assertions. The business world *is* often characterized by moral lawlessness. It is a lawlessness which stems largely from the impersonality of economic relationships. Older societies depended upon religious and social obligation, and were, therefore, out-going; in economic society we take account of others only in so far as they can serve our interests. In is indeed, *not* out of regard for our interest that the baker bakes our bread. Any explanation of the contemporary importance of business morality inevitably relies upon a coincidence of interest implicit in economic relationships, the baker bakes good bread because it is in his interest to serve his customers well. But that statement would go too far, in fact. The baker does not have to bake 'good' bread or serve his customers 'well'; he has to avoid serving his customers so badly that he drives them away. The coincidence of interest becomes a matter of precise calculation and the development of a market economy enables us all to take part in the calculation.

Moral lawlessness in the business environment extends at two levels. At the level of social relationships, the co-operation which impressed Durkheim is based upon enlightened greed. At the level of work, the further extension of the division of labour promotes co-operation in the sense that each must perform his work with the 'unfailing regularity of parts of a machine', but the orchestration and cohesion of this activity is in no sense voluntary and it promotes no mutual good-will among the 'co-operative workers'. Some evidence seems to suggest that potential for social co-operation declines. Hospital workers were once powerful dissuaded from engaging in strikes because of their responsibility for patient care when they worked at general tasks, closely related to visible patients in relatively small hospitals. Now that their tasks have been divided and they are separated from patients in large, 'industrial' medical units, they suffer no such disadvantage.

The complaint that the division of labour leads to demoralization has become very familiar in twentieth-century social commentary. Much of it takes the form of Cassandra-like wailing, a kind of perpetual cultural anodyne which helps to assure us that our worrying demonstrates us to be not quite so venal and materialist as our behaviour suggests. Some of the most hysterical and familiar complaints have been provided by Erich Fromm who has argued that the division of labour (among several other causes) has produced meaningless work which is accompanied by meaningless life and that the result is a society which is not sane. It would take us a very great deal of time to analyse Fromm's case and it is doubtful if our time would be well spent. He uses technical terms, or terms with pretentions to be technical, like fragmentation bombs in order to scatter indiscriminate destruction on generalized targets: 'whenever he feels that something is not as it should be, he characterises it in terms of alienation. He does this in connection with such different things as "love", "thought", "hope", "work", "language", man's relation to "the world", contemporary "culture" or "society", and the processes of "consumption" and "production".' Schacht (1971 : 116) adds that 'Fromm seems to refer to almost everything of which he disapproves as an instance of "alienation". He disapproves of a great deal, so it is not surprising that he finds alienation to be "all-pervasive"' (1971 : 139).

Fromm's difficulties may be explained by a double handicap which hinders his approach to work, he is influenced by the theories of both Marx and Freud. His allegiance to Marx makes him allocate central importance to work in the life of man. 'Work is not only an inescapable necessity for man. Work is also his liberator from nature, his creator as a social and independent being. In the process of work, that is, the moulding and changing of nature outside of himself, man moulds and changes himself ... The more his work develops, the more his individuality develops' (Fromm 1956 : 177). We have tried to suggest, in the last chapter, that such exaggerated, one might say, unnatural expectations of work are bound to find the real world a disappointment, alienated and unfulfilling.

As far as Freud is concerned, he provides the very setting for *The Sane Society* in that Fromm takes up his suggestion 'that one day someone will venture upon this research into the pathology of civilized communities'. Fromm's account (1956 : 296) of the pathological state of contemporary society is largely stated in Freudian terms. More specifically he is operationally committed to a Freudian psychoanalytic approach in answering such questions as whether people are, in fact, dissatisfied with their work. In order to find an answer, says Fromm 'we must differentiate between what people *consciously think* about their satisfaction, and what they feel unconsciously'. The difficulties surrounding the reliability of such answers when we get them are well known.

Friedman (1961 : 135), like Fromm, stresses 'the vital importance of work in maintaining or restoring the balance of the personality'. Friedmann describes the effects of loss of work as a consequence of unemployment.

'The unemployed person shows signs of an emotional instability which increases more or less rapidly and intensely in accordance with his occupational history and the successes or failures he has previously experienced during his working life ... after a first period of shock when the personality resists and remains almost unchanged, there comes a second in which there is a more or less active search for work, the worker's demands constantly decreasing until a paid job of any sort would be accepted. Finally a stage of depression ensues. The loss of the settled framework provided by a job and its daily routine, combined with a decreased awareness of the passage of time and a kind of apathetic attitude towards it, unite with family complications to produce in the unemployed man a growing unfriendly complex as regards the members of his family and particularly his wife and children.'

Friedmann (1961 : 129) concludes that 'Loss of work ... produces after a while a "toxic condition".'

The similarity of this passage to descriptions of drug dependency and withdrawal symptoms is quite striking. Retired workers, particularly retired managers, frequently speak in the same terms of missing the urgency, the demands, the tensions imposed by work. So, it seems, we are trapped in a gloomy dilemma: work demoralizes; the loss of work demoralizes.

In one sense it is quite possible that both statements are true. If we are taught that work is all important, that it reflects our personality and expresses our importance and if all our experiences in society reinforce this teaching, then we can hardly be blamed for discovering that the actual work we have to do and its withdrawal are both demoralizing. The paradox of the contemporary situation is that it embodies unrealistically high expectations of work and very low probabilities of fulfilment.

The most significant element of Fromm's approach is that it seems to stress the importance of achieving some sort of congruence between expectation and reality. Our examination of developments of the ideology of work suggest that incongruence is almost an inevitable result of the organization of work on a large or mass scale. We do not mean to suggest by this that the large-scale organization of work leads to the division of labour, that the division of labour leads to anomy or alienation. This is a fallacy which we have tried to counter. Incongruence arises because the large-scale organization of work separates out the functions of the control, co-ordination, and supervision of labour. Labour management becomes a specialized activity,[10] as soon as labour becomes a distinct and organized commodity in the production or distribution process. As labour becomes more important, its commitment to its task becomes more necessary. Testimony for the accuracy of this description comes appropriately enough, from Fromm (1956 : 80) himself: for industrial society to have developed, he says, 'Man had to be moulded into a person who was eager to spend most of his energy for the purpose of work, who acquired discipline, particularly orderliness and punctuality, to a degree unknown in most other cultures ... The *necessity* for work, for punctuality and orderliness had to be transformed into an inner *drive* for these aims. This means that society had to produce a social character in which these strivings were inherent'.

In a sense, concepts of alienation, anomy, the demoralization associated with mass production, all *accompany* developments in the division of labour, they are not produced by them. They are both phenomena which accompany the productive development and extension of labour. As labour comes to be managed more effectively it is both subjected to greater specialization and division on the one hand and to ideological exhortation on the other. It is an inevitable consequence of the ideological exaggeration of the importance of work that the reality of work will fall short of its promises and that the worker will not meet his expectations. It is an understandable mis-reading of the resulting 'problem' that it is the specialization and division of labour which causes the 'problem of work' and the 'demoralization of the worker'. It is more likely in fact that both phenomena have little or no objective reality but they are both perceptual accompaniments of the same cause. We might express the argument in this way. The drive for the more effective management of labour (A), leads to the extension of the division of labour (B), and to the ideological appeal for labour to be committed to its work (C). The development of the ideology results in the realities of work appearing to be pathological or debased and to conclusions concerning alienation (D). So, A → B and C, C → D. The process is more usually misrepresented as A → B → D.

There are various ways in which we might attempt to bring about a greater degree of congruence between reality and expectations in work. By far the most usual approach among writers about work is to suggest that work must be changed in order to make it match their expectations of its importance more closely: work should be made more inherently satisfying by applying to it a variety of techniques (of job rotation, job enlargement, job enrichment, partnership, and participation). This is the standard text around which libraries of British and American volumes are woven. It is the view taken by Friedmann. Erich Fromm sees that it is a view with suspect intentions. We have suggested that it is an outlook which is entailed by an essentially managerial ideology of work because it rests upon a view of work that is exaggerated and unreal, a view that accompanies the control of labour. In this view the expectations of work are given, work is a terminal value, reality is almost by definition a disappointment, so reality must be improved.

A second approach is to suggest that congruence can be achieved by adjustments to our expectations, to bring them nearer to what appear to be the experiences of work. Once we begin to make this adjustment we see that the 'problems' attending the division of labour begin to recede with a change in our own perceptions. Not only do we cease to be confronted with the necessity of solving unreal problems, but we are also given the further advantage of being able to avoid constructing, upon the shoddy foundations of work, moral and social systems which they are quite incapable of supporting. Durkheim was driven to attempt to square the circle by acknowledging in the first instance that the world of economic relationships was, at best, morally neutral, and asserting, in the second place, that work was the most socially significant force because it provided the only basis for co-operation. We suggested that the contradictions in Durkheim's approach are almost unbridgeable. Not only does work fail to form the basis of any adequate moral and social system but any attempt to build them upon it is likely to debase the society in which it takes place because it confines, as we have tried to show, educational and social values to those that are required in the world of work and it regards as dangerous any which continue to transcend it.

In practical terms, there is a much greater preoccupation with the first course than with the second. This is not only because of a managerial concern that work should be taken more seriously and the worker more completely immersed in it. The radical view, forms of which we have been examining, encourages us to take the same course because it places work and the worker at the centre of the world.

Part III
The Integration of Work

9. Integration by the State

Marx succeeded in changing the world partly because he changed its understanding of work. After Marx there has been a continual pre-occupation with the problem of work (recently formulated as the problem of alienation) persistently presented in terms of labour's actual or potential hostility.

The problem has occupied society at two levels. One is represented by a purely managerial response; the worker's hostility or his disengagement from his work is an obstacle to economic goals concerning productivity and profit, it is an impediment to the effective control of the production process. The problem has received massive attention in Europe, Britain, and the United States; we shall examine it in chapter 11.

The second level concerns the worker's disengagement from his work and, more particularly, from his political society. This is essentially a political, not a managerial, problem but it arises in one of two sets of circumstances. It arises, in the first instance, when the worker's hostility, which results from the conditions of his work, is such as to provoke him to revolutionary activity against his state. The revolution which is feared is believed usually to be based upon a communist theory of class antagonism and a communist interpretation of the worker's position, but those who fear the revolution are not likely to share any other understanding of communist theory; they are normally afraid of the consequences of a theory which they totally reject. It leads to one of a number of political solutions which are essentially designed to fend off revolution. The second set of conditions in which work emerges as a problem in political terms concerns the very different circumstances in which the revolution has actually happened. When the post-revolutionary state has been established the relationship of the state to the worker is seen as a problem of dominating importance. This is because (always assuming that the successful revolution was a communist revolution) the worker has a position of supreme importance in the *raison d'être* of the state and in its political ideology; the worker *is* the state. In more mundane terms, the communist state is always highly centralized and devoted to economic planning. This means that the political apparatus of the state and its administrative machinery is unavoidably involved in managerial problems, problems of managing, not simply the economy, but of managing the labour force. A content analysis of the speeches of Soviet leaders and of the discussions of party conferences would surely show a greater preoccupation with, for example, power production or output in the machine-tool industry than has become fashionable even in our own society.

In this chapter we shall examine these responses, in which formulations of an ideology of work have come to be almost indistinguishable from political theories. They illustrate the way in which the perceived need to integrate or to reintegrate the worker looms so large in a society pre-occupied with economic and technological questions that it becomes the major political problem so that its solution dominates politics. The integration of the worker by the state implies a largely political solution to the perceived problem of the workers' alienation.

I *Democratic Socialism*

The first example of a political approach which we shall take is the least doctrinaire and the least obtrusive in the political landscape. Democratic socialism, perhaps because of its advantages of flexibility and compromise, rarely presents a unified and consistent ideological appeal. It is, at least in the context of British politics, an empirical (or even, in a word which came to be closely associated with Sir Harold Wilson's leadership of the British Labour Party, 'pragmatic') position in which, at any particular time, a variety of widely different influences can be discerned.[11] But democratic socialism is always likely to be influenced by a Marxist theoretical approach to the extent that it involves a class analysis of society and social problems although the analysis is seen as requiring parliamentary representation and pressure-group activity for the working class and its institutions (among which free trade unions take an important position) rather than revolutionary activity. Democratic socialists are, in short, democrats as well as socialists.

Their commitment to socialism goes further than the requirement for representation of the working class, it leads to intentions for the achievement of social change. Whatever the precise formulation of these objectives at any particular time, democratic socialists are likely to be perpetually concerned with the need to engage in economic planning by government in order to bring about a more just and equitable distribution of wealth. The means involved in such a process of planning are likely to include the nationalization of industry and this is sometimes accorded the emphasis of a separate objective rather than a means. Nationalization is often regarded as an inseparable part of a socialist programme because it directly concerns the position of the worker and because it represents a socialist's inherent antipathy to private enterprise and private profit. Burns (1963 : 181) summarizes socialism as 'the abolition of private enterprise and the substitution of collective ownership and control, for the benefit of the whole society, of at least the principal instruments of production, distribution and exchange ... the destruction of private investment and the profit system and the adoption of a new standard for the distribution of wealth.'

The essential problem for all democratic socialists is that they must somehow reconcile their long-term objectives for achieving social change, and their middle-range economic plans when they are in office, with the constant possibility of the opposition being returned to power. How is a socialist party to transform and organize the new society when a very different government can always intervene in the process? The alternative problems that accompany the absence of any alternative government are obvious to everyone — except revolutionaries.

There are, however, essentially political problems or problems of political theory; as such they do not directly concern us.

The means or the ends of democratic socialists (the emphasis changes from time to time) concern planning and nationalization. The intention is that the worker should be accorded a 'fairer share' of what he produces (his living standard should be improved), he should be protected from the effects of unemployment and poverty and he should be allowed more authority in the direction of his work. It is a matter of interpretation whether such intentions are seen as directed at establishing a different society or whether they are seen as improvements to a society which remains essentially unchanged. Democratic socialists would undoubtedly claim that their activities had led to considerable improvements in the condition of the workers and that this improvement was a necessary alternative to revolution.

The major impact of democratic socialism, on the worker's relationship to his work (at least in Britain) has been in terms of the issue of nationalization. Yet, the British Labour Party hardly achieved a final commitment to nationalization, as it was established in the nationalization acts of the Attlee Government, until the 1940s. Some form of joint control or worker control seemed to be the preferred alternative for the previous thirty years of the party's history and development. The demand for some form of joint control, after 1910, became more and more continual and vociferous. It was given particularly powerful and coherent expression by the Mineworkers Unions and in *The Miners' Next Step*, a famous publication by the Miners' Unofficial Reform Committee in Tonypandy in 1912, which declared itself against nationalization because it simply created a national trust which would be backed by government power and would extract profits in order to relieve other landowners and capitalists. The miners, in this document, were as much concerned with problems of authority as with the redistribution of economic resources.

Six years later, in 1918, the Conference of the Miners' Federation of Great Britain, decided that nationalization without joint control of the industry would be useless. The miners drew up a draft Parliamentary Bill for nationalization and for joint control which Pribićević (1959 : 8) has called 'the most important document produced by British workers in their struggle for worker control'. The miners drew up a programme of demands including a wage increase, a six-hour day, state ownership, and joint control of the industry. The government responded with the offer of a Commission which the Miners' Executive Committee narrowly decided to accept, as the alternative to a coalfield strike. The Chairman's report of what became known as the Sankey Commission, recommended nationalization with a strong element of joint control. Local Mining Councils were to be set up to advise the manager on all questions concerning the direction and safety of the mine. The Local Councils were to consist of three management representatives, four elected workers, and three men appointed by the District Council. The District Council was, in effect, to run the industry and to appoint colliery managers; it was to be composed of equal representatives of miners, consumers, and managers.

The Labour Party Conference of 1918 demanded increasing participation in central and local management for railwaymen and miners. A memorandum by the Labour Party, the TUC, and the Miners' Federation demanded nationalization of the coal industry and an effective programme of worker participation in its management;

the demand was endorsed by the Labour Party Conference in the same year.

Outside the Labour Party, but in close proximity to it, the National Guilds League, under the powerful, intellectual leadership of Cole, argued incessantly for a programme of social change based on worker control. The programme, outlined both in general terms and by reference to specific industries, in a stream of pamphlets, advocated nationalization simply as a first step in a process of 'encroaching control' which would begin with the demand of industrial unions for full recognition and would go on to their achievement of the right to challenge disciplinary decisions, to the right to elect foremen and managers and, finally, to incorporate technicians and managers in the union which would then effectively control the industry.

The Shop Stewards' movement, centred on Clydeside, and the Clyde Workers' Committee began as a defence against the union restrictions in the Munition Act but became quickly concerned to establish one Clydeside industrial union which 'would take and hold the region's industries for the working class'. Attempts to widen the organization of the Shop Stewards' movement were partially successful. An engineering strike beginning at Rochdale in April, 1917, achieved massive proportions in the north west of England and was brought to an end by an inconsistent but practical combination of a royal tour of the north with the arrest of the strike leaders. The strike led to a Commission of Enquiry into Industrial Discontent which reported evidence of discontent with food prices and profiteering, a 'breakaway from faith in Parliamentary representation' (Kendall 1969 : 163) and the likelihood of drastic attempts by the working classes to secure direct control of particular industries. The considerable power which the shop stewards had succeeded in organizing was not effectively directed at the achievement of political ends. This was because of ineradicable contradictions associated with the syndicalist influences on the movement. As Kendall (1969 : 165) puts it, 'The shop stewards were victims of a hidden contradiction in their own thought and action ... Events drove the shop stewards towards centralised leadership, ideology made them hesitate and step back ... Whilst the mass waited for an initiative from its leaders, the leaders in turn waited for the movement of the mass.'

Whatever theoretical inconsistencies prevented the achievement of the shop stewards' objectives, their activities certainly contribute to a picture of a widespread commitment in working-class movements to a degree of worker control in industry. The movement was influential both outside the Labour Party and within it and it cannot be dismissed (as it was often dismissed until recently) as the concern only of an insignificant minority. The movement for joint control seems to have dominated discussion of the left between 1915 and 1930, to have found its way into formal expressions of Labour Party policy and in the policy decisions of major trade unions. It is all the more mysterious, therefore, that the theme of joint control disappeared so completely from the deliberations of the Labour Party.

There are a number of explanations for this disappearance. The most practical is the trade recession of 1921. By July one quarter of the members of the engineering union were out of work. By the end of the year, the employers' demands for substantial wage cuts had been conceded by the union. In 1922 the employers insisted on managerial rights to determine overtime and to change workshop rules and practice. The employers demands were rejected (against the advice of the executive) by a ballot vote and the consequential lock-out lasted from March to June. The men returned to work to meet further reductions in wages. Four years later, the collapse of the general strike meant, as Pribićević (1959 : 3) put it, that 'any such bold demands as nationalization and workers' control had to be dropped'; the unions were concerned with survival.

The enormity of the gulf that had opened between employers and labour, culminating in the general strike, contributed to a change in relationships. Both sides may have sensed that things had gone dangerously far in the direction of total breakdown. The initiative of Sir Alfred Mond (Lord Melchett) in calling the Mond-Turner talks in 1926 pointed to a new and less hostile spirit on the employers' side. Mond offered the concept of 'rationalization', represented in the image of the big, efficient, and benevolent employer. The change in attitude seemed to be reflected in a new emphasis from representatives of the Labour Government who stressed a new kind of 'scientific socialism' in which a labour government presented its advantages in terms of the improvement of industrial efficiency. *The Times* referred to a speech by Herbert Morrison in July, 1929, in which 'He appealed to business men to look upon the members of the Government not as enemies but as men and brothers, who were out to do their best to help make their enterprises more successful, though not at the expense of the workers' (quoted in Barry 1965 : 307f). This reassurance to businessmen and the emphasis on socialism as a more rational alternative accompanied the Labour Party's new responsibilities in government. The Party's close association with the trade unions took the unions into a relationship of greater responsibility. The objectives of both the party and the unions were modified by a decision to work within the system. The decision is always likely to be rewarded by considerable influence but the framework inevitably modifies the objectives of the party taking the decision.

One further and important part of the explanation of the disappearance of the commitment to joint control is the peculiar part played by Morrison. In an administration which was short of experienced administrators, he enjoyed the influence and the reputation of having established the London Passenger Transport Board. Morrison concluded that the industries to be nationalized were to be controlled by boards in the same way. He was also very unsympathetic to any notion of worker control. He wrote in the *New Clarion* in 1932, 'This buses for the busmen and dust for the dustmen stuff is not *socialism* at all ... it isn't a busman's idea; it's middle-class syndicalist romanticism' (*New Clarion* September 17, 1932, quoted in Barry 1963 : 325). Morrison's view prevailed and in his book *Government and Parliament*, (1954 : 248) he dismisses the whole controversy in a sentence or two. When the TUC came to publish its Interim Report on Post-War Reconstruction in 1943, there was no mention of joint or worker control. Industries were to be nationalized and the rights of management to exercise control were to be absolute, subject only to the recognition of unions for bargaining and consultative purposes. When the coalmining industry came to be nationalized in 1946, the provisions for joint consultation were remarkably similar to those made by the coalowners on the Sankey Commission in 1919.

This may be a reasonably accurate illustration of the extent to which the British Labour Party had evolved an effective strategy in relation to industrial employees. However comprehensive the machinery of planning, full employment, and of the welfare state, its impact on workers as such was confined to programmes of limited nationalization and for the extension of joint consultative arrangements. It is fair to conclude that their ideological impact on workers has been almost nil. There is no evidence to suggest that the morale or the commitment to work of employees in nationalized industries is either greater or less than those of employees elsewhere. Nationalization, whatever its other advantages, provides a classic illustration of the proposition that ownership is irrelevant to questions of authority in industry. As the apocryphal miner was quoted as saying the day after his colliery was nationalized, 'it's the same face behind the manager's desk'.

There is considerable evidence, on the other hand, to suggest that joint consultation has been a failure. It is a failure, at least, in so far as its purpose was originally conceived as advancing the participation of workers in their enterprises, of enhancing joint decision-making or promoting a sense of partnership. Joint consultation may, in some cases, have provided a useful management communication channel but the channel was not used for ideological purposes. If industrial workers are alienated, neither nationalization nor joint consultation has changed their situation. In an extensive study of consultative minutes of a nationalized industry covering a period of twenty years it appeared that 62 per cent of all items were raised by management, a third of the items raised by management concerned the comparison of production records on an historical basis and in 90 per cent of the issues raised by management its purpose was to use the committees as a channel of communication to employees. There was comparatively little discussion of any circumstances of change in relation to the industry. Even more significantly, in a structure designed to facilitate the meeting of different groups and the reconciliation of different interests, there was an astonishing absence of conflict of any kind. In this, as in other industries, management intended joint consultation to bring about a sense of unity. But the consultative channel was choked with historical data and items were selected to concern subjects likely to be free from conflicts of interest or of values.

These consequences did not stem from any malicious intention on the part of managers but rather on the mistaken theory that 'effective' communication is sufficient to achieve a sense of commitment. Dahrendorf (1959 : 71) has warned that 'the attempt to obliterate lines of conflict by ready ideologies of harmony and unity in effect serve to increase rather than decrease the violence of conflict manifestations'. He regards co-determination in the German steel and coal industries as 'an ill-conceived pattern that contradicts rather than supports a general trend toward the reduction of violence and intensity of industrial conflict' (Dahrendorf 1959 : 267). This conclusion is related to the familiar argument that influential worker representatives who become associated in the process of management become associated with management's objectives and so are perverted from their original objectives. The argument can be extended to joint consultation because, although less influential, 'entanglement' and its dire consequences depends not upon the effectiveness of the representatives' association with management but upon their belief in the strength of this association. The irony of joint consultation is that while it affords worker representatives no significant influence on the direction of their enterprise, it sets out to deprive them of the influence which they might have exerted from a position of independence. If it succeeds then it is open to Dahrendorf's objections; if it fails then it wastes management's resources and is ineffective.

Management regarded joint consultation as a means of increasing 'psychological' participation; by means of improved communication it intended to achieve a sense of unity, a commitment to the organization that would result in a reduction of conflict. But management confused ends with means: because conflict was intended to be reduced or eliminated by the consultative process its expression was discouraged so that joint consultation could be shown to be effective by its characteristic absence of conflict. Managers were encouraged to believe that consultation would avoid conflict, that conflict was the result of mistaken attitudes and poor communications. So managers did avoid it, particularly in the channels designed to obviate it. The result was that consultation could not become a forum for the meeting and adjustment of different attitudes and interests.

Joint consultation does not justify the attention we have given it and, in so far as it represents a managerial approach, it is out of place in this present discussion. But it illustrates the poverty of the ideology of the British Labour movement. Its original preoccupation with joint control was replaced by two concepts designed, in part, to capture and hold the allegiance of workers; nationalization and joint consultation. The former seems to have been abandoned for all practical purposes, and any current reference to it in Party discussions is guaranteed to produce a horrified reaction from a substantial section of the British Labour Party, convinced that to revive the issue of nationalization will lose the next election. The latter has given way to the appointment of worker directors in the steel industry, an innovation which has been greeted with more enthusiasm by management than by unions or their members and which has, in any case, been overtaken by the necessity of achieving arrangments for the participation required by Britain's European partners under the European Commission's Fifth Directive. Participation has been taken much further in Europe than in Britain, with the legal requirement to establish works councils in France, the inclusion of worker representatives on supervisory boards in Germany, and the appointment of worker directors with considerable authority in the German steel and coal industries. These arrangements are more constitutionally complex and legally entrenched than anything that has been attempted in Britain but there is nothing to suggest that they have been any more successful in achieving either the influence or the commitment of workers. The search for the philosopher's store of commitment to work by means of participation continues but with more zeal by managements' representatives than by workers', and with no more prospect of success than was won by joint consultation.

At the political level neither the British Labour Party nor the trade union movement have succeeded in making a significant contribution to the ideology of work. It would still be possible that the trade union movement had evolved a practical ideological approach for its membership in their work rather than in their political relationship. The trade unions could have developed a consistent explanation of the relationship of their members to their employment and that explanation could have taken a positive form or it could have been an outright rejection of work ideologies directed by employers at their members. A trade union ideology could, in other words, have rested upon an explanation of the affiliation of the worker to his work or on his alienation from it.

British trade unions have done neither. No one answered Woodcock's pathetic question, when he was Secretary of the TUC, 'Why are we here?'.

The failure stems in part from the British unions' boredom with affairs of such intellectual abstraction and partly from a deliberate decision which the unions have undertaken concerning the separation of functions. The trade unions are convinced that their industrial activities must be confined to matters concerning the economic interests of their members and that political matters are the affair of Parliament in which the trade unions have adequate means of representation by way of the Labour Party, in which the trade unions have considerable influence. The Webbs (1920 : 672) issued a magisterial pronouncement on this subject to the effect that only the most lunatic and unthinkable measures could provoke the unions into a political general strike.

'We imagine occasions that might, in the eyes of the Trade Union World, fully justify a general strike of non-economic or political character. If, for instance, a reactionary Parliament were to pass a measure disfranchising the bulk of the manual workers ... then, indeed, we might see the Trades Union Congress recommending a general strike; and it would be supported not only by the wage-earning class, but also by a large section of the middle class, and even by some members of the House of Lords. That is one reason why, short of madness, no such act would be committed by the Government or by Parliament.'

The division of functions is a trade-union doctrine for which we all have reason to be thankful. The Webbs argue that it is not only a revolutionary provocation which would cause a political strike but also that a political strike would cause a revolutionary situation. The trade unions are a slumbering giant content to have their power respected by political institutions which are concerned not to arouse it.

So any direct contribution of an ideological nature emerging from the trade union movement is likely to be expressed in the internal debates of the Labour Party, just as the case for joint control was once expressed in political forums. The activities of trade unions as such, in the industrial context is likely to be confined to economic issues. In this context the unions are very much constrained by the economic framework if only because they are organizations of employees; considerable hostility to the employer or a commitment to the long-term overturning of the employment relationship and of private enterprise, runs the risk of doing short-term damage to the employees' interests. Trade unions are bound to be conservative bodies because any well-directed attack against the *status quo* is likely to result in unemployment of the membership. Trade unions may constitute a permanent opposition to management, as they are often described, but, unlike a political opposition, they never wish to bring down the government or to replace it.

The non-political, economic, and industrial activities of trade unions consist, very largely, of collective bargaining and collective bargaining is widely recognized as a mixed relationship of both hostility and co-operation, however aggressive the posture of one party towards the other, there is a shared assumption that their relationship will continue and will improve. If this assumption does not exist then the agents are not party to a collective bargaining relationship at all. The ambivalence is always present in collective bargaining and the more militant or hostile is the trade-union bargaining strategy the more poignant is the conflict entailed in its position. This is illustrated very well by the complex manoeuvres which Allen has to conduct in defence of *Militant Trade Unionism* (1966 : 164):

'Militant tactical bargaining is a positive policy in that it benefits both unions through extracting the utmost from market advantages and the community through encouraging the use of more efficient methods. It is, therefore, economically good for the system itself. How, it may be asked, can unions reconcile an aim to alter the system to make it more equitable and with an activity which makes it more viable and resilient and thus more capable of resisting pressures to alter it. The answer is twofold. Firstly, it is not the purpose of unions to change the capitalist system through disrupting its operation and creating depression. Unions must extract as much as the system will permit and the more efficient it is the greater will this be. This function is forced on unions in a capitalist system by their very nature irrespective of their long-term intentions. The question of reconciliation never comes up.'

It is just as well, perhaps, that it does not, for Allen has done nothing to lead unions out of the dilemma in which he found them, indeed, his comments simply illustrate rather than resolve it. Trade unions, he continues, can only watch and wait, they could 'assist in the analysis' of the 'forces which produce and resolve revolutionary situations'. This is just the kind of theological obeisance to dogma to which 'militant' trade unions are driven while they continue to play the market.

The dilemma is inescapable, unions, by their very involvement in collective bargaining, are tacitly accepting the economic environment and the more active their negotiating strategy the more likely they are to contribute to its efficiency and improvement. The collective bargaining relationship is a market relationship and trade unions engaged in it are commited to market behaviour. This is why trade unions cannot make any contribution to an ideological exchange, at least within their economic and industrial role. The British trade unions have never engaged in an ideological examination of the society in which they operate because the contradictory conceptual framework on which they are founded forbids it. British trade unions, on the contrary, usually regard any emerging ideology within its own ranks (as in the Clydeside movement or in *The Miners' Next Step*) as an incipient revolt against their own authority; the normal reaction of a British trade union to a developing ideology is to put it down.

This is not a problem in the United States where trade unions do not set off with any political objectives nor with any close political ties. American unions are business unions and the ideological commitment which they share is, for the most part, to a business ideology. This means, paradoxically, that they can behave with much greater bargaining zeal than their British brothers, they are not constrained by any commitment to society or to a government. Because they share ideological assumptions with their business opponents they are permitted by the ideology which binds them to behave with great hostility towards them.

Our purpose here, however, is not an examination of trade unions as such but, in the context of British politics to examine their contribution to an ideology of work. We suggest that the existence of a political channel for the presentation of union views helps to prevent the expression of ideological views by industrial means. In any case, whether it is the result of an absence of opinions or of means for their expression, the net result seems to be that the contribution either of the British Labour Party or the British trade unions, to an ideology of work has been negligible. This may not be the case in every example of democratic socialism but it is likely that the major influences are likely to emerge from Marxism or from syndicalism or from some other ideological route that we have already examined. Democratic socialist movements, particularly where they are associated with government, are likely to be preoccupied with and greatly influenced by problems of practical politics and administration. They are likely to be distinguished from other political groups not so much in terms of ideology (to this extent a process of convergence is probably at work on all parties) but in terms of the distinct practical and short-term interest of the class they represent.

But the defence of practical and short-term interests entails the formulation of judgements and the articulation of values. The defender may begin with no sense of direction but he will usually find himself driven into positions which have to be defended with ideology. The drift of a great deal of left wing criticism of the trade unions has been that their pragmatism has involved a refusal to advance the cause of the Labour movement as a whole, that their conflicts have been narrow, sectional, and short-term and that they have been incorporated in the administrative machinery of the State. Thus Lane (1974 : 291) writing of British industrial relations in the 1960s says,

'The Labour Party became a more or less perfect expression of the sort of politics embodied in trade unionism. Creating no socialist consciousness amongst the working class, it ensured that the class remained locked up in the factory consciousness that developed out of collective action in the workplace. With the dominant institutions of the Labour "movement" as a whole bereft of any clear and coherent understanding of the historical process of capitalism, it produced *ad hoc* "solutions" to *ad hoc* problems and left the working class wide open to such reactionary mystifications as nationalism, racism, and "benevolent" capitalism.'

Lane does not entirely despair because, he believes, the rank and file exert pressure on their leadership and because the 'wage militancy of the working class ... stopped the unions from becoming part of the appparatus of a corporate state' (1974 : 292). But in April 1976, Mr Healey's budget involved the trade unions in negotiations over public taxation policy related to a level of acceptable wage increases. Most of the worries expressed about this unique departure from previous practice concerned issues of a constitutional and parliamentary nature but the more important question may concern an unprecedented step in the incorporation of the unions in government. The defence of practical and short-term interests may involve the unions finding themselves, as The *Guardian* put it, with a heavy responsibility for the maintenance of a Labour government. The unions end up in an ideological position which they had not sought to establish.

Lane probably sees trade unions as either advancing the cause of the workers in a political class war or as taking a position subordinate to the ruling institutions in capitalist society. Democrats or pluralists might take the different view that trade unions are a vital part of the complex process of control and representation in an industrial society. The difficulty they have in performing this function is that while it demands that they should be independent and representative, they are constantly under pressure to control their members rather than represent them. They are required to serve the national interest and this constantly threatens to incorporate them in the State.

II *Fascism*

The most extreme statement of the paradoxes that may inhere in democratic socialism, and the most pessimistic conclusions from them, were expressed in Michels's 'iron law of oligarchy'.[12] Michels argued that the leaders of big organizations always had an unique advantage, they were better informed than anyone else, they controlled the channels of communication within the organizations and experience contributed to their superior administrative and political skill. The same centralizing tendencies can be observed in labour organizations but they are emphasized by the division of labour among the members which fractionalizes the experience, interest, and knowledge of the members. These characteristics encourage the need for and the emergence of leaders who will continue to depend upon mass support but who will 'replace the power of one minority with that of another'. Criticism of their leadership will merely serve to make the leaders protect themselves by reducing the means of democratic control in the organization, emphasizing the hostility of its external enemies and defining its internal critics as traitors.

A socialist revolution would give rise to a 'dictatorship in the hands of those leaders who have been sufficiently astute and sufficiently powerful to grasp the sceptre of dominion in the name of socialism ... Thus the social revolution would not effect any real modification of the internal structure of the mass. The socialists might conquer, but not socialism, which would perish in the moment of its adherents' triumph' (Lipsett 1969 : 416).

Michels concluded grimly that democracy and socialism were not compatible and he was forced to abandon democracy. He chose, as alternative, Mussolini. The only way of resisting bureaucratic centralizing tendencies which lead to an élite, controlling in its own interest, the only way of introducing effective change is to find strong charismatic leaders, men like Mussolini. Michels's construction is an iron paradox rather than an iron law; democratic socialism leads to totalitarianism; the only alternative to totalitarianism is fascism.

Fascism or national socialism can take one of a number of attitudes to work and to the worker. This is because it is not possible to look for any essential consistency in fascist positions. Fascist doctrine is sometimes associated with left wing movements which emerge from syndicalism. Fascist doctrine can also be based on the more obscure corners of nineteenth-century romanticism in which case it may deliberately repudiate rationality and will not develop any consistent outlook towards work or towards economic affairs of any kind. This basic inconsistency may arise from the fact that Italian fascism and German National Socialism have been wrongly identified on the basis of a similarity in the methods of the governments (although based upon quite different ideologies) and, of course, because of their political and military alliance from 1940 to 1944.

On the other hand, Woolf (1968) argues that particular conditions of economic development are always likely to be propitious for the achievement of any fascist form of government. These phases are likely to be those in which a relatively under-industrialized society is subjected to a rapid process of modernization and industrialization which is accompanied by large-scale mobilization of the population and the movement of rural populations to the towns. Previously unorganized sections of the population find themselves, for the first time, with access to political power, by virtue of their greater knowledge, wealth, proximity to each other, industrial power, and union membership. They are newcomers to the political system and 'once in the political system the new entrants wield their political power to gain more acceptable treatment in the economic and social system as well' (Woolf 1968 : 28).

If their demands are not met there is the prospect of continued agitation and conflict. If they are met, an established system based on domination by an élite has to be quickly changed into a mass system. The élite will tend to defend itself by resisting change and there is the likelihood of civil disorder and a great deal of talk of the imminence of revolution. This provokes an attempt to dismantle the emergent organization of workers and of the left while there may also be an attempt to slow down the rate of economic growth. Woolf points out in support of this explanation that, after the Fascists gained power in Italy, laws of 1931 and 1939 prohibited rural workers from moving to large towns, wages were held down and economic development slowed in the 1920s and almost stopped in the 1930s. Prior to the Fascists' capture of power, however, just such a process of industrial development had been taking place. The Socialist General Confederation of Labour had grown from 327 members in 1913 to 2.2 million in 1921, Catholic unions had increased by 2 million and other unions had a membership of 700,000. The electorate had expanded, socialist parties had greatly increased in size, there were many strikes and lock-outs and a great deal of civil disorder.

While steps are taken to slow down the development of industrialization or to impede the growth of an urban proletariat, alternative defences are constructed against it, by attempting to integrate it in the political fabric of the state. The integration that

Fascists seek as an alternative to industrial alienation is to reduce the consciousness of alienation in the worker and to reduce his consciousness of class. Fascism represents, often, the attempt to replace the economic institutions of society by essentially political means of association, it represents the 'triumph of politics' over economics. In this sense fascist governments, along with the survival of theocratic regimes, are the isolated exceptions to the consistent development of economic values that has characterized the western world since the seventeenth century. Fascism stresses the importance of the state as the alternative to class and it attempts to destroy or reduce in importance any faction within the state that is likely to militate against its unity. Woolf suggests that while social mobilization of new groups in society is reduced their political mobilization is deliberately encouraged. While institutions like trade unions are destroyed, new forms of political association are established to extend membership to groups previously excluded from political activity, e.g. youth, the middle classes, and women. But the political activity is of a symbolic kind with no real involvement in decision-making and a great deal of marching, singing, and rallying. In this way, 'fascism attempts to permit the nation to be both modern and non-modern, to modernise economically without the socio-political consequences of such modernisation' (Woolf 1968 : 33).

In some senses fascism represents one of the very few alternatives to capitalism, it really is outside the consensus over economic values which we have described as encompassing capitalists and their communist critics. Fascist government are often anti-business, the programmes of early fascist governments in Italy, Germany, and Japan were all described as anti-capitalist, demanding heavy capital levies, heavy tax on profits, the establishment of minimum wage rates, and workers participation in management, (but not by means of independent trade unions). Woolf (1968 : 127) commented that a 'Deep mistrust of "big capital" permeates the economic philosophy of the early fascists. Italian fascists distinguished between productive and parasitic bourgeoisie; Nazies between rapacious and creative (or industrial) capital.' This attitude did not necessarily accompany, however, any great affection for the industrial worker.

Antagonism to capital was modified because capitalists formed an important part of the élite on which fascists depended to come to power; it was, in part, the fear felt by capitalists which enabled fascists to emerge. 'Fascism arose in all countries as an anti-socialist movement and continually reiterated its determination to replace class-conflict by class collaboration in the national interest' (Woolf 1968 : 128). But fascist parties do harbour socialist aspirations of a kind. Mussolini started his political life on the extreme, syndicalist wing of the socialist movement and was strongly influenced by Sorel. The Nazies' name, 'national socialists', was not entirely without meaning.

In order to achieve the supremacy of the state, workers must be converted from class consciousness or, perhaps as in Spain and some South American regimes, class consciousness must be prevented from developing. Workers' institutions have to be ruthlessly suppressed or totally controlled and workers have to be integrated within the state. But this process cannot be achieved by symbols and sacrifice alone, there must be some genuine concern for their welfare. It is not as workers but as 'the people' that the proletariat takes on an existence and a meaning in fascist societies.

The solution to this problem of how the workers are to be both destroyed and nurtured is ingenious and it takes us back to the thinking of Saint-Simon. He believed, along with Robert Owen and other associative socialists, that political institutions were moribund and that government based on political processes and institutions was irrelevant. He argued that society would have to be ordered by the arrangement of economic institutions and relationships. Later syndicalists also saw industrial and economic institutions as alternatives to the established, national, and political institutions. Industry was to be transformed by means of the *syndicats,* to become a means of revolutionary change in society and, thereafter, a means of its administration by the workers.

The fascists took this process and stood it on its head. The theory of corporatism was developed by Mussolini, partly as an answer to successive capitalist crises and partly as a means of subordinating economic to political criteria. Syndicalism, or a version of it, became the means of subordinating industry to the state, instead of, as it was conceived, of subordinating the state to industry. Spearman (1939) describes the way in which Italian industry was organized with a network of twenty-two industrial organizations designed to incorporate the functions of both employers' associations and trade unions. All aspects of an industry were subsumed in the corporation with equal representation for employers and employees (a total of some 500 for the textile industry) along with three representatives of the party. These industrial corporations were set up initially with fairly limited responsibilities for the regulation of apprenticeship and of employ-ment exchanges. They finally became responsible for regulating economic conditions in the industry, controlling production, regulat-ing wages, and prices. They were subject to the overall control of the political body, and general assembly and, in this sense, they were finally subordinated to the state. Corporatism as it developed in Italy and, to some extent in Spain, was believed to result in the elimination of class antagonism. It was also regarded as a means of extending collective bargaining. Mussolini believed that industrial corporations would gradually reduce the distance that separated the very rich from the very poor.

But the control exercised by the state was absolute and arbitrary. Independent trade unions are re-integrated within the corporations. Whereas Saint-Simon and other collectivists had seen the economic institutions and the workers permeating the state, the fascist state organized the institutions and the workers so that the state could the more easily permeate them. In Germany, the Labour Front was 'given the task of winning over the workers to National Socialism, and nothing, not even the smooth running of the arms economy was allowed to impede the efforts' (Woolf 1968 : 183).

The early fascist proposals were described as directed at achieving 'vast and subversive reforms: workers participation in the management of industry, partial expropriation of wealth ... a yearning for dictatorship by a bold, resolute minority to be expressed in workers associations' (Woolf 1968 : 229).

None of this can be regarded as having any relationship to an ideology of work, however, because that would be a conception totally alien to the foundation of a fascist outlook. Fascism responded to industrialism by rejecting it. In its more sinister versions it represents the hunting society in which work is a despised activity carried out by women or slaves, the virtues it valued were military rather than economic. Even where the worker was treated with any respect or benevolence it was not out of regard for his role as worker so much as his citizenship of the state. This respect, where it existed, might shade into an acknowledgement of his power as worker but to this extent the respect was based on fear and the worker's integration was partly a defensive response. Fascism is perhaps the only genuine alternative to the transcendence of economic values and of a dominant work ideology that has been seen in modern times.

This is an account that would certainly not be acceptable to

Marxists. The Marxist explanation of fascism is that it represents the final corrupted form of the capitalist state, it is capitalism in its penultimate stage of decline. Capitalism in its phase of economic expansionism can afford, even requires, the trappings of bourgeois, liberal democracy and the provision of comforts to ameliorate the situation of the proletariat. But, as expansion comes to an end, profits fall, the cyclical crises that accompany capitalism become more and more severe, the regime must enforce subordination. Capitalism in decay can no longer afford democracy, as it cannot any longer secure the approval of the proletariat it must now organize its regimentation.

The problem remains, within this explanation, as to how, in these harrowing circumstances, fascism manages to find sufficient support to bolster its authority, 'where does the bourgeoisie find its troops'. It finds them, say communists, from the middle class who are afraid, in these trying times, of falling into the ranks of the proletariat and it finds them from Marx's greatly despised 'lumpen proletariat', the ignorant workers so benighted as to have no true consciousness of their position, the lackeys. Unfortunately, fascist support, in fact, sometimes seem to be much more broadly based than this. It may include demobilized war veterans, the unemployed, peasants, and youths. George Orwell added intellectuals who are often sympathetic to an apparent return to the past and who are likely to defect from the left as soon as the fascists have won. 'The intelligentsia are the people who squeal loudest against fascism, and yet a respectable proportion of them collapse into defeatism when the pinch comes. They are farsighted enough to see the odds against them and, moreover, they can be bribed' (1970 : Vol.2, 299).[13] There is some evidence for his contention: Mussolini's government, in 1931, required all university teachers to take an oath of allegiance. Apparently, out of 1,250 teachers throughout Italian universities, only twelve refused (Woolf 1968 : 229).

Orwell believed that the most obdurate resistance to fascism, and to any other imposed ideology, would come from the great unorganized mass of the workers. It is this sullen resistance which an ideology of work is aimed at reducing. Fascism attempts to circumvent it by denying the workers' existence as a proletariat and emphasizing their relationship to the state. It may also be of some significance that organized slavery re-appears in the western world under a nazi regime. We began the examination of the development of an ideology of work by suggesting that it was unnecessary in a society that depended upon slavery but that it became a necessary intellectual preoccupation once slavery disappeared. Is it coincidental that in a regime in which there is a rejection of an ideology of work as unnecessary slavery returns in the form of the concentration camp and the regimentation of the forced labour of conquered nations?

The German government introduced forced labour for all Jews between the ages of 14 and 60 in 1939 (Krausnick and Broszat 1970 : 75). Subsequently the Nazis were to provide a further hideous illustration of the antipathy between slavery and economic values: in 1941 a Government department pronounced that 'The rules relating to the problem require that the demands of the economy be ignored' (Krausnick and Broszat 1970 : 88). The problem was the extermination of the Jews. The solution to this problem, however, did not rob the concentration camps of labour, particularly after the territorial expansion of Germany had begun. In a very real sense, the German Empire was to be built upon slave labour because the grandiose architectural plans of Albert Speer were to be given real form in brick and granite produced in SS enterprises manned by slave labour. The camps at Flossenburg and Mauthausen were established in order to serve neighbouring quarries. Conditions in the quarries at Mauthausen were so bad as to be fearful even by comparison with other Nazi punishments. 'One of the forms of punishing prisoners in Auschwitz was to send them to the quarries of Mauthausen. Buchenwald had its own quarries; nevertheless its prisoners were in mortal fear of being transferred to Mauthausen' (Le Chêne 1971 : 64). Between its establishment in 1938 and its liberation in 1945, at least 1,244 prisoners were executed at Mauthausen, 54,299 died at the camp or in the quarries during the same period.

III *Communism*

If democratic socialism is characterized, in relation to work, by an absence of a distinctive ideology, the opposite is true of communist states. Communist governments are occupied at both the levels which we began by distinguishing. Their foundation and the reason for their existence rests in an ideology of work and they are so closely engaged in the direction of a planned economy that they are practically involved with an ideology of work as managers of labour.

The evolution (or, as some might prefer to put it, the corruption) of Marxist theory into the ideological foundation of a government, is a process in which Marx's original theory has been successively interpreted in order to meet practical political problems in the government of the Soviet Union, first by Lenin, then by Stalin, and now by Stalin's successors, and as evolving within a particularly demanding and inflexible environment.

Lenin's essential contribution was practical, he brought about a revolution. Carr (1952) has argued that one of the principle developments contributed by Lenin was to substitute the concept of 'party' for 'class' as the main agent of change. Lichteim (1966) has explained that while one interpretation of Marx's theory pointed to the inevitability of class struggle and revolution, Lenin had very special problems to wrestle with, of a kind that were not foreseen in Marx's analysis. They included.

'the imminent approach of a revolution in a backward country with an immature proletariat ... Lenin's elitism was the outcome of a situation in which socialist consciousness was incorporated, not in the actual empirical labour movement, not even in a sizeable minority of that movement as in the West, but in the "classless" intellengentsia. The Menshevicks had drawn back when they perceived the implications of this fact; they were prepared to wait. Lenin was not. His understanding of Marxism did not exclude action designed to force the pace of history.'

Forcing the pace of history meant, it has been said, the creation of an industrial state in order to make it theoretically possible, within Marxist terms, for a socialist revolution to take place, thus Robert Conquest: 'From a Marxist point of view the proletarian party which had achieved power without an adequate proletariat was an anomaly. But it was an anomaly which some communists hoped to correct by creating *ex post facto* the necessary industry and proletariat' (Conquest, 1967 : 10). There is, of course, a considerable debate as to how industrialized Russia was before the Revolution. Russia was making considerable progress in industrialization and in economic growth but was probably falling behind other European countries. Nove (1972 : 28) concludes, with qualifications, that 'if the growth rates characteristic of the period 1890-1913 for industry and agriculture were simply projected over the succeeding fifty years, no doubt citizens would be leading a reasonably comfortable life and would have been spared many dreadful convulsions'. In some ways the early government went about the task of creating the proletarian state in a strange way. The proletariat was actually *reduced* in size by the revolution, it fell from 2.6 million workers in 1917 to 1.2 million in 1920. Gross output of all industry fell by 1921 to one-third of the level of 1913 and large-scale industry to about one fifth. Nove (1972 : 71) adds that a plan for the electrification of Russia was illustrated by a vast map lit by electric light bulbs. Unfortunately, Moscow's electricity supply had almost to be cut off in order to light the map.

It was the urgent requirement of survival in the face of unemployment, foreign and civil wars, famine, inflation, complete industrial chaos, and economic breakdown which largely influenced early Soviet policies. But ideology was also influential. In the first phase of what has been called 'war communism'. Nove (1972 : 74) distinguishes the essential features as including:

1. an attempt to ban private manufacturing, extended nationalization. State control of stocks
2. a ban on private trade
3. seizure of all peasant surpluses
4. the partial elimination of money
5. terror, arbitrations, expropriation — 'a siege economy with a communist ideology. A partly organized chaos.'

A second phase set in with the New Economic Policy, after 1921, when Lenin agreed to the re-introduction of limited, private trading. Industry was reorganized into industrial trusts which were expected to operate commercially. 'Profit-making and the avoidance of losses were to be the operational criteria'. By 1922-3, 75 per cent of all retail trade was private (Nove 1972 : 88).

There was another reaction against private trading which set in after 1926-7 with a drive to achieve the more complete control of production and distribution. Stalin gained control; Nove (1972 : 143) writes that 'whether in literature or in philosophy, in the party's own internal arrangements or in the sphere of economics, the line became one of stern imposition of conformity, centralized authority, suppression of uncontrolled initiatives'. In 1926 the 15th Party Conference decided to strengthen the control of socialist industry over the whole of the economy and spoke of the need to catch up with and pass the advanced capitalist countries quickly. The first five-year plan was formulated in 1928. Thereafter the events were forced to take account of Stalin's despotism and the privations of the war. After Stalin died in 1953 there seems to have been a gradual relaxation and a re-examination of previously established policies, including labour policy and labour law.

This superficial summary of some of the stages in Soviet economic development is really meant only to suggest that the generalizations about Soviet attitudes and policies towards work and workers have to be qualified by the different circumstances through which the Soviet Union passed and the different policies which it adopted. There is probably even less consistency in this respect in the Soviet Union than one might find in Britain or in the USA over a period of similar length.

But one thing is constant in Russia and that is something in the official attitude to work and the worker. Whatever the changes in the worker's actual conditions, however brutal his condition, whether he prospers or starves, the official ideology remains broadly fixed; the Soviet Union is a workers' state. As Conquest (1967 : 7) puts it:

'In any advanced society, the relationship between the government and the industrial proletariat is a major element in the political and social scene. But in the U.S.S.R. this is particularly so. For it is there a matter not merely of the practical conduct of a large part of the nation's affairs, but also of doctrinal issues crucial to the entire position of the ruling party ... the industrial working class in Russia although it lacks any real voice in deciding issues has always been "theoretically" speaking, the ruling element in the Soviet Union.'

In the early stages of the Soviet Union the establishment of the first workers' state was believed to be sufficient cause for the abolition of any labour discipline imposed on the workers from above. In this early, idealist stage, labour discipline was to be a matter of conscience, a voluntary acceptance of the need to work hard and well. The belief in 'comradely labour discipline' is probably an inseparable part of Soviet ideology and of the complex of political and social concepts that underlie the state. The belief has survived the most strenuous attempts to impose an actual discipline of a most coercive kind, as we shall see. Bukharin and Preobrazhensky (1969 : 339) emphasize the new moral code in many passages:

'The period of the destruction of the old discipline is over. There is now being inaugurated a new, comradely labour discipline, not imposed and sustained by the masters, not imposed and sustained by the capitalist whip, but by the labour organizations themselves, by the factory committees, the workshop committees and the trade unions.'

'Labour discipline must be based upon the feeling and *the consciousness that every worker is responsible to his class*, upon the consciousness that slackness and carelessness are treason to the common cause of the workers'. (1969 : 339)

'We must control one another mutually. He betrays the workers' cause who fails now to help in getting the workers' cart out of the mire; such a one is a blackleg'. (1969 : 340) (Notice the capturing of perjorative terms like 'blackleg' for official usage).

'We must establish a workers' code of honour, so that any worker who, without good reason, fails to contribute his quota to the common cause, shall be regarded as a contemptible loafer'. (1969 : 342)

But the problems facing the Soviet Union were so urgent that there was not sufficient time to rely on the transformation of men, on the internalization of the drive to work. In theory, as Carr (1952 : 199) says, 'Labour was a form of service to society' but as early as 1918 the party congress demanded 'the most energetic, unsparingly decisive, draconian measures to raise the self-discipline and discipline of workers and peasants'. In October 1918 labour books were introduced (they seem to have remained a permanent feature of Soviet society) which had to be produced to get ration cards and travel permits and which had to demonstrate that the holder was performing useful work. Disciplinary labour courts were established in 1919 to raise productivity and discipline in enterprises. They were composed of representatives of management, trade unions, and the workers and they were to try all violations of discipline, they could impose penalties ranging from public reprimand to direction to hard labour.

The re-introduction of discipline on the workers, even though it was ostensibly conducted by the workers themselves, was a significant step. Conquest (1967 : 8) argues that after the suppression of the sailors' and workers' rebellion at Kronstadt in 1921, 'Henceforward the Party, cut off from genuine working class roots, rested on its ideas alone. Its justification came no longer from the politics of actuality but from the politics of prophecy.' Labour discipline certainly demanded special efforts to explain its necessity and its purpose because it must have seemed a break with the essential ideology of a socialist state. The explanation lay in the threatening environment, in the practical necessities of war communism. Conquest quotes a contemporary and authoritative voice which suggests that there was a considerable degree of worker hostility to the workers' state and that the Party was emerging as the representative of the best interest of the workers even though they did not know it. Karl Radek, in a speech in 1921, said that the workers' 'state of mind is at present frankly reactionary. But the Party has decided that we must *not* yield, that we must impose our will to victory on our exhausted and dispirited followers' (quoted in Conquest 1967 : 8).

The transformation was opposed from left and right. Trotsky emerged as the strong man of the labour front who could whip the disintegrating railway system into some sort of shape and who could impose discipline by forceful means. The labour front did in fact emerge as a realistic concept in an actual and a metaphorical war that was being waged against a hostile, bourgeois environment. Armies were converted into labour armies and Trotsky advocated 'the militarization of the working class'. (Carr (1952) : 213) quotes Karl Radek as making '"an appeal to organized labour to overcome the bourgeois prejudice" of "freedom of labour" so dear to the hearts of Mensheviks and compromisers'. Trotsky defended the new, and anything but comradely, labour discipline against the Mensheviks' arguments for freedom of labour.

> 'We are now advancing towards a type of labour socially regulated on the basis of an economic plan which is obligatory for the whole country, i.e. compulsory for every worker. That is the foundation of socialism. And once we have recognised this, we thereby recognise fundamentally ... the right of the workers' state to send each working man and woman to the place where they are needed for the fulfilment of economic tasks. We thereby recognise the right of the state, the workers' state, to punish the working man or woman who refuses to carry out the order of the state, who do not subordinate their will to the will of the working class and to its economic tasks ... We know that all labour is socially compulsory labour. Man must work in order not to die. He does not want to work. But the social organization compels and whips him in that direction.' (quoted in Carr 1952 : 214-16)

There is a characteristic appeal incorporated in this passage. It justifies what the state can do to the worker by using the phrase 'the workers' state' — although this claim to legitimacy must be very suspect in the light of Radek's confession as to the extent of the workers' opposition. It is also worth noticing that Trotsky here takes a very realistic view of work as something that we would all avoid if we were not compelled to it.

Lenin, in 1929, justified coercion in similar terms; the worker was being disciplined by the workers. The first attempt was to introduce conscious self-discipline, comradely discipline, the second attempt was, we might say, the collectivization of this self-discipline.

> 'We are introducing labour service and are uniting the working people without in any way fearing to use coercion, since no revolution was ever made without coercion, and the proletariat has the right to use coercion so as to hold its own at any cost ... Now the task is to apply to the peaceful tasks of economic construction ... everything that can concentrate the proletariat, its absolute unity. Here iron discipline is necessary.' (quoted in Conquest 1967 : 96)

So a campaign was launched against labour deserters, that is, those who tried to better their conditions by changing their jobs. Workers wishing to leave their jobs had to give reasons to a factory committee. A decree of 1920 ordered absentees to forfeit pay and to work off absence in overtime and in holiday work. Fifty years later, in *One Day in the Life of Ivan Denisovitch*, Solzhenitsyn (1973) described how interruptions to work in a labour camp by blizzards were officially regarded as absenteeism and had to be made up, but they were still welcomed by the prisoners.

Labour discipline after 1922 seems to have come to be regarded more as a managerial function. The Rules of Internal Labour Order established that penalties were to be imposed by management and also established a machinery for reviewing dismissals before a Rates and Conflicts Commission. Managerial action to improve discipline replaced the former 'Comrades Disciplinary Court'. The drive against absenteeism was intensified with further measures to strengthen labour discipline in 1932. The USSR Procurator-General ordered his subordinates to prosecute managers who were failing to carry out sufficiently vigorous disciplinary measures, managers were accused of being feeble in the use of their right to enforce discipline and they were encouraged to use the full range of penalties available to them (Conquest 1967). Discipline was further tightened during the war. The working day was extended with the explanation that 'If in capitalist countries the worker is compelled to work 10-12 hours for the bourgeoisie, then our Soviet worker can and must work longer than at present, at least 8 hours, since he works for himself, for his socialist state, for the good of the people' (quoted in Conquest 1967 : 119).

After the war, and after Stalin, there was another shift in emphasis, a return to the 1920s attempt to legitimize and enforce discipline by the more complete involvement of the workers and by re-emphasizing the anti-social character of indiscipline in work. Conquest (1967 : 108) writes that 'the years 1957-60 witnessed the increasing involvement of the public in maintaining public order in general and labour discipline in particular. The passing of anti-parasite laws and the parallel revival of the Comrades Courts are two main examples of this.'

The Comrades Courts were re-established in 1959. 'The campaign against parasites appeared to lapse temporarily after the first drive of 1957 ... It was conducted with resumed violence after the Conference of the Movement of Communist Labour in May 1960 which resolved:

"It is essential ... to become more intolerant ... towards drones, hooligans and wreckers"' (Conquest 1967 : 110).

Amalrik in *Involuntary Journey to Siberia* (1971) provides an account of what it is to be a victim of this new intolerance. He does not make the point explicitly but the reader gets the strong impression that the refusal to work becomes a major aspect of political rebellion for the individual, almost a matter of an inalienable right to refuse to do anything useful. If this impression is correct, it is an interesting development as one of the few forms of self-assertion left to the individual in a society which has emphasized work as incorporating its most important values.

The contemporary embodiment of Soviet law and attitudes to work and to labour discipline is set out in the Model Rules of Internal Labour Order which serve as the basis for work rules which are agreed with the trade unions. The obligations for management indicate a requirement 'to strengthen labour and production discipline'. The obligation for workers is 'to work honestly and conscientiously, to observe labour discipline, arrive at work on time, utilise all working time exclusively for production work and official duties, execute punctually and accurately orders by the management, fulfil output norms and strive to over-fulfil them' (quoted in Conquest 1967 : 112). The Rules lay down that any violation of labour discipline requires a disciplinary penalty which is graded as follows: first a reproof, followed by a reprimand, a severe reprimand and then a transfer to other and lower paid work for up to three months. As in the best

British or American industrial practice, the slate is wiped clean after a period of good behaviour, 'reproofs and reprimands are lifted if a year passes without the commission of another offence'.

The injunction to 'over-fulfil' production targets indicates an aspect of another important means of achieving the integration of the worker in the Soviet Unionism. This has been referred to at various times as 'socialist competition', 'emulation', the employment of 'shock brigades' and Stakhanovism. All these terms refer to an attempt at the positive integration of the worker rather than the attempt to coerce him. Following the introduction of the first five-year plan in 1928, workers in factories and collectives were encouraged to produce 'counter-plans' in which they undertook to exceed plans and norms imposed on them from above. Great publicity was given to workers who succeeded in continuing to exceed targets that had been raised as the result of their past performances. The drive to encourage socialist competition is founded upon the concept of the heroic quality in work, it marks the most complete transformation by communism of previous attitudes to work. It would not be an exaggeration to say that a great deal of Soviet pronouncements and a significant part of Soviet literature and art has been directed at romanticizing work and at capturing both the individual's commitment and, even more powerfully, at mobilizing the pressure for asserting norms and values in the working group. To this extent modern Soviet and American managerial practice are often similar; what is different, of course, is the underlying legitimizing foundation.

The most colourful manifestation of socialist competition emerged in the Stakhanovite movement. In 1935 Alexei Stakhanov a collier, produced fourteen times the production norm. Whereas in the West he would have been regarded by his fellow workers as a contemptible rate-buster (in fact, a war-time effort was made in Britain to establish a version of Stakhanovism in the coal industry: it failed), in the Soviet Union Stakhanov not only became a hero, his name became associated with an order of heroism. 'The emulation movement of communist work teams and shock workers' is described as inducing Soviet workers 'continuously to raise their trade, educational, cultural, and technical standards, and teaches them to work, acquire knowledge, and live in a communist way' (Yovchuk 1966 : 173). By 1960, 312,000 people were said to have joined the movement. Apart from the drive for technical efficiency and production, 'communist consciousness' or moral purity are claimed to be essential ingredients, the rise in technical standards 'is organically linked up with the moulding and development of communist consciousness and morals, and with the struggle against survivals of the past' (1966 : 176). The intention is to direct public opinion and focus the pressure of the group so as to rebuke the malingerer: 'at the Serov Iron and Steel Plant, a blast-furnace gas watchman and State Prize winner, E. Fukabov, and other leading workers sharply criticized people who had formerly been outstanding but had failed to keep themselves abreast of progress in the smelting of pig-iron' (1966 : 177).

Successive waves of ideological appeals have been launched in the Soviet Union. After the Twenty-First Party Congress in 1958, the 'Communist Labour Movement' was established in which labour teams competed to fulfill the national plan and to 'raise their cultural and technical level, participate in public activity and behave in a model way in social and private life' (Fidlon, 1973 : 329). 'Spontaneous' suggestions proposed that the competition should be extended from teams to individuals who could compete for the title 'Shock-worker of Communist Labour'; in the Urals, 'the title was awarded to a boring lathe operator' (sic) who fulfilled the requirements of the first 12 months of the plan in 3 months. It has been claimed that 'the mass scale of the movement reflected the general rise in the cultural and technical level of the working people, their high political consciousness' (1973 : 331).

Perhaps one of the most poignant illustrations of the formidable difficulties in the way of establishing a truly effective ideology of work in modern production conditions is to be found in the reports attending the results of Stakhanovism. It is not that it did not work, it did, workers were persuaded, or persuaded themselves, to produce more. 'Following a series of conferences held early in 1936 work norms were very sharply raised: by 30-40 per cent in engineering, 34 per cent in chemicals, 51 per cent in electricity generation, 26 per cent in coal mining, 25-29 per cent in the oil industry, and so on'. But Nove (1972 : 233) continues, 'speed-up and higher work norms caused much strain in sectors in which there was no easy way in increasing output per man. Many a "Stakhanovite" team was given favourable treatment by managers, who expected to benefit from the publicity which accompanied record-breaking, at the cost of neglecting the interests of the rest of the workers.' Berliner (1957 : 274) reported that managements' opposition to Stakhanovism was based on 'the disorganizing effect of the movement on the total production process ... The rhythm of production was interfered with, overwork of machines led to breakdown and overwork of men led to increased subquality output.' The problem as many British managers will instantly understand, is that in complex and integrated production processes, unusually high performance is a nuisance and to maintain it may require fairly serious dislocation. What is necessary is a steady and predictable achievement of a norm. The sad fact is that in conditions of modern integrated production systems the requirements of the work's organization discourage hard work. This is perhaps one of the most alienating and contradictory characteristics of modern production processes.

But socialist competition had considerable results and it is still an inseparable part of the general Soviet injunction that its citizens should work. Conquest says of the Model Rules of Internal Labour Order that they do not specifically mention socialist competition as part of a worker's duty because it is part of the moral, not judicial, expectation from him.

Competition of a more general kind was encouraged by the New Economic Policy when Lenin was defending himself against charges of introducing state capitalism. We are not concerned with the labyrinthine shifts in Soviet economic policy but there is one aspect that is worth attention in this context and that concerns the development of an official Soviet view concerning managerial functions. The defence of managerial functions (as against some form of syndicalist structure) rested partly, once again, upon the practical demands of the moment, but it went beyond it when Lenin described the essential character of modern industry.

> 'Neither railways, nor transport, nor large-scale machinery and enterprises in general can function correctly without a single will linking the entire working personnel into an economic organ operating with the precision of clockwork. Socialism owes its origin to large-scale machine industry. If the masses of the working people in introducing Socialism prove incapable of adopting their institutions in the way that large-scale machine industry should work, then there can be no question of introducing Socialism ... The slogan of practical ability and business-like methods has enjoyed little popularity among revolutionaries.' (quoted by Nove 1972 : 57)

Bukharin and Preobrazhensky suggested the urgent need for certain innovations in Soviet industry, including the introduction of methods of accounting and of standards concerning a normal working day and

normal intensity of effort. Lenin saw the need and expressed it with
force and clarity. In *The Immediate Tasks of the Soviet Government*
Lenin (1969 : 401) outlined the tasks of administration and
organization that had to be accomplished and went on to catalogue
the unpalatable items that would have to be swallowed, an income
tax, compulsory labour service, organized accounting and control, and,
not least, the raising of labour productivity. A successful revolution is
easy, he says, in that it can be accomplished in a few days; improving
labour productivity is much more difficult because it will take years to
accomplish. In the passage that follows he goes on to illustrate the
obstacle of an inexperienced and untrained proletariat that must be
overcome and he clearly identifies the solutions that production
problems demand:

'The Russian is a bad worker compared with people in advanced
countries. It could not be otherwise under the Tsarist regime and in
view of the persistence of the hangover from serfdom. The tasks that
the Soviet government must set the people in all its scope is — learn
to work. The Taylor system, the last word of capitalism in this
respect, like all capitalist progress is a combination of the refined
brutality of bourgeois exploitation and a number of the greatest
scientific achievements in the field of analysing mechanical motions
during work, the elimination of superfluous and awkward motions,
the elaboration of correct methods of work, the introduction of the
best system of accounting and control, etc. The Soviet Republic
must at all costs adopt all that is valuable in the achievements of
science and technology in this field. The possibility of building
socialism depends exactly upon our success in combining the Soviet
power and the Soviet organisation of administration with the up-to-
date achievements of capitalism. We must organise in Russia the
study and teaching of the Taylor system and systematically try it out
and adapt it to our own ends. At the same time, in working to raise
the productivity of labour, we must take into account the specific
features of the transition period from capitalism to socialism, which,
on the one hand require that the foundations be laid of the socialist
organisation of competition, and, on the other hand, require the
use of compulsion, so that the slogan of the dictatorship of the
proletariat shall not be desecrated by the practice of a lily-livered
proletarian government.' (Lenin 1969 : 417)

Lenin went on to emphasize that industrial organization required absolute obedience to authority, *'unquestionable subordination* to a single will is absolutely necessary for the success of processes organised on the pattern of large-scale machine industry. On the railways it is twice and three times as necessary' (Lenin 1969 : 425).

Bendix (1970) describes the work of the Time League in introducing a respect for standards necessary to industrialization and the enthusiasm shown for American methods of management control represented in the movement for Communist Americanism. Conquest's (1967) descriptions of the changes in Labour policy after the abandonment of the early devotion to equality of payment reads in terms very similar to British or American management accounts of wage-structure administration and job evaluation.

One of the most intense debates over this process of evolving attitudes more appropriate to industrialization concerned the role of the trade unions. It provides an excellent illustration of Sturmthal's comments concerning the difficulty of accommodating trade unions within socialist theory. The conflict, as Carr (1952 : 219) put it, was over whether the union function 'was to stimulate production or to defend the immediate and sectional interests of their members, whether they should mobilize and organize labour by compulsory or solely by voluntary methods and whether they should take orders from the state on matters of policy or maintain some degree of independence'. Bukharin (1969 : 333) put the party's view, or rather, that of the victorious faction: 'the trade unions and the co-operatives must develop in such a way that they will be transformed into economic departments and instruments of the state authority; they must be "statified".'

The lines of early conflict were drawn between those who saw the unions as agents of the workers' state and freed from any requirement to represent the workers (since independent representation against a workers' state was no longer necessary) and those who believed that the revolution should be followed by workers' control. Lenin launched an attack on the syndicalists. In *'Left-Wing' Communism — an Infantile Disorder*, published in 1920, Lenin (1969 : 588) gives a short history of the Revolution explaining the victory of the Bolsheviks and, in passing, emphasizing 'that absolute centralisation and rigorous discipline in the proletariat are an essential condition of victory over the bourgeoisie'. Lenin also tried to enlighten his followers on the distinction between good and bad compromises, a problem that has surely remained a testing one for communists unless and until it has been resolved for them by their party leadership. In effect, Lenin's advice seems to amount to saying that a valuable compromise is one necessary to survival while one that is not is a 'concrete' compromise or treachery.

Lenin's attitude to trade unions was, to say the least, equivocal. 'The trade unions were a tremendous step forward for the working class in the early days of capitalist development ... When the *revolutionary party of the proletariat, the highest* form of proletarian class organisation, began to take shape ... the trade unions inevitably began to reveal *certain* reactionary features, a certain craft narrow-mindedness, a certain tendency to be non-political, a certain inertness, etc.' (Lenin 1969 : 539). The trade unions are a 'school of communism', but in capitalist society trade unions are so contempt-ible as to deserve a truly Marxist stream of abuse, 'narrow-minded, selfish, case-hardened, covetous, and petty-bourgeois "labour aristo-cracy", imperialist-minded, and imperialist-corrupted' (Lenin 1969 : 540).

'Left-Wing' Communism provides an example of Lenin's tactics as a propagandist. The argument he conducts over the trade unions really resembles a boxer's feint with the left, followed by a knock-out with the right. Having generally castigated trade unions in capitalist countries he then proceeds to criticize the 'left' communists, who presumably agreed with the attack, for upholding the 'ridiculous "theory" that Communists should not work in reactionary trade unions'. This is nonsense, they must 'work wherever the masses are to be found' (Lenin 1969 : 541). In this way Lenin first establishes a groundwork of criticism of the trade unions and so establishes his credentials, as it were, for attacking a group which might otherwise claim a more purely communist policy than his own.

If the argument with foreign communists concerned their refusal to work with trade unions in capitalist society, at home it turned upon the relationship of trade unions to a socialist state. At one extreme, the syndicalist element saw the unions, already based on an industrial structure in Russia and therefore exempt from criticisms of craft-élitism, as suitable to provide the framework of government. This view was represented by the Railway Union which, in 1917, claimed absolute self-government for the railway industry, 'It was syndicalism in its most extreme form'. Carr (1952 : 395) explains that, in order to regain control of a powerful and independent industrial organization, the Soviet government had itself to adopt a syndicalist policy in order to construct a new railway organization which could capture control 'from labour'. 'The Railways', he suggests, 'were a microcosm of Russian industry' and 'The policy adopted in dealing with them was the prototype of industrial policy as a whole. Workers control successively served two purposes. It broke up the old order that was hostile to the revolution and when pursued to its own logical conclusion, it demonstrated beyond possibility of contradiction the need for new forms of control, more rigid and more centralized' (Carr 1952 : 397).

Lenin's understanding that the trade unions had a transitional role and were training grounds for communists was at least accurate in that it took no clear account of their position within a communist state. Their claim to authority in the early years of war communism had been rejected and subsequently the party had established its control over the central Council of Trade Unions. With the establishment of state capitalism, the trade unions began to be seen in something like their role in capitalist societies. 'Membership was voluntary, although encouraged', and 'even strikes ... were not prohibited, though the trade unions were to make it clear to the workers that "strike action in a state with a proletarian government can be explained and justified only by bureaucratic perversions in that state and by survivals of capitalism"' (Carr 1952 : 327). The trade unions were expected to behave with a degree of independence of the state, dependent upon their members dues, negotiating wages above national minimum, entering conciliation machinery for the resolution of disputes, but their independence was neutralized by the absolute control which the party asserted over them when 'the eleventh party congress formally adopted the resolution ... that only party members of several years standing could be elected to leading posts in the trade union organization' (Carr 1952 : 328).

The illusion of independence which was represented in the changed expectations of trade union behaviour could not be maintained for very long. Despite the emergence of the collective contract negotiated by the union, their involvement in the management of state enterprises, and their responsibility for the establishment of factory committees, the unions could not escape from reminders of their duty to the wider society, to the workers' state of which they were a part. They were allowed to strike, but expected to see to

'the "speedy liquidation" of any strike which broke out "spontaneously or against the wishes of the unions"', they were to represent
their members' interest but also to maintain the production targets
expected of their members. The problem of coexistence between
independence and responsibility was an exaggerated version of the
conflict we see in our own society whenever the state require
adherence to an income policy or any other aspect of economic
planning. "Labour and trade union policy was an integral part of
the whole problem of the efficiency of national economy. Whatever
forms might seem to be dictated by the logic of N.E.P., to stimulate
industrial production was still the basic need of the Soviet
economy.' (Carr 1952 : 331)

The replacement of NEP by the commitment to planning meant
that even the illusions of trade union independence were no longer
useful. The favourite image used to illustrate the role of the trade
unions became the 'transmission belt' which related the state to the
worker. The trade unions increasingly came to be seen as agents for
ensuring that the state's production targets were met and that other
labour policies and labour discipline were effectively implemented in
the place of work. Conquest (1967 : 153) suggests that the trade
unions' relationship to the state have been too unequivocally
established even for the state, '... the unions have been so dependent
on the State and the Party that the latter has on occasion had to
remind the unions of their function as defenders of the workers'
interest'. He quotes 'Trud' in 1952, describing the trade unions
functions in terms which clearly identify them as the enforcers of
comradely labour discipline;

> 'the essential duty of the economic and trade union executives is to
> see to it that every worker and employee labours productively all the
> 480 minutes of his working day ... It is necessary to educate the
> masses in the spirit of intolerance even to the slightest violations of
> the [production] schedule ... It is necessary ... to expose the hack-
> workers, the slovenly workers, the people who have lost the feeling
> of responsibility for the job entrusted to them.' (Carr 1967 : 157)

There seems to have been a return, more recently, to the principles
of economic competition, or at least, to profit as an indicator of
efficiency. Parry attributes the return to the influence of the
'Liberman Reforms'. Professor Liberman waged a theoretical battle to

establish that the pursuit of profit and freedom from the dictatorship of a national plan were not anti-Marxist heresy. Parry suggests that the theoretical struggle is over, that the economists have won and that, by 1965, 'the Party merely waited to be told by Liberman and others what to do next'. By 1965, the Central Committee of the Party had accepted the principles of economic reform. Economic reform provided socialist emulation with an economic basis. Reductions in the length of the working week brought about by shorter hours, longer holidays and, apparently, an increase of 13 per cent in absenteeism, meant that 'each working hour had to be used with the utmost efficiency' (Fidlar, 1973 : 360) — precisely Marx's conclusion about the behaviour of capitalist employers similarly pressed to intensify production. Bonus systems of payment were introduced for workers and the activity of industrial enterprises was assessed on the basis of the fulfilment of sales and on profit plans. The language in which these innovations are described is almost indistinguishable from managerial texts in the USA or Western Europe; the purpose of the innovations is also concerned with reaching the same objectives, production, technical improvement, productivity, even profit. But the ideological derivations of these common objectives remain distinct. Pravda said 'Everybody needs money ... life is life [but] in our society money is not filthy lucre. It merits every respect for it emits the noble gleam of labour' (Fidlar, 1973 : 362). The final ideological justification is to be found in Lenin. 'Lenin pointed out that each enterprise should be a paying one. Its income should be able to cover all its expenditures and ensure a profit. The economic reform creates favourable conditions for this' (Fidlar, 1973 : 362).

So we see confused and sometimes contradictory aspects of Soviet labour policy. The attempt at developing a socialist conscience, socialist competition, comradely labour discipline, was never entirely successful although it has never been abandoned. In this sense, the attempt at the political integration of the worker failed, he had to be managed, encouraged, controlled and coerced as in every other industrial society. In that the whole of Soviet society was directed at achieving a process of rapid industrialization the Soviet worker has probably been more managed, encouraged, controlled, and coerced than most. It may be that, in the early days, the appeals to worker co-operation based on his integration in a socialist state were genuine in that they were believed to be sufficient; they were entailed by the theory that had established the state. The appeals have continued because no manager can avoid exhorting his subordinates in order to achieve his own objectives and because communism provides a legitimate and acceptable foundation on which to base such appeals. They may also have continued because, whether they are effective or not, they no longer relate simply to a work ideology but are, by now, a part of the mythology of a communist state.

In this sense it may be that the original *raison d'être* of communism is that it seems to provide a means of integrating an industrial proletariat in a well-ordered society. It explains the role of the proletariat in heroic terms, it assures the worker of justice, it takes the accomplishment of his every-day tasks very seriously, in short, it offers a political means of avoiding what has often been perceived as the almost intractable problem of an industrialized society, the social and political alienation of the workers. The suggestions are that it fails to do this in terms of establishing a relationship between the worker, his work, and his society. Writing in 1966, Nagy said that ' ... in societies which are officially described as "people's democracies", where "the ruling class is composed of workers", and where the workers "own" the enterprises in which they labour, alienation has not only failed to disappear, but has grown into a social problem of considerable proportions. Indeed, recent evidence from Hungary ... suggests that the average worker feels much more estranged, powerless and alienated from his society than his Western "capitalist" counterpart.' Nagy quotes a Hungarian, Peter Veres, to the effect that the alienated western workers at least have money to comfort them, they have 'something to turn to in their alienation'.

If such reports are true, and the continued exhortations and attacks on parasites in the Soviet Union suggest at least a grain of truth in them, then the workers' society has not succeeded in integrating the worker. But even if the communist state does not meet its early promises in this respect it has, at least, succeeded in establishing itself as a state. The apparatus of government exists and therefore has to be defended. Having failed in the integration of the worker *per se*, in a workers' society, the state now has to meet the original problem which it was brought into being to resolve, it must integrate him as a citizen. The more centralized the state becomes, the more committed to planning, the more the party justifies itself as ruling in the interests of the people, then the more frequently coercion has to replace attempts to achieve the workers' commitment to his work. The official adoption of an ideology of work pushes back the frontier that delineates treasonable conduct because the refusal to work becomes treachery to the state. Capitalist societies have the great advantage, for their occupants, of being relatively inefficient in their control of the worker and of being incapable of succeeding in capturing his commitment. Capitalism rests upon self-interest and, however vulgar or enlightened it becomes, it provides a poor basis for capturing the zeal of others in the pursuit of one's own enterprise. Capitalists, therefore, make a virtue out of the necessity of having to leave people alone.

Communist societies are more demanding. This is why we suggested that Amalrik implies idleness as an act of political opposition. Whereas in the western countries the idler is regarded at worst as lazy and at best as a fellow of infinite cunning, in a communist country he is condemned as a traitor to his fellows and as holding in contempt the values upon which his society is founded. What is more, because of the manifold ways, ideological and practical, in which the state is involved in work, the idler begins to be seen as a threat to the state and as justifying the most 'draconian measures' to correct him.

The first labour camps were set up in 1919 although 'the system had not, in this initial stage, the sinister significance which it later acquired as a major economic asset' (Conquest 1971 : 211). The population of the labour camps is estimated to have reached eight million in 1938 and forced labour came to play a very significant part in the Soviet economy. The labour camp work force is said to have been distributed in 1941 between one million in mining, 200,000 in agriculture, one million in a variety of state enterprises, three and a half million in general construction work and 600,000 in the maintenance and construction of the camps themselves. However important to the economy, Conquest (1971 : 482-3) argues that, because slave labour is inefficient, 'the mass arrests remain basically a political phenomenon. The slave labour motive can only have been secondary ... once arrested the extraction of physical labour ensured at least some contribution to the economy.'

Just as the Nazies distinguished between categories of concentration-camp prisoners, regarding the political prisoner as the most serious 'offender', so the Russian Corrective Labour Codex distinguishes between three kinds of labour camp; factory and farm colonies for training and disciplinary prisoners, camps for 'class-dangerous elements requiring a more severe regime in distant regions', and 'Punitive camps for the strict isolation of those previously detained in other colonies and showing persistent insubordination'. Both the

Russians and the Nazies seem to have treated those who would elsewhere be regarded as criminals, comparatively leniently, to the extent that they were often made 'trustees' and given disciplinary responsibilities to exercise over the 'politicals' (Conquest 1971 : 450).

Discipline and working conditions in the Russian labour camps were originally controlled by rules laid down in the general labour code governing the conditions of all Soviet workers, but these rules came to have no relevance in the camps and the rules that did operate within them serve as a grim and ironic contrast with any limitations on hours of work and permitted overtime. In the huge camps of the Kolyma gold fields, outside work was prohibited when the temperature reached -50°C (Solzhenitsyn's Ivan Denisovitch speaks of -40°C as prohibiting outside work).

Incentives to work took the form of a scale of deprivations rather than rewards. In one camp the prisoners had to work a twelve-hour day to earn a food ration of 800 grammes, failure to reach their work norms reduced the ration to 500 grammes, further punishment reduced it to 300 grammes, a level which meant death. A grim cycle was set up in which a man literally worked himself to death in order to avoid starvation. 'A very active man would sometimes remain healthy by producing 120 or 150 per cent of his quota for a year or 18 months and then one night would be found dead of heart failure in his bunk ... when worn down, debilitated to the degree that no serious work could any longer be got out of them, prisoners were put on sub-starvation rations and allowed to hang around the camp doing odd jobs till they died' (Conquest 1971 : 472). Ivan Denisovitch realizes that the outsider must wonder why they worked in such conditions: 'we work in order to survive', he says.

Many did not survive. One estimate suggests that two million eight hundred thousand people died in the labour camps between 1936 and 1939, and a further one million eight hundred thousand from 1939 to 1941. The death rate in mining camps and in lumber camps is estimated to have been about thirty per cent per year (Conquest 1971 : 493).

Forced labour did not necessarily imply manual labour. The Soviet government eventually grew concerned at the gross inefficiency of employing physicists and economists to fell trees and began to establish a policy of selective deployment of its slaves. The result was Mavrino, the 'special prison' of Solzhenitsyn's *The First Cirlce*.

'They first set up a special prison in 1930 ... they wanted to see how scientists and technicians would work in prison ... The experiment worked out very well. In normal conditions you could never have two top engineers or scientists on the same project — one would always oust the other in the fight over who was to get all the credit and the Stalin Prize. That's why all ordinary research teams consist of a colourless group around one brilliant head. But in prison it's another thing ... You can have a dozen academic lions living together peacefully in one den, because they've nowhere else to go. They soon get bored just playing chess or sitting around smoking. So they set about inventing something. No end of original work has been done like that.' (Solzhenitsyn 1970 : 82)

The First Circle is a very apt commentary of the extension of Marx's intensification of work to the last remaining independents in the labour force, the intellectuals. It may also illustrate the final acknowledgement of failure to develop an effective ideology of work even within a workers' state. The scientists at Mavrino are slaves, however comfortable their conditions compared with those of the labour camps from which they were recruited and to which they will return. And yet slavery is inefficient. The engineer Bobynin explains the intransigent inefficiency of slavery when he is being bullied by a Minister who says he can deal with men like Bobynin:

'"No you can't" Bobynin's piercing eyes flashed with hatred. "I've got nothing, see? Nothing! You can't touch my wife and child — they were killed by a bomb. My parents are dead. I own nothing in this world except a handkerchief. These denims and this underwear — which haven't even got any buttons" — he bared his chest to show what he meant — "is government issue. You took my freedom away a long time ago and you can't give it back to me because you haven't got it yourself. I'm forty-two years old. You gave me twenty-five years. I've done hard labour. I know what it is to have a number instead of a name, to be handcuffed, to be guarded by dogs, to work in a punitive brigade — what more can you do to me? Take me off this special project? You'd be the loser. I need a smoke".' (Solzhenitsyn 1970 : 105)

The awful significance of the labour camps is probably greatest in terms of the apparatus of political control. Their miserable inhabitants also, no doubt, contributed by their labour to the Soviet economy as a whole but this was a by-product. Berliner (1957 : 313) has suggested that the punitive threat of imprisonment has not, since the thirties, 'played a crucial role in the organization of Soviet industry' and that 'the inhumane features of Stalin's system, ranging from the barbarism of prison labour camps to the petty annoyance of night work, were a dismal overlay and not an integral element in managerial behaviour'.

Management's need to appeal, by practical and ideological means, for the co-operation of workers is of the same nature as it is in the West. The result is much the same mixture, in different proportions, of coercion, incentive, and moral exhortation, but there are two essential differences. The social context within which management operates is different in that the State is inextricably involved in the management process; the whole relationships of management and authority in work are political questions. Partly as a result of this association, the problem of legitimating managerial authority over workers is an easier one than in the West; appeals to work will carry the whole weight of loyalty to class, country, and the fundamental doctrine underlying the workers' own state.

For this reason appeals for the workers' active co-operation in comradely discipline or in socialist competition are frequent and the appeal for the worker's help can be carried further into arrangements for his participation in the management of his enterprise. Granick (1954 : 233) concludes that four basic methods have been used to achieve 'mass participation' in Soviet industry;

> 'One of these is supervision by the employees in a firm over the work of the management, and their strict criticism of all its deficiencies. A second is the offering of suggestions — particularly through employee conferences. A third is the direct performance of administrative tasks by workers who do this in addition to their regular work. Finally, and as important as any of the other three forms, is the movement upward of rank-and-file workers into posts in management and into leading positions in Party and trade union organizations.'

Six years later, Granick (1960 : 57) had concluded that 'occupational mobility seems much the same in the Soviet Union as in the United States' so that the last form of participation may be no more advantageous to the worker than it is in the West.

Other forms of participation seem to offer a real opportunity of countering management's plans and of criticizing management's performance. The trade union can exercise some control over management although in practice this may not appear to management as a serious threat. 'It is quite another matter when mass participation takes the form of criticism and conferences. Such forms of mass participation pose a real threat to management by the possibility of disclosure of its inefficiency.' Professor Berliner (1957 : 272-4) goes on to explain that the political circumstances at these conferences and the publicity that can attend disclosures by a workman in the interests of the state 'are such that the man attacking the enemy of the state speaks with a voice amplified many times ... The temptation is great, which is as the state means it to be, the ardent people fall under the temptation sufficiently often to have caused the large production conference to become a source of great unrest to management' (Berliner 1957 : 276). Nothing so embarrassing can be imagined as emerging from our own attempts at 'participative' management; they usually aim at, and succeed in promoting, resonance.

The most complete and widely publicized attempts at promoting worker participation are to be found in Yugoslavia. The electoral bases of the workers' councils and their very considerable responsibilities and powers have been described by Sturmthal (1964), by Kolaja (1965) and others. Very broadly, management of the Yugoslav enterprise has to pursue objectives determined by a process of national economic planning within a framework of constraints set by an elected workers' council, the trade union, the League of Communists, and the local commune. The director of the enterprise is appointed by representatives of workers and of the commune and he is responsible, apart from the fulfilment of planned objectives, to the workers' council and to the commune. The responsibilities of the workers' council extend to the appointment of the management board, the approval of production, marketing and wage policies, and the distribution of those earnings which are within the discretion of the enterprise. 'In general, the workers' council is entitled to be concerned with every problem of the enterprise. It is also the highest authority in the enterprise to which persons can appeal' (Kolaja 1965 : 6).

In this context, we are not interested in management structure *per se*, only to the extent that it seeks to legitimate management's authority over workers in order to achieve their more complete co-operation. The Yugoslav system of management was conceived, in part, in order to break down the division between management and workers. While it has attracted great attention and some enthusiasm there are also some more critical accounts of its achievements (to be measured against the great goals at which it has been directed). Kolaja (1965 : 72) concludes that while the workers' councils may have reduced hostility between management and workers, its 'close co-operation with management precluded its becoming a genuine workers' body. The workers' council tended to be identified with management because of the overlap between the two bodies.' More significantly perhaps, in terms of our later discussion of the nature of participation in western business enterprise, Kolaja (1965 : 75) concludes that 'essentially, the new workers' council legislation has primarily benefited management, giving it more freedom and room for initiative. On the other hand, workers' labour unions have remained more dependent, not only upon management, but also upon direction from outside. On that count the workers have obtained less independence.'

Perhaps the explanation lies in Dahrendorf's (1959 : 254) words: 'The replacement of functioning owners or capitalists by propertyless functionaries or managers does not abolish class conflict, but merely changes its empirical patterns. Independent of the particular personnel of positions of authority, industrial enterprises remain imperatively co-ordinated associations the structures of which generate quasi-groups and conflicting latent interests.'

Industrial enterprises are imperatively co-ordinated associations under capitalism or communism. Communism may have discovered ways of emphasizing the imperatives more effectively because the authority that is exercised over the worker appears to be more legitimate in that it is said to derive from the worker himself. Whether this emphasis is, in fact, any more effective is questionable. What it does seem to entail is the emergence in practical form of the paradox of alienation that we identified in the Marxist outlook as a whole. The question is not an empirical one concerning the extent to which the Russian worker is integrated or is alienated. The question is, rather, how far are the managers (political and industrial) of Soviet society driven to a preoccupation with the workers' alienation by their own ideological perceptions? Russian factories, like those in the USA, are imperatively co-ordinated associations, but where factories, the tasks performed in them and the workers who carry them out, are accorded the greatest political significance, the imperatives become much more significant. Perhaps any centralized, autocratic regime is driven to perceive conspiratorial threats against its survival, only communist regimes can perceive the worker's withdrawl of total commitment to his work as involving such a threat. Alienation is likely to be a more serious problem in the Soviet Union than it is in the West, not because the Russian worker *is* more alienated but because the extent to which his integration is required is more total. The more work is idealized the more the worker's performance may be seen as a disappointment or as a threat; the more work is idealized the more passionate and coercive are likely to be the attempts to integrate him. The 'problem' of alienation is magnified by a communist perception of work; the existence of the problem intensifies the significance with which work is perceived; this in turn magnifies the problem of alienation.

Parry suggests that a new tension has grown between the managers of a society (so founded in industrial values that it has promoted management to an élite of critical importance) and the Party which controls the society. The modern Soviet manager, he says, is 'a much more assured and demanding man than was the harried factory administrator and the hectic Red executive' described by Granick and Berliner in the 1950s (Parry 1966 : 160). The managers, scientists, and technologists, are more powerful because they are necessary to an industrial society which the Party has made for them. Now that they are necessary they will, Parry argues, erode the control of the Party by importing their own culture and education and by countering the incompetence of the Party apparatus. If this is so then the Soviet Union may become a manager's rather than a worker's state, but it is unlikely to abandon the ideological framework intended to convince the worker that it is he, rather than the Party or the manager, who is in control.

10. The Enlightened Employer

We have just examined some aspects of the attempt to integrate the industrial proletariat by political means. We shall now return to the main theme in which we are concerned with ideological appeals made to the worker by his employer or by management. These involve attempts to integrate the worker in his work and they may go beyond it in an attempt to relate him to the wider society outside it.

To regard these approaches to political and to industrial integration, as clear alternatives is, of course, unreal. The political response entails policies towards work and workers. It may be less obvious to suggest that the technical response often entails political assumptions. This convergence may continue to the extent that the process of directing industry and controlling its labour begins to subsume politics entirely. The last occasion on which we discussed the replacement of politics by some form of corporate management was when this process was presented as a left-wing or syndicalist programme emerging from Saint-Simon's industrialism. The Fascists showed that the process could emerge both from the right and from the left and that in some respects, the extreme left and the extreme right may become difficult to distinguish.

The replacement of politics by corporatism may come about gradually, not as the result of an overt political programme. It may be the result of economic or managerial tendencies rather than deliberate political intentions. The argument has been presented in various forms. One of the earlier statements was in Belloc's 'The Servile State':

> 'the future of industrial society, and in particular of English society, left to its own direction, is a future in which subsistence and security shall be guaranteed for the Proletariat, but shall be guaranteed at the expense of the old political freedom and by the establishment of that Proletariat in a status really, though not nominally, servile. At the same time, the Owners will be guaranteed in their profits, the whole machinery of production in the smoothness of its working, and that stability which has been lost under the Capitalist phase of society will be found once more.' (Belloc, 1912 : 183)

The threat of collectivism or corporatism was vividly described by Hayek in *The Road to Serfdom* (1944). Burnham (1941) advanced a specifically managerial version in which he concluded that management had emerged as a distinguishable group exercising power in its own interests, supported by a specific ideology, threatening democracy with its replacement by a totalitarianism sympathetic to industrial management.

Current versions suggest that the corporate state is emerging all over the industrially developed world. While there are some who see the established nation state as becoming more and more preoccupied with economic and industrial concerns, others see the process going further, to the extent that the government of the state begins to take a subordinate role in the direction of the large, inter-linked multinational corporations. In this situation, more may usefully be said by way of describing the individual as employee of Ford Motors than as citizen of the United States or Great Britain. The process of corporate management may finally require that the sovereignty of the old nation states may have to be dismantled in order to create larger trading areas with fewer boundaries to hinder market development and labour recruitment.

'In terms of investment, many "multinational" companies seemed much more powerful than any of the host governments in whose territory they operated. The State was equally being superseded by efforts to establish wider markets, wider regions of economic control. Capitalism, having used individual States to cut the wings of the mass of small capitalists, now seemed set to abandon even the state and large national capital. The very largest companies were disentangling themselves from association with particular nationalisms ... The rise of the international company and the creation of the European Common Market directly threatened British capitalism and the British State, yet it also offered ways of survival for the largest business concentrations in Britain ... The survival of Britain seemed to depend upon the liquidation of Britain.' (Harris 1972 : 253)

A less extreme version of what is essentially the same argument is that whether the corporate state will emerge or not is hardly important because we are all learning to think in managerial terms. In this sense politics is not replaced and neither is the state; they are both invested by managerial assumptions and managerial values. This state of affairs, in which problems are set in managerial terms so that they require solutions as the result of the application of managerial techniques, is one which some would argue has long been estabished in the United States, Germany, or Britain. It is a state of affairs that requires the general acceptance of what, for the moment, may be loosely called a managerial ideology. One of the latest adherents to this view is Harris who argues that the extraordinary powers of survival of the Conservative Party is explained by its constant readiness to accommodate the holders of power and this ability is now demonstrated by its allegiance to managerialism.

Does it make sense to speak of a managerial ideology and if it does, what does a managerial ideology mean?

There are at least two sides to the examination of these questions. The first concerns the 'facts' in so far as they can be observed in such an area. The emergence of a managerial ideology is believed to be related to a phenomenon in advanced capitalist countries concerning the separation of the ownership of industrial and commercial enterprises from their control. This is a familiar argument that, it seems fair to say, has won more and more adherents. It was advanced as long ago as the 1930s by Berle and Means, its more recent champions include Ralf Dahrendorf (1959), Andrew Shonfield (1965), and Kenneth Galbraith (1970).

The separation of ownership from control has led to consequences about which there is more debate. Dahrendorf (1959 : 44) takes one view concerning the consequential 'change in the basis of legitimacy of entrepreneurial authority. The old-style capitalist exercised authority because he owned the instruments of production. The exercise of authority was part and parcel of his property rights, as indeed property may always be regarded from one point of view as simply an institutionalised form of authority over others. By contrast to this legitimation by property, the authority of the manager resembles in many ways that of the heads of political institutions.' Conceding that the manager's right to command continues to derive, in part, from property rights delegated by shareholders, Dahrendorf (1959 : 45) argues that the manager now 'has to seek a second, and often more important, basis of legitimacy for his authority, namely some kind of consensus among those who are bound to obey his commands ... the manager, unlike "the full capitalist", can ill-afford to exercise his authority in direct and deliberate contravention to the wishes and interests of his subordinates.'

Nicholls (1969 : 141) takes another view. He concedes that the hired manager has gained in status and power but he holds that,

> '*de jure*, his function is still to serve the shareholder interest and, in practice, there is little reason to suppose that his outlook is much different from that of properties directors. Certainly we think it doubtful that he has developed a distinctive professional or techno-cratic normative orientation. The norms which govern his conduct derive in part from the shareholder interest and in normative, relational, and to some degree, economic terms, his position approximates to that of the propertied director. Managerialists have written of a "divorce" or "separation" of ownership and control. In this content we find it more fitting to write of a "marriage of convenience".'

Sutton *et al*. (1956 : 33) also distinguish between what they regard as two versions, classical and managerial, of the business creed. In the classical version the emphasis is on 'a decentralized, private competitive capitalism, in which the forces of supply and demand, operating through the price mechanism, regulate the economy in detail and in aggregate'. The enterprise is viewed 'as an exercise of the owners' right to dispose of their property as they see fit. It is expected, and it is deemed entirely proper, that the owners of business property will see fit to employ it to their own maximum profit'. The managerial version, on the other hand, emphasizes the importance of 'professional' managers, who have little or no stake in the ownership but considerable authority and power in the direction of the business enterprise. (Sutton *et al*. 1956 : 57).

To some extent this controversy is arid, at least within the context of our own immediate concern. Nicholls may contend that the managers' prime concern remains that of the shareholder but we are not greatly interested in the consequence of any difference of interest between managers and owners, important though this difference may be for the sociology of the enterprise or for the economic theory of the firm. Our chief concern is in any difference between the basis of legitimacy of managerial as opposed to purely business enterprise. In other words, our concern is in differences in the bases from which ideological appeals are launched.

Immediately, we seem to find a distinction between quite different arguments for different forms of legitimacy and the distinction adds considerable confusion. On the one hand, it is capitalism, private ownership, and business enterprise, that persist as a model. Galbraith

(1970) points to the continued power of the myth of American capitalism in the face of quite contrary facts. Shonfield speaks of continued references to free competition as 'the authentic expression of the nostalgia for the automatic checks and balances which used to keep management in its place' (1965 : 381). Sutton *et al.* (1956 : 254) say that the classical creed is 'an argument for the social virtues arising from the pursuit of individual self-interest'. Harris (1972 : 260) argues in terms of influence upon the Conservative Party 'the rhetoric of competition and free enterprise continues to this day, yet it is constantly contradicted by the party's practice in office'.

On the other hand, it is sometimes the newer managerial version that is presented as typical and that is claimed to be capable of capturing general allegiance. The two versions are quite different, they may even be, as Sutton says, mutually contradictory. Why is it that appeals for legitimacy are sometimes made to rest on the one, and sometimes on the other?

The most reasonable explanation is that the ideological ground shifts with a change in the direction of the attack. When the enemy of business takes the form of constraints which are to be imposed by the state then the legitimacy of the business enterprise is made to rest on classical foundations. In these circumstances we are reminded of the 'automatic checks and balances' which contribute to an ordering of affairs as they should be ordered; it is, once again, Adam Smith's invisible hand at work.

But attacks come from other quarters in the form of organized labour and there is the apparently intransigent refusal of workers to share with enthusiasm in the pursuit of managerial and business objectives. In the repulse of these attacks the foundation of legitimacy in ownership and self-interest is hardly sufficient, it may even be a burden to be quickly jettisoned. Capitalism, as Dahrendorf (1959 : 37) says, is an economic concept, 'the notion of a capitalist society is an extrapolation from economic to social relations; it assumes some formative power on the part of economic structures'. But capitalism is constrained by its own assumptions, its appeals can only be economic and they can be effectively directed only at those who are amenable to economic appeals, to those who will succeed or who can be deluded into believing in their own economic success.

In business enterprises that depend upon the co-operative effort, or at least, upon the avoidance of a withdrawal of effort, of many thousands of people, some effective appeal is necessary. Whether it can be found or not is another question but it seems likely that management is inescapably committed to the pursuit of co-operation or to overcoming what it perceives as alienation. This process of winning approval, or at least tolerance, of the employment relationship requires that the tasks to be performed should be accepted (with all the performance implications in terms of quantity, quality, cost, and time), that the relationship of subordination in work should be accepted and that, therefore, authority should be regarded as legitimate by those over whom it is exercised. Child (1969 : 227-31) makes the important distinction between legitimatery and the technical function of management. The legitimatery function, he says, is primarily directed at securing recognition and approval for managerial authority and the way in which it is used; it is concerned to achieve social approval and it is associated with claims advanced in management thought that it is based on socially acceptable values. In particular, Child continues, management is concerned, within its legitimatery function, to achieve approval for managerial authority by those over whom it is exercised.

Our point is that in this latter respect, the basis of legitimacy may have to be different and it may, in fact, require the dismantling of the previously established basis. It may require establishing the belief that the employer has vanished. The employment relationship, with all its implictions of authority and subordination, poses problems more particularly for managers than for owners. It is managers (once they have been appointed) who are expected to control labour and finding a legitimate basis for authority becomes more urgent for them than for the employer. For this reason the solutions to the problem are likely to be centred around the managers' authority, rather than that of the owners. In short, the specific form of the problem of legitimacy is one that lends itself to an emphasis on the role and importance of the manager. It coincides also with a separate recognition of the inadequacy of capitalist theory and self-help ideology as the basis for any kind of moral appeal or exhortation directed at the subordinate. The capitalist cannot break out of his own ideology so the manager, the real controller of labour, has to construct a new ideology.

It is possible that the whole concept of managerialism is a construction created to meet this need. From this point of view, managerialism may be not so much the result of objective changes in the nature of business control but rather that the notion of managerialism is developed to meet ideological requirements. While

Dahrendorf and Bendix have argued that human relations and consensus theories are symptoms of managerialism and of a changing basis for authority, it is also possible that managerialism is the outcome of the need to provide a more legitimate basis for authority in industry. Capitalism is incapable of providing an ideological framework so capitalism is reconstructed to meet ideological needs.

Some testimony (although it may be unwilling) for this view comes from Nicholls (1969 : 67). He points out that the belief in managerialism was given great credence by Labour Party apologists in 1945:

> 'for the Labour Party leadership, the belief that Britain had a management-controlled economy was confirmation that industry itself could be "managed" by government. And since the belief that managers are more manageable than capitalists has become evidence to the thinking of the Labour Party's leadership we may infer that their acceptance of the separation of the ownership and control thesis has served to complement and corroborate their wider politic-economic theories and policies. For them, the removal of the capitalist from capitalism has been a factor in legitimating policy.'

A belief in a 'managerial revolution', he adds, is also useful in dealing with left-wing critics of the Labour Party because it can be used to justify the view 'that public ownership was no longer a prerequisite to a socialist society and that the economy was manageable'.

An example of this view, advanced by a Labour Party apologist rather more recently than 1945 is provided by Moonman, one time lecturer in management and a labour Member of Parliament, in his book *The Manager and the Organization*. Addressing himself to his erstwhile trade-union colleagues about the need for the recognition of management principles in the trade unions, Moonman (1965 : 26) urged that a 'worthwhile start would be for executive committees of unions to rid themselves of the notion that the term "manager" should be regarded with the same emotional over-tones as the term "boss".'

Nicholls refers to the political convenience of such views in order to cast some doubt on the reliability of the case for a division between a management group and capitalists. We are arguing that the very convenience of managerialism is a powerful explanation of the emergence of a managerial ideology as distinct from the ideology of capitalism. It is not only for the Labour Party that managerialism has ideological advantages. While private ownership and the pursuit of profit and self-interest may furnish a basis in legitimacy for defence against the state and other institutions and while it may provide a purely legal defence of authority, it cannot provide the basis of compliance, rather than coercion, which integrated industrial processes must have. The process of providing for compliance is assisted by establishing the belief that the employer has gone. Whether the leopard has changed his spots or not, or whether he has been replaced by the lamb or not, it is believed to be an advantage to spread the belief that the change has taken place. In other words, whether the facts point to the replacement of an ownership structure by a management structure or not, the claim that the replacement has taken place has great ideological advantages. And it is not only for the Labour Party that these advantages are apparent; the managerial view is most particularly suited to the convenience of managers and seems much more conducive to the construction of an effective ideology of work.

One of the elements in the construction of a foundation for a new ideology of work was the development of scientific management in the United States by F.W. Taylor. Child has pointed out that it involved an approach to work that was essentially at odds with the indifference shown by *laissez-faire* to planning and control. It involved, he says (1969 : 38) 'a search for optimum principles of industrial operation and a conscious endeavour to inject a new philosophy of relationships in industry'. This philosophy was further developed by the psychologists' reactions — often critical — to scientific management. The search for a new basis of control of labour had become more urgent when the extremity of left-wing attacks on the traditional authority of the employer coincided with unprecedented levels of industrial disputes and the critical need for production in the first world war. Although the urgency of the crisis diminished with the post-war return of unemployment, the search for a new moral authority in work was not abandoned and it achieved a new importance in Britain with the general strike.

The idea of service was not new but it was given a new emphasis. Even the toughest of the new industrialists, Henry Ford, (1922 : 13) tempered (or disguised) his materialism with an emphasis on the importance of service: 'Money comes naturally as the result of service. And it is absolutely necessary to have money. But we do not want to forget that the end of money is not ease but the opportunity to perform some service.' Production for consumption implies the provision of service — if there is no service then there is no production, no business, no profit. In this sense, the idea of service is subsumed in capitalist theory in any form and it partly explains the constant coincidence in business apologists between the good and the profitable. 'There is a most intimate connection between decency and good business', as Ford put it (1922 : 100). Ford, however, extended the notion of service to a second level in which the business institution can be expected to take on wide community responsibilities, 'everyone who is connected with us, either as a manager, worker or purchaser — is the better for our existence. The institution that we have erected is performing a service' (1922 : 19). This meant, said Ford, that factories should be cross-sections of the community and should employ a due proportion of disabled people. Service and materialism continue to be inseparably linked for this policy is not to be carried out in a spirit of charity; to give one-armed men jobs out of good will would be both bad business and bad rehabilitation.

There is nothing new in such attitudes, of course. Robert Owen had expressed and practised them at New Lanark. They were at last ceasing to be eccentric or radical; they were coming to be recognized as good business. In Britain, Lord Melchett's emphasis on rationalization and the potential for happier employee relations offered by the big, benign, and profitable enterprise, began to make considerable headway, not least among the old labour critics. The old idea of paternalism, of a reciprocal relationship of rights and obligations binding owners and employees, was introduced again. Benevolence and responsibility were stressed as duties of the employer if he was to expect loyalty, obedience, and work. But paternalism, as we suggested earlier, meets or creates an almost inevitable challenge to its authority as it teaches its employees sturdy independence. It also faces, in large and complex industrial enterprises, a challenge from the managers whose role is to intervene in the employment relationship between the owner and the worker. The theoretical *coup de grace* of paternalism was probably delivered by Alan Fox (1961) in his demolition of the 'unitary frame of reference'.[14] It is worth observing that this assault achieved enormous support from managers and those institutions, the staff colleges, in which managers are taught togetherness. Managers were taught to apply and rely upon control techniques rather than paternalist appeals for loyalty to men other than themselves.

At the same time as techniques of management control were being developed, the belief that 'business as a trust or profession implied that the right to industrial authority was now being derived on the basis of effectiveness and capacity in the administrative function' (Child 1969 : 46). Saint-Simon's age of rule by industrials, experts in what is to be administered, seemed to be dawning at last. The title of the effective manager was to be grounded in his expertise, in his superior knowledge of the 'law of the situation'. Taylor claimed that scientific management 'substitutes joint obedience to fact and laws for obedience to personal authority. No such democracy has ever existed in industry before.' Ford said that 'the work and the work alone controls us' (1922 : 93).

The manager's posture towards labour was not simple and sometimes it involved attitudes that were contradictory. The very widespread influence of Elton Mayo's work and the apparent scientific respectability of the Hawthorn experiments had established a reaction to the belief in the techniques of scientific management as sufficient in themselves. The techniques and the 'management principles' with which they were associated were rarely questioned but a belief began to spread that they could be taken too far, that there were other influences. It was as though a romantic movement in management was beginning to follow the age of reason; reason was never entirely discredited but it began to be recognized that other forces, some of them dark and mysterious, had to be accounted for in exploring and influencing human behaviour.

Hawthorn emphasized the importance of non-rational feelings among workers (their importance among managers has taken longer to recognize), the strength of group pressures in influencing the behaviour of individuals and in subverting the directions of management, the importance of communication and supervision. The emphasis was taken to the point at which the worker seemed to be regarded as incapable of rational action so that it required an entirely therapeutic reaction from management in order to control him. Coser (1956 : 49) distinguished between realistic conflicts (which are means to an end, 'which arise from frustration of specific demands within the relationship and from estimates of gains of the participants') and non-realistic conflicts (which 'are not occasioned by the rival ends of the antagonists, but by the need for tension release of one of them'). Coser concluded that 'the studies in industrial sociology inspired by Elton Mayo show no recognition of the existence of realistic conflict or of its functions. Behaviour which is the outcome of a conflict situation is almost exclusively dealt with as non-realistic behaviour' (1956 : 52).

Human relations theorists and their disciples continued, for several decades, to stress that conflict was the result of a fault which could be corrected by improved management performance and understanding. In most cases communication was isolated as the cause of conflict and it was usually deemed sufficient to supplement improved communication by a recognition of the social system of groups which, in the 'informal system', ran through and under the formal organization of a factory. If the informal system of primary groups could be recognized and, better still, infiltrated by management's lower levels, e.g. the foremen, then all causes of conflict should disappear.

If conflict ceased, then those institutions, the unions, which existed to channel it in confrontations with management should have a lot less work to do. This attitude goes a long way to explain the often-noted silence of human relations theorists concerning trade unions and industrial relations. They could not have any significance in such a view. Their virtual removal from a position of importance also facilitated, and was required by, the new position to be adopted by management. Management was expected to achieve a representative role in relationship to its workers. This objective was rarely stated but it is certainly the ultimate conclusion of the injunction that the social system is to be invested by managers and their appointees. This is the supreme objective of management which, recognizing that its own position is defined by its dependence upon subordinates, must claim a totally effective control of its relationship with them.

The large-scale development of such claims is seen in microcosm in the complicated evolution of those specialists in management who were regarded as especially expert in attaining this control. The personnel managers had begun their existence as welfare workers. Paradoxically enough, they really did begin by seeing themselves as having a genuine welfare interest in their 'clients', the workers. At most they might acknowledge that they owed dual allegiance to management and workers, or that they were neutral as between the two sides. There is no doubt that they were, in the early days, motivated by goodwill and good intentions, strongly controlled by ethical considerations and genuinely concerned to improve the condition of the workers whose interest they believed they were appointed to serve.

Welfare workers, where they have survived, are now generally despised for these same characteristics by the personnel managers whose 'profession' (rigorously purged of any professional ethic) has now engulfed them. The concern with workers' interests manifested by the welfare workers was altogether too genuine to survive incorporation in a managerial movement which demanded control rather than improvement. Self-respecting personnel managers now identify themselves squarely with other managers in their devoted pursuit of efficiency, profit, and survival. Paradoxically, while personnel managers have excluded the genuinely professional elements found in their progenitors they have embarked on a ceaseless quest for their own 'professionalization', almost entirely in order to enhance their status in the eyes of other managers. In this sense, personnel managers have been in continuous retreat from the position of close proximity to real professionalism which they once occupied. The professional, it has been said 'adheres to a service ideal — devotion to the clients' interests more than personal or commercial profit should guide decisions when the two are in conflict' (Wilensky, quoted in Crichton 1968 : 260).

Who are the personnel managers' clients? Certainly not the workers. For many years personnel managers comforted themselves with a belief in the old happy coincidence, that by contributing to the happiness of employees they were also ensuring the success of the employer. In the Institution of Personnel Management's Jubilee Year statement in 1963, the objective of the personnel manager was given as to develop an organization that gives individuals satisfying work while enabling them to make the best contribution to the success of the whole enterprise. Such ambivalence has now been abandoned. In the most recent policy statement published by the Institute of Personnel Management (Barber, 1970), the personnel manager's role is defined as deriving from the fundamental problem of the enterprise, 'how the efforts of the people who make up the enterprise can be organised and developed in order to attain the highest levels of efficiency adaptability and productivity'. In a paper drawn up by the Institute of Personnel Management's National Committee for Organization and Manpower Planning, the Committee announced that effective planning would 'take into account the needs, aspirations and abilities of the people who are to develop and execute the plan. Since the personnel manager is the specialist in matching the human resources available to the work to be done and vice versa, he can contribute to the decisions which are translated into action' (IPM 1972).

This more single minded concern with the pursuit of the organizations' business goals will not preclude the personnel manager continuing to interest himself in the workers' well-being; he claims, after all, to have special expertise in the management of human resources and this is the area in which his own contribution to business efficiency can be made. The personnel specialist's cultivation of this area may require that he develops sympathetic understanding of workers' problems and a concern for their welfare, but he certainly no longer regards this concern as a major preoccupation.[15]

The personnel manager is one of the most vocal representatives of management's attempt to establish a new relationship with employees. The approach seems to have taken different forms in the USA and in Britain. Sutton, *et al.* (1956) certainly suggest that, into the 1960s, the American appeal for co-operation and legitimacy was based on traditional 'classical' capitalist lines. The appeal, as they describe it, is essentially that business works, produces the goods assures prospertiy, offers opportunity, and is associated with political democracy. Many writers have, like Mills and Galbraith, pointed out the appeal is largely mythical, but this is never a sufficient or effective ground from which to attack an ideology. The American appeal for worker co-operation is essentially based on ownership; the appeal is sufficiently powerful to maintain unparalleled levels of consumption and productivity, and it is sufficiently flexible to incorporate a vigorous 'business' trade unionism which acknowledges capitalist ideology to the extent of joining with businessmen in a ruthless struggle for higher wages.

British attempts at achieving worker co-operation are now rarely based on a capitalist ideological framework. For reasons that reside in political and social history, British workers are rarely subjected to an appeal concerning allegiance to the owners of business enterprise. The emphasis is rather on a managerial exhortation to work hard or consistently, often mixed with references to the need for a patriotic response to the current economic crisis.

A managerial appeal stresses features in the employment structures which have been judged to be acceptable or attractive. The first of these is the very contention that the owner is dead. In one form or another this underlies the announcement that it is old-fashioned to think of industry as composed of two sides because the old divisions of interest have vanished. One element in the disappearance concerns the end of ownership (a particularly appropriate and repetitive appeal in in the early years of the nationalized industries). Another element includes the assertion that managers are virtually indistinguishable from employees 'we are all workers now', to which the ideological counter is, presumably, 'we are all bosses now'. A third element in the managerial appeal is the emphasis on the common interests involved in any employment situation. The emphasis given to this particular approach will vary; in circumstances of industrial conflict or of a commercial crisis in the enterprise, it will be essentially negative and intended to induce fear, it will concern the consequences of closure and unemployment if co-operation is withheld. In other circumstances the appeal is more positive, the only way to higher wages is a more profitable industry, the only way to bigger slices is to bake bigger cakes.

An additional element in the managerial appeal is the emphasis which it often contains on management's expertise. Managers are, thus, not only freed of the prejudice against owners, but they have additional claims to legitimacy, they know what they are doing, they are, in some way, expert.

The general effect is of a benevolent, capable and well-intentioned management exercising authority in the best interests of all. Management claims the position of assessing and balancing claims for consideration (from shareholders, consumers, workers, suppliers) and, as the result of its objective and rational decisions, of being able to govern in the best interests of all. But the claim to authority by the enlightened manager does not succeed. In the first place, it meets the continuing challenge of organized labour, the trade unions claim to be the best representative of employees' interests and this claim has the unanswerable appeal of winning the apparent support of the workers. In the second place, where it is possible to take measurements of worker dissent from management's views (in, for example, strike statistics) the results show that conflict does not diminish and, in some respects, it tends to increase. Other indices of the extent to which workers are preapred to co-operate in the pursuit of managerial goals show no great improvement or, at least, there is not much evidence of managers becoming more satisfied with the result. Managers' speeches and writing continue to be filled with complaints of the withholding of energy and co-operation by employees.

Personnel managers, who could be expected to be most sensitive to the reactions of labour, have shown signs of changing their approach in seeking a more co-operative attitude. The deluge of appeals for unity, claims to rationality and fairness, and exhortations have given way to a more 'scientific' approach. The old naivety of the exhortative approach has given way to an attempt to influence the worker, to change him and certainly to change the job that he is required to do. In a sense we could almost conclude that there *has* been an end to ideology in the industrial context, in that there seems to be an acknowledgement of the futility of simple appeals for commitment, effort, and co-operation. This conclusion may be deceptively attractive, what is more likely is that managers now see the necessity of introducing changes in work and its organization in order to make appeals more likely to succeed. If we look at the brief analysis of the subjects of articles in *Personnel Management* it is noticeable that while a number are concerned with managerial responses to problems (in industrial relations, for example), a considerable number are concerned with introducing change in the environment of work: training (13), manpower planning and organizational change (9), management training, education and development (9), the application of social science, etc. (9).

The language in which some of these managerial pieces are written illustrates both this new concern and their complete unsuitability as ideological appeals to employees. Thus:

'Personnel officers should become more aware of the needs of the workers who form their manpower source. Knowledge of the predictability, the variety and the lack of fragmentation of sub tasks preferred by the majority of the labour force, should enable production systems to be designed which are more likely to satisfy the needs of the workers and lead to behaviour more in keeping with the company objectives.' (Dickinson 1971)

These two sentences incorporate many of the current concerns of management. They also express them in a style which illustrates an attempt to influence managers, not workers, by creating the belief that they are being asked to share in the application of scientific truths. The personnel manager has been frequently exhorted to acquire some scientific authority for himself, as a matter of urgency, so that he can make predictions about the behaviour of employees (a tacit admission that they will not listen to preaching) and in order to enhance his status and prestige among other managers who, it is said, have long ago acquired the legitimacy of experts:

'The recognition of the policy making role of the personnel manager depends upon the extent to which he can demonstrate that he possesses a degree of expertise in the systematic analysis of the social consequences of economic and technological decisions which other members of top management do not possess. When his colleagues turn to him for professional advice in the same way as they would turn to an accountant, an engineer, a market research man or an expert in operational research, and he is able to give such advice, he has become the new style personnel manager to whom I have been referring. I am arguing that only if he has a good working knowledge of the theories of the behavioural sciences and an ability to apply this knowledge to the analysis of the problems of organization, will he generate confidence in his ability as a professional'.
(Lupton 1964 : 57)

11. Integration by the Social Scientist

The science to which there is an allusion in so much of current management literature is no longer the science of F.W. Taylor, it is now social or behavioural science.

Bendix (1956 : 338) makes the simplest possible statement of management's concern: 'The management of large scale enterprises will be greatly facilitated if workers as well as managers regard their daily work as a token of their allegiance. Since non-co-operation in any form presents a problem to management, it is reasonable to expect a constant and perhaps an increasing concern with inducing a co-operative attitude among the employees.' Benevolence was not enough and human relations approaches have been largely discredited, because they are not well-founded in theory, have not always been rigorously applied, and have been subjected to very damaging criticisms.

The first of the behavioural scientists to be recruited to the assistance of management was the psychologist. The first task of the psychologist was to assist in the development of reliable methods of selection and to help to develop methods of learning which could be used in industrial training. But Bendix (1956 : 293) comments, 'Employers found that tests of performance or of aptitude were not enough; it was necessary to concern oneself with the factors that determined the industrial worker as a whole man rather than merely as a bundle of skills and aptitudes'. Most of the techniques described by Baritz (1965) in his vivid account of the recruitment of social sciences by management are psychological techniques concerning selection, training, personality assessment, and counselling. After the second world war they are accompanied by techniques directed at groups rather than individuals, sociometry, role playing, and group dynamics.

The psychologist was first concerned to measure, monitor or control the individual employee. Latterly, as part of a general attempt to facilitate the development of more co-operative employee attitudes (other than by simply appealing for them), the psychologist has begun to recommend changes in job structures and organization, so as to bring about the achievement of fuller co-operation. One of the most influential examples of this approach to work can be found in Argyris and we shall set out now with an account of the case he presents in a work significantly entitled *Integrating the Individual and the Organization* (1964).

The problem is clearly stated: 'Our problem is to understand the changes that the organization (and the individual) will have to make if it is to obtain the most possible energy for productive effort' (Argyris 1964 : 11).

Organizations were constructed in order to meet specific objectives, they 'have an initial or intended structure which is simply a static picture of the units as planned by the creators in order for people to achieve the objectives' (Argyris 1964 : 35). The assumptions underlying this structure are usually those of scientific management and they lead to behaviour that has consequences other than those intended by the organization's designers. This is because they 'create work situations having requirements counter to those for psychological success and self-esteem' (Argyris 1964 : 36).

A process of adaptation has to take place in which individual members begin to modify the structure of the organization. The individual worker finds himself in a work-world that is unsympathetic and he is almost required to make modifications to it. The main characteristics of this work-world are that work is highly specialized, on the assumption that the simpler it is the higher is productivity and the lower are costs; responsibility for planning, manning, scheduling, and evaluating performance rests entirely with management and not with the worker. The demands of work are reduced to the point where so few of the employee's abilities are used that he becomes dependent upon and submissive towards his superiors. This tendency is encourged by the pyramidal shape of the organization which is designed to concentrate information and influence at the top so that the worker enjoys less and less opportunity to exercise any control over his own activities.

These conditions, says Argyris, are not consonant with those necessary for psychological success and self-esteem. Psychological success is an important concept in the development of the argument and Argyris defines it as the mechanism for increasing self-esteem, which increases with opportunities for defining one's own goals when the goals are related to central needs or values, when the individual can define the path to these goals, and when the achievement of these goals represents a realistic level of aspiration for the individual. The argument, at this point, is perilously close to tautology because the approved value is built into the definition. Psychological success is defined to equal self-esteem. Self-esteem is defined to incorporate certain 'participative' work characteristics. Therefore, non-participative work conditions must produce psychological failure.

Argyris concludes this argument with three propositions. The first is that 'there is a lack of congruency between the needs of individuals aspiring for psychological success and the demands of the (initial) formal organisation' (Argyris 1964 : 40). The second is that the results of this disturbance are frustration, failure, and conflict. The third is that in certain conditions these characteristics will become more marked.

Employees are capable of making some limited defensive adjustments to incongruent conditions. 'One way to resolve these activities is to institutionalise some of them by developing a new organization that has equal power — a trade union for example' (Argyris 1964 : 59). There are alternatives which involve various forms of psychological withdrawal, symptoms which may include absence, turnover, restrictive working, and aggression against management. Workers may try to reduce the extent of their dependence upon management by joining trade unions 'which will not only represent their interest and back them up with appropriate weapons (for example, strikes), but will tend to ask for some voice in such practices as job rating, job changes, layoffs, discharges, and so on' (Argyris 1964 : 61).

Another form of defensive or adoptive reaction is to ask for more money, 'the greater the dissatisfaction, the greater the reward.' Argyris mentions a study which found that employees who did desire self-actualization were not highly motivated by increased cash. 'They preferred opportunities for challenge and satisfaction while at work' (1964 : 63). Hence an attractive aspect of this particular argument to managers is, no doubt, that the kind of policies advocated by Argyris will be cheaper.

Returning to the main objective, Argyris sums up, 'The problem of ineffectiveness is to increase the amount of psychological energy available for work' (1964 : 89). And the problem can be solved only by bringing about changes in organizations and, to some extent, in their inhabitants. Argyris refers to research by Likert, McGregor, Shepard, Bennis, Blake and Mouton, Burns and Stalker, Barnes and Litwak (almost a complete pantheon of management orientated 'behavioural scientists') which suggests important similarities. Likert (1961) for example, distinguishes between authoritative and participative systems. Authoritative systems are exploitative, benevolent, consultative and demonstrate unilaterial control. Participative systems demonstrate mutually shared control. Burns and Stalker (1961) distinguish between mechanistic and organic systems. McGregor (1960) distinguishes between his typical constructs represented by Theory X and Theory Y. Argyris concludes that all this research suggests that self-expression and self-actualization are best achieved in the organic systems.

He goes on bravely to face certain practical difficulties that the manager has to confront and which might be difficult to tackle in the kind of organization of which he approves. Termination of employment, for example, can be accommodated in a truly participative style. He paints a worrying picture of democracy in action as the tumbrils roll to popular applause. Termination 'could be initiated by an individual or groups assigned such responsibility ... Anyone who is to be terminated must have the opportunity to participate in all the discussions ... the line supervisor of the employee could raise the question about the employee's capacity to meet the standards he accepted upon entrance. The employee's own peers could also raise the same question ...' (Argyris 1964 : 210).

In respect of more pleasant relationships, Argyris is enthusiastic about the possibilities. 'The concept of directive authority or power will be expanded to include the influence of individuals through rewards and penalties that minimize dependence, through internal commitments and the process of confirmation.' The organizations will incorporate job enlargement and there will be considerable changes in policies and practices. 'Thus employees (at all levels) may meet in small groups to constantly diagnose organisational strengths and weaknesses' (Argyris 1964 : 274).

Argyris makes one of the most comprehensive and consistent statements of a view that is now shared by a wide range of psychologists and sociologists working in industry, by many consultants to industry, and by many managers. Managers are more usually introduced to this approach in the writings of people like Blake and Mouton (1964), or Herzberg (1968), who tell them what is to be done rather than engaging in theoretical discussion. Blake's grid is one of the most influential of these approaches.

Blake is concerned to change the individual in the organization, although some adjustment of the organization may also be necessary. The grid is a matrix in which manager's concern with achieving production is compared with their concern with people. Thus:

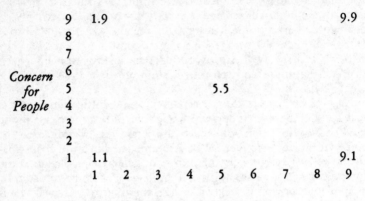

Concern for Production

To illustrate these correlations let us take five positions in the grid:

1.1 has a minimum of concern for both production and people.
1.9 has minimum concern for production, maximum concern for people.
9.1 has maximum concern for production, minimum for people.
9.9 has maximum concern for production and maximum concern for people.
5.5 has 'an intermediate amount of both kinds of concern'.

Each position classifies a particular managerial approach and Blake adds description to some of them. The description of the 9.1 position is filled with noxious characteristics; it is accompanied by reliance on formal authority, discipline and aggression, managers characterized by a 9.1 approach believe that people dislike work. What begins as a description of mixed characteristics in the grid ends as a description of almost pathological personality characteristics. The other positions are similarly described in terms of characteristics which belong to some quite different and unspecified method of analysis. The ideal position is the 9.9 square.

'Unlike the other basic approaches it is assumed in the 9.1 managerial style that there is no necessary and inherent conflict between organization purpose of requirements and the needs of a people. The 9.9 approach is oriented towards discovering the best and most effective solution in any given situation ... By utilizing both the mental *and* execution skills of people, this approach aims at the highest attainable level of production. This highest level is only possible through work situations that meet mature needs of people ... accomplishment and contribution are seen as the critical aspect of organization performance and individual motivation. When one is met the other is gratified.' (Blake and Mouton 1964 : 142-3)

Blake emphasizes the importance of 'genuine', 'sound', participation. 'Under 9.9, direction and control are achieved, first by working for understanding and of agreement by subordinates concerning organization purpose and how to contribute to it' (Blake and Mouton 1964 : 144). The approach requires 'a fundamental reorientation of management practices. Far greater attention is required through education, to the feelings and thoughts of people than has yet been considered except in a few experiments'. Blake goes on to explain the methods and purposes of 'education' and, incidentally, to assert the inadequacy of capitalist ideology in motivating employees. 'It can no longer be taken for granted, for example, that people accept profit as a legitimate organization purpose. Rather, it is inevitable that the concept of profit be "thought through" studied and understood in depth.' It is no accident that Blake puts 'thought through' in inverted commas because he goes on to make it clear that people who are to participate in this process are to have little opportunity of influencing management's understanding of its purpose or practice and that the 'educational' process to which they are to be subjected is to be more concerned with attitude and emotional adjustment than with intellectual comprehension. Having re-established the necessity of profit 'as an organizing concept, as a measuring tool and as a source of motivation' he goes on to say that 'ordinary methods of education are relatively worthless for aiding understanding of concepts such as these which are difficult to comprehend and shrouded with emotions. Other educational methods, themselves consistent with 9.9 are available and have successfully been used, however' (Blake and Mouton 1964 : 145).

At this point a footnote refers to five references on human relations and group dynamics training so we know what he means by education.

Perhaps sufficient has been quoted to suggest the effectiveness of Blake's style and its affinity to what seems to be his conception of education. One of the most noticeable characteristics of many of these writers on management is that their style is propagandist, designed to have an effect, to persuade. To be sure, in that the approach is supposed to be grounded in the behavioural sciences, there is often a great paraphernalia of proof, validation, and experiment. Blake, for example, has a whole chapter headed 'Career Accomplishment and Managerial Style' in which he sets out to prove his position. The assembly of pseudo-science includes the 'Managerial Achievement Quotient' (MAQ) which is a measure of individual performance. Blake presents the following example:

$$\text{MAQ} \quad = \quad \frac{5 \ (9\text{-L})}{\text{Age to 50-20}} \quad \text{x 100}$$

in which, 9-L is the actual managerial level subtracted from a constant, 9, which is based on 8 levels in a hierarchy. 5 is a 'constant progression factor' showing intervals of time in moving an individual from the bottom to the top in 40 years (Blake and Mouton 1964 : 229).

So, 'with an effective formula permitting comparison in achievement among managerial members' it is possible to investigate factors responsible for individual differences. The formula is effective because it has been validated; thus, 716 managers, after thirty hours at the Managerial Grid Seminar assessed each other's grid styles. Results were discussed and 'consensual rankings' were agreed. The most prominent managerial theory, or position, was 5.5, but the rank order for those in the highest MAQ group showed the 9.9 position to be more prominent, '9.9 becomes a progressively more prominent theory as MAQ increases'.

The reader might well have concluded by now that managers would be better (and more cheaply) employed studying the entrails of chickens and he might also have entertained the passing thought that we were all wasting our time on such ponderous nonsense. The truth is that it probably represents one of the strongest influences on current management thinking, it is solemnly (and uncritically) taught in many management centres and universities and it has influenced the policies and structure of companies such as BP and ICI. It would take a considerable programme of research to validate the hypothesis that all 'behavioural science' management teaching is rubbish, so we shall have to content ourselves with the unproved assertion that most of it seems to be so.

We cannot dispose of it so easily, however, because it is influential and because it has significant characteristics in terms of the new ideology of work. One of these is that, although it is now fashionable to approve of conflict in work and to reproach Elton Mayo and his colleagues for their naive view that it could be abolished, the behavioural scientist's view is still clouded with prejudice. Blake, for example, outlining the probable reactions to a 9.1 approach (that is, a preoccupation with production with small concern for people) said that they would include (1) low compliance, doing the minimum required, withdrawal; (2) joining unions to act against the organization; and (3) sabotage. So unionization, as it does in Argyris, comes to have some unsavoury associations. McGregor (1960 : 4) also puts industrial disputes in revealing company: 'Many of the important social problems of our time reflect the inadequacy [of prediction and control of human behaviour]; juvenile delinquency, crime, the high traffic fatality rate, management labour conflict, the cold war.'

Argyris (whose treatment is much more rational and intellectually respectable) paints a vivid and often accurate picture of the inhuman consequences of modern industrial employment. His approach, like that of McGregor, emphasizes the damage done to the individual by inadequacies of organization rather than those with which we have become more familiar and which derive from the nature of manual production tasks. The problem to which we are asked to turn our attention is, in fact, the subordinate manager rather than the assembly line worker. Argyris's approach is part of a shift in the focus of managerial concern, from workers to staff. This could be seen as a recognition of the truth of Marx's prediction that the staff functionaries of the capitalist would become proletarianized and that this area is becoming an important battle ground as the subordinate managers become both more hostile and more important to production. It could equally be a recognition that the workers are so recalcitrant, so steeped in 'strategies of independence' as Bendix puts it, or so reliably incorrigible as Orwell regarded them, that managerial attempts to achieve their commitment are finally, after several centuries of effort, to be abandoned.

Argyris almost admits to this conclusion. He admits that the pathological effects of incongruence between the individuals' needs and the organizational structure will not arise where 'the individual has decided not to aspire toward psychological success, *where it is a cultural norm not to be involved in work*' (Argyris 1964 : 41). [my emphasis] This seems to be a most important concession in that only those in a culture demanding involvement in work will suffer from *not* being involved in work. In other words, the worker may not suffer psychological deprivation as the result of his 'inhuman' work unless he shares his manager's view of its importance. One bitter conclusion is that managerial exhortation has, in the past, been directed at making the worker suffer while management refuses to change work so that it could become satisfying. The workers' 'strategies of independence' would, thus, seem to have considerable survival value for them.

Blake and other consultants are almost entirely occupied with an approach directed at managers rather than at manual employees. Blake admits that 'less direct change has taken place at this level' and reaches a 'general conclusion that bargainable people continue to need a strong union to act in their behalf. Another way of saying it is that the integration of people into the organization through more effective supervision has not as yet been as fully realized as it might have been' (Blake and Mouton 1964 : 300).

The outlook of the behavioural scientists who have been recruited to the assistance of managers thus frankly asserts that trade unions are countervailing organizations, that employee membership in them is evidence of managerial failure to adopt the right policies and to construct the right kind of organization. The consequential withdrawal of managerial concern with labour and the redirection of the ideological appeal towards its own ranks is beginning to find some expression in managerial personnel policies: 'the most important problem for personnel management today is the management of scientific, professional and technical, and managerial manpower' (Crichton 1968 : 284), 'the personnel manager is now also concerned with personnel management of managers' (Lupton 1964 : 56). This would not be invalidated by the considerable attention that is being currently given to the field of industrial relations management. The explanations for this activity lie jointly in changes in the law and in the increasing power of trade unions, neither these phenomena nor management's response to them is an indicator of management's wish to 'control' labour or to commit it to the employer. Indeed, one could argue that management's defensive attention to labour and industrial relations has increased as the optimism of its belief in winning labour's commitment has declined. The development of industrial relations management may well have been paralleled by the redirection of the more 'positive' aspects of personnel management to staff employees. An illustration of this concern with the application of the less defensive aspects of personnel management to staff in the USA is given in the following table: (Whisler and Harper 1962 : 429).

	Percentage of surveyed companies formally appraising performance of industrial employees	Percentage of surveyed companies formally appraising performance of managers and executives
1940	95.3	45.6
1947	80.8	43.7
1953	77.5	47.5
1957	77.0	58.0

It seems likely that the contrast is still more marked in Britain where union resistance to appraisal and merit-rating schemes has been fairly consistent. We could not maintain, however, that management has entirely abandoned any ideological approach designed to capture the commitment of manual workers to its own objectives. It may be necessary to distinguish two current managerial approaches which have replaced the older and less effective appeal based simply on capitalist, self-help premises.

The first of these, represented by Argyris, Blake and Mouton, Hertzberg, and others is aimed at emphasizing the psychological damage done by work in its usual form and demands that work should be changed so that the workers' potential for co-operative effort can be released; work must become the medium through which the individual seeks the satisfaction of basic needs. Argyris is, essentially, giving an updated and more scientifically based description of the causes and consequences of alienation (in one passage he actually discusses alienative effects although he makes no reference to any Marxist associations of the term).

What we arrive at as the result of this analysis, largely in psychological terms, is one of the most total statements of a managerial ideology yet advanced. It is designed not only to 'increase the amount of psychological energy available for work', to induce co-operative attitudes among workers; it also provides an ethical foundation for the legitimation of managerial authority in work, a foundation that has been lacking in capitalist formulations.

The ethic rests on the demonstration of the benign intentions of management in promoting the psychological health of the employee. The argument rests on the essential premise that work and its institutions form the only reality in our lives, a premise shared, as we have seen, by other observers with very different intentions for change. The premise entails that those who are in a controlling position in work are the only ones able to provide psychological well-being for their subordinates, the workers. Management thus comes to be presented as controlling the allocation, not only of material comfort, but of sanity. This is surely the strongest bid for legitimate control that has ever been made. Its strength is demonstrated by the peculiar difficulty that any critic has in distinguishing his criticisms from association with a wish to reduce the worker's well-being, or to promote his misery. The difficulty illustrates the illegitimacy of attacks upon a position which is so well established.

However, it is an approach to the achievement of commitment to work which is constrained by the context of the work itself. There is a tendency to direct attention to those jobs and at the occupants who are likely to respond most readily. Those workers who have been 'taught' that work is not important, as Blake puts it, are more likely to reject an approach so thoroughly grounded in its value. Those workers whose jobs can more easily be enlarged, enriched, or rotated are the more likely targets of appeal. Those workers who are the more ready to seek their own psychological capital in the achievement of their managers' objectives are more frequently incorporated in group therapy and 'educational' programmes of reform.

What about the great unwashed whose sins cannot be so easily ritually cleansed? It is here that it may be possible to distinguish a second branch in the contemporary ideological approach to the worker. The first approach concerns the individual and the content of his job, and to a lesser extent, the structure of the organization surrounding him. The second approach is more directly concerned with relationships of authority in the organization and with the mechanisms of control. The first approach is concerned largely with the psychology of the individual, the second with his relationship to the enterprise, it is frequently referred to as concerned to establish participation.

Baritz (1965 : 186) describes the enthusiasm with which this approach has been greeted:

'Making it possible for employees to participate in decisions affecting their behaviour was frequently said to be the final and democratic industrial answer to personnel problems. Here at last, argued several companies, was the way to humanize and democratize industry. Of course, management pointed out, employee participation increased productivity, reduced costs, reduced grievances and resistance to change and increased morale. But these were supposedly less meaningful than the sense of importance and belonging felt by participating employees. One company, a subsidiary of Bethlehem Steel, reported that employee participation in management decisions actually converted radical workers into ''sound'' management-oriented employees ... American Telephone and Telegraph said that its members accepted ''restrictions'' more willingly when they had a hand in formulating them.

Atlantic Refinery was more explicit. The advantage of participation, according to this Company, was that an individual tended to accept the decision of a group of which he was a member. Group pressures were so relentless that, regardless of personal convictions, conformity to a group decision was virtually guaranteed.'

Baritz (1964 : 209) concludes that industrial social scientists 'have put themselves on auction ... Time was when a man knew that his freedoms were being curtailed. Social scientists, however, are too sophisticated for that. The fires of pressure and control on a man are now kindled in his own thinking. Control need no longer be imposed. It can be encouraged to come from within.'

In his description of the production of these pressures, Baritz is primarily concerned with the work of the psychologist and social-psychologist in the service of business. Where he refers specifically to sociologists he suggests that they have behaved with greater discretion and detachment. But sociologists have not escaped criticism, some of it by sociologists. Coser pointed out that the first generation of American sociologists 'saw themselves as reformers and addressed themselves to an audience of reformers, (Coser 1956 : 16) but that, 'as university research oriented itself to the demands of outside agencies, the public of the sociologist tended to shift' (Coser

1956 : 19). Contemporary sociologists address either academic audiences or 'have attempted to find a hearing among decision-makers in public or private bureaucracies'. They have concerned themselves primarily with 'the maintenance of existing structures and the ways and means of ensuring their smooth functioning. They have focussed upon maladjustments and tensions which interfere with consensus' (Coser 1956 : 20). He explains that the sociologist's outlook has come about partly because of the rise of applied sociology; as they have turned to applied research so 'they have relinquished to a large extent the freedom to choose their own problems, substituting the problems of their clients for those which might have interested them on purely theoretical grounds'. The audience of the sociologist becomes, at the same time, his employer, so he is required to examine his employer's problems which are likely to concern 'the preservation of existing institutional arrangements' (Coser 1956 : 27).

Sociologists may have corrected the balance to some extent but the indictment has some justification: it is true that not all sociologists work for business management, but business management has certainly recruited some of them. And the recruitment of sociology has certainly complicated the outlook of managers; the ideological appeal of management is now more effective largely because it has advanced in subtlety and comprehension.

One change which illustrates this advance is the more complex attitude adopted by managers to conflict. Once committed to the view that conflict was damaging and should be avoided, that organizations were like football teams in which every member was trying to get the ball into the same net, managers have now been carefully taught by sociologists to recite that it is more realistic to see an organization as 'a pluralistic system or a coalition of interests'. Managers now understand, so they say, that conflict is legitimate and unavoidable and that their own role in relation to it is concerned with its dynamic management rather than with its removal.

Of course, this begs several questions. To begin with the sociologist (or a particularly influential school of sociologists, the functionalists and those concerned with systems theory) is often committed to a kind of institutional conservatism quite apart from the politics of his employer. The funcationalist tends to subsume all goals under that of the survival of the structure itself and those committed to a systems approach are concerned with its continuance. Once systems are defined they tend to be defended, there is some preoccupation with the *status quo*. As Child puts it, the tendency to see the business enterprise as a social organism 'is neither necessary nor particularly satisfactory. It presents the danger of reifying what is only an analytic construct — the "system". Similarly, there has been an equally unnecessary and misleading tendency for the systems frame of reference to be used to cloak a kind of latter-day structural determinism. That is, the functional requirements of the business enterprise as a system are presumed to be inviolate, and are assumed to be behavioural determinants to the exclusion of other influencing factors' (1969 : 182).

The argument over industrial conflict concerns different theoretical approaches to industrial conflict and the reaction against Mayo's consensus theory which has been heavily attacked by Sheppard (1954), Coser (1956), Dahrendorf (1959), and Fox (1966). Many of these critics have made the point that a consensus view is both unrealistic and damaging to the organization that adopts it and its relevance does not depend on the acceptance or rejection of a Marxist view of class-conflict and divided material interest. Industrial conflict, they assert, does not depend upon an unequal distribution of economic resources nor will the more equal distribution of resources end it. Industrial conflict is largely concerned with the distribution of authority and power. Dahrendorf, in particular, argues that interest groups are differentiated in terms of their relative positions on an authority-subordination continuum. Having disposed of a purely material source of conflict, this reaction to consensus and to human relations theory goes on to assert two basic propositions. The first is that conflict may be 'functional' and may contribute to the stability of the structure in which it takes place. The second is that it is possible to outline the steps necessary to institutionalize conflict so that it may act as a social dynamic or, at least, so that its affects are not too damaging to the structure.

Some of Coser's reformulations of Simnel's arguments, support the first of these propositions. 'Conflict serves to establish and maintain the identity and boundary lines of societies and groups' (1956 : 38), 'conflict is a mechanism through which adjustment to new conditions can be brought about' (1956 : 128). Coser also supports the second proposition; rigid, totalitarian systems redirect conflict and utilize safety valves but they cannot adjust to change; flexible systems allow occasion for conflict and are not likely to meet the danger of basic consensual breakdown. Parties in conflict have an interest in the organization of the enemy, they prefer the opponent to be organized as long as the parties have reached a rough equality of strength.

Dahrendorf is also concerned to maintain this, second, proposition. He examines various possible attitudes to conflict; conflict resolution, which he rejects because the elimination of conflict is neither desirable nor possible; conflict suppression, which he rejects because it may lead to violent consequences and breakdown; conflict regulation, which he accepts because it permits 'such forms of conflict control as address themselves to the expression of conflict rather than their causes' (Dahrendorf 1959 : 225). Regulation depends upon both parties recognizing the necessity and reality of the conflict situation — this is not possible where too great an emphasis is laid upon a common interest. Regulation also depends upon organization, 'organization presupposes the legitimacy of conflict groups and it thereby removes the permanent and uncalculable threat of guerilla warfare' (Dahrendorf 1959 : 225).

So far so good. Among the criticisms of Elton Mayo's outlook one of the most frequent has been that it represented a bosses' philosophy, that his concern with peace and stability was essentially in the employers' interest. The reaction against Elton Mayo seems to restore the balance, to establish the legitimacy of conflict. Conflict is restored and a variety of recommendations are made about the need to establish machinery for its expression. Fox's paper (1966) for the Donovan Commission has done a great deal, by the fluency of its language and the persuasiveness of its argument, to make this the received view in current management thinking and it represents a totally orthodox outlook in all well-founded Staff Colleges. It seems open to challenge only by those whom it has overthrown. The view is worth examination, however.

The first of the two general propositions contained the word 'functional'. Functionalism, is, of course, a system of concepts which embraces much more than attitudes to conflict but, in this context, conflict is said to be functional if it maintains the institutions in which it takes place and, in these circumstances, conflict is to be approved and recognized. Mayoists have been criticized because of their failure to see that to ignore or suppress conflict would inflict damage on the institution; organizational health, on the other hand, is promoted by coming to terms with conflict and even welcoming it as a social dynamic.

But would it not be relevant to ask some questions about the nature of the organization whose health and persistence in time of conflict is being recruited to serve? Emmett puts this question clearly (1966 : 28):

> 'The conclusion can be drawn that while terms like "stability", "harmony", "integration", even "social health" may sometimes be used descriptively to denote a state of society in which there is absnece of conflicts, or successful resolution of conflicts, they may also sometimes be "value laden" as implying that such a state is desirable. But is it always desirable? Should we approve of "integration" in a Nazi Germany, or "stability" in an apartheid South Africa?'

Kornhauser, Dubin, and Ross (1954 : 17) were also concerned to determine the 'functions of group conflict in a free society'. They asked, 'Is continued industrial conflict threatening to the interests of the larger society?' and come to the general conclusion that 'when conflict becomes institutionalised it becomes an integral part of the society's way of daily functioning'. This reply is, of course, tautologus, but it is also a reply to an unanswerable question. We cannot say whether a conflict is 'functional' or not without saying something concerning what it is about.

It may be possible to draw up lists of characteristics of conflict which are functional, to produce categories of the circumstances in which it may be functional, but none of this will help us to recognize a 'functional' conflict and to distinguish it from a dysfunctional conflict when we meet one. The difficulty lies partly in the unpredictable outcome of many situations and partly in the impossibility of off-loading questions of value from conflict issues. Judgements about the functionality of conflict are complicated by the object of conflict and by the relative position of the authority who is making the judgement about the particular conflict.

We could easily set up an exhaustive, logical categorization in terms of the functionality of conflict in a business enterprise and the wider social environment:

1. Conflict is functional for the enterprise   positive/
    Conflict is functional for the wider society   positive
2. Conflict is functional for the enterprise   positive/
    Conflict is dysfunctional for the wider society   negative
3. Conflict is dysfunctional for the enterprise   negative/
    Conflict is dysfunctional for the wider society   negative

4. Conflict is dysfunctional for the enterprise   negative/
    Conflict is functional for the wider society   positive

In only two out of these four possibilities would there be agreement about the functional value of conflict by judges representing the two different positions. The parties to a conflict situation within the enterprise, employers, and unions, let us say, have been left out of this elementary scheme, and they might well be expected to disagree about the functional value of a conflict in which they had engaged dependent upon the way the result had affected their futures. The judgement about whether any particular conflict is functional or not will depend upon the viewpoint of the judge.

There are at least three levels of interest concerned in judgements about conflicts. There is the level of judgement of one of the parties to a particular conflict, the union, for example. There is the level of the institution or environment within which the conflict has taken place, the company or the industry, for example. There is the level of the total society, the economic or the political system. One of the inescapable difficulties in judging the value of conflicts is the difficulty of identifying the level at which a judgement is made. Perhaps, just as logicians have constructed a hierarchy of meta-languages to avoid paradoxes of the type 'Parmenides, who is a liar, says all men are liars', so the sociologists should construct a hierarchy of interests before judgements about the functional value of conflicts become permissible.

Management is, of course, particularly prone to confusion in this matter. Managers are much given to speaking of managing conflict in the interests of the enterprise and they are often, in these circumstances, speaking as representatives of parties to a conflict situation. Any adverse comment they make upon the 'value' of their opponent's case is perfectly legitimate at this level; anyone whose purpose is opposed and who maintains his purpose can be expected to label the opposition's behaviour as damaging or dysfunctional. Confusion begins to arise when managers see themselves not only as parties to the conflict but as representatives of the environment within which it takes place. They have some justification for this view. In a real and a legal sense, they represent the shareholding ownership of joint stock undertakings, but they do not represent the consumers, whose interests the economist recognizes as reflected in a kind of market place conflict, they do not represent the employees, and they do not represent the community.

Of course, they will often claim to do so, indeed, they can be expected to do so because this sort of role trespass is a posture that parties to conflict find it useful to adopt; managers in an industrial dispute will often rally the wider community to their side.

There is considerable evidence to suggest that management is being advised to take part in a process of moral aggrandisement, in which it claims to be the arbiter of the value of conflict of which, because of its new realism, it approves. Dahrendorf's advocacy of conflict regulation and Fox's case for the acceptance of a pluralistic frame of reference, despite their enlightened realism, point in this direction. Conflict regulation is to be preferred because it reduces the risk of guerrilla warfare; industrial conflict in 'post-capitalist' societies has become less violent because its existence has been recognized and its manifestations have been socially regulated. Now this neatly illustrates that, in many respects, the only thing that distinguishes the new sociology from the old human relations is a greater degree of sophistication. While Elton Mayo naively advocated the removal of conflict the sociologists recommend its regulation in order to ensure that its effects are less damaging by controlling it within institutionalized channels. But control, regulation, and institutionalization might well be seen by one of the parties to conflict as effective methods of controlling his own power and could therefore be, as far as he was concerned, a powerful weapon in his opponent's armoury. Society and its institutions are warned of the dreadful dangers of guerilla warfare but guerilla warfare may be the only effective strategy for one of the combatants in a variety of situations. One interpretation of the sociologists' current attitude to conflict is that it is designed, by its very realism, to afford better protection to the institutions of employment. Perhaps one reason that the established institutions have survived is that they have had the benefit of sociologists' advice; reformist or revolutionary movements are most likely to be diverted from the pursuit of their objectives when the conflict in which they engage is institutionalized, recognized, and regulated.

There is some support for this view in the field of collective bargaining. The entire social purpose of disputes procedure is to 'take the dispute away from the shop floor' where feelings are most involved and pass it up to a level where those concerned have a professional interest in its settlement. This was the point made so clearly in *The Miners' Next Step* and the reason why workers were exhorted by its authors to have nothing to do with any conciliation machinery. In the history of industrial relations there are many events which suggest that an instant and militant reaction would have been appropriate and effective but that it was avoided by chanelling the conflict into institutionalized levels. A national miners' strike was prevented in 1918 by the appointment of the Sankey Commission. When the strike came in 1921, economic circumstances had changed and it failed. It is conceivable that, had the miners struck earlier and more successfully, the terrible disputes of 1921 and 1926 might not have occurred and necessary reforms in the coal industry might have been introduced earlier than 1946 — but this is to apply the very functionalist hindsight of which we have already disapproved.

Attempts to come to terms with industrial conflict by stressing the importance of regulating, controlling, or managing it are in fact part of the posture which one of the parties has adopted in order to reduce the effectiveness of his opponent. Enlightened managements are now constantly exhorted to manage conflict rather than run from it. The truth is that you can only manage a conflict by winning it; the victory is, of course, much easier to achieve if you can claim to be disinterested or even to represent the other side.

But what if the claim to represent the other side is in some sense genuine? Is the claim to have established a legitimate basis of managerial authority legitimate?

One way in which legitimacy is established is by claiming that managerial authority is founded in the subordinates' consent and agreement. This is precisely the same process that we observed developing in a communist or workers' state but we noticed that despite considerable advantages in the political framework upon which managerial authority was established, it failed. How then can Western business management succeed? The first essential is to bury the boss, to claim that capitalism has ended, because authority based upon ownership can hardly be shared with those who own nothing.[16] This is the great ideological usefulness of 'managerialism', quite apart from questions concerning its objective reality.

The second essential is to establish management's authority upon the consent of the subordinate by claiming the establishment, at last, of industrial democracy. The claim is advanced under various titles: democracy, participation, joint control, consultation, and it is now frequently advanced with enthusiasm by the Conservative Party, the Labour Party, the Church, managers and trade unionists. Where there is so much agreement there must surely be clarity and finality.

In fact, there are few areas of human affairs where there can be more ambiguity than in the field of industrial democracy. The case for it has been advanced in terms of political action directed against all capitalist parties and aimed at the establishment of a central production board which would 'issue its demands on the different departments of industry, leaving to the men themselves to determine under what conditions and how the work should be done. This would mean real democracy in real life ...' (1912 : 30). If that is industrial democracy it is most certainly not what is meant by Anglican Bishops, Harold Wilson, and the CBI. The version in the quotation represents syndicalism, of course. How is it that terms coined on the far left have come to be acceptable currency amongst managers and their associates?

The process of terminological exchange which took place between 1912 (the date of *The Miners' Next Step*) and 1944 (the date of publication of the TUC's Interim Report on Post War Reconstruction) is fascinating, but we cannot follow it here. Certainly the British Labour Party contributed to taking the venom out of the words 'industrial democracy' and, by establishing their neutrality, made them available for use by those against whom they were originally directed. Worker control has evolved or degenerated into worker participation.[17] The current preoccupation was formulated as long ago as 1952, 'There has not yet been any broad and effective attack on the problem of how to create a true sense of participation in a common purpose while preserving proper scope for the exercise of leadership and authority' (NIIP 1952 : 8).

This quotation illustrates the problem exactly; how to achieve participation without damaging managerial rights[18], how does the manager share control with others without reducing the degree of control he retains himself? Has management succeeded in solving the old problem of defending its own authority by abdicating it? Or is it in the position of Shaw's King Magnus who promises to abdicate and then threatens to stand for Parliament?

One of the most subtle explanations of the process of shared control is advanced by Tannenbaum. He argues that it is a mistake to regard the amount of control that is available to an organization as a fixed sum to be differentially distributed between its members, so that the more that goes to management, the less is available for subordinates. On the contrary, he says, the total amount of control can be increased so that 'the total amount of power in a social system may grow and leaders and followers may therefore enhance their power jointly' (1968 : 12).

The prospects of more of anything for everyone is always appealing but one of the problems which might limit the pleasure of the subordinate is that he may not decide the extent of any increase in his power to exercise control, it may not even be decided jointly, it is, apparently, to be decided by managers. Their decision is influenced by the extent to which superordinates judge that their own control will be increased by increasing the amount of control available to subordinates. In other words, management controls the distribution of control.

The notion advanced by Tannenbaum of a quantity of 'total control' which can be increased by giving more both to subordinates and superordinates is, not, in itself, very convincing. One important questions which it avoids concerns the *relative* distribution of this new and increased total sum of control. There is after all, no one in any organization who is totally devoid of influence but any increase in that influence is not necessarily significant because what determines the subordinate's position as a subordinate is the relative distribution of control. We may, for example, give the typist more control by allowing her to choose her typewriter, office carpet, and the time of commencement of her lunch-hour, but none of this would enhance her position greatly, particularly if we require her to work twice as hard for half the money. When Tannenbaum illustrates his argument by a hypothetical control graph it is significant that the curve illustrating increased total control shifts to the right, it does not change its shape.

It seems certain that the intention in enlarging the amount of total control and the amount of control available to subordinates is to increase their commitment to the organization, as indeed our typist might become more committed by being allowed more influence, particularly if she was stupid. Tannenbaum says that the more traditional management methods, in which control was restricted to management, represent the phenomenon of partial inclusion and he comments on them that:

'There are limitations to the range of activities that are subject to influence, excluded from influence is that large segment of the person that does not belong to the organization ... Anything that enhances members' personal commitment to or identification with the organization is implicitly including them more fully within the organization, and hence is increasing the possibility of an expanded

total amount of control. Human relations approaches that are designed to increase the identification of members may therefore result in
greater inclusion and greater control.' (Tannenbaum 1968 : 16)

Tannenbaum thus seeks to establish that there is no contradiction
between increased control for subordinates and for their managers;
both can be increased without detriment to either so that the result is
an increase in the total quantity. The argument seems to rest, yet
again, on the assumption of an identity of interest between the two
and upon a unitary frame of reference. Presumably, in circumstances
where interests are not shared, an increase of control for the one is
likely to result in a decrease for the other.

Tannenbaum's argument barely conceals the fact that the increase
in total control is brought about as the result of management's
effective control becoming more absolute. He gives the game away in
the passage we have just quoted where 'anything that enhances the
members' commitment to the organization includes them more fully
within it'. In other words, the attempt to 'share' control is designed
simply to secure a greater degree of commitment to the organization's
goals. The attempt to achieve the greater commitment of subordinates
must, of course, be a thoroughly respectable goal from the
management position. The need for management to legitimize its
objectives and its authority is probably a need which it is incapable of
resisting; any process that gives its commands moral authority is
bound to be pursued.

Moral authority has several advantages. The search for it is made
partly in an attempt to shift the organization towards a basis in the
normative compliance of subordinates. If it can be achieved,
management believes that it can pre-empt opposition, which may
otherwise be expensive to overcome and which can be self-
perpetuating and hostile. Moral authority means greater efficiency.

Moral authority is also attractive to management because it is
important in terms of the motivation and control of managers
themselves. Managerial effectiveness requires a degree of zeal and
enthusiasm which may be beyond what can be established by the
application of remunerative power. Etzioni (1961), arguing his case for
the existence of three essential bases of compliance in organizations,
pointed out that managerial sub-systems of organizations, themselves
resemble normative organization which, like hospitals or university,
are more entirely based on moral compliance. Managers, in other

words, have to believe in what they are doing and this requirement encourages them to search for legitimization.

Thus they attempt to extend this moral basis for compliance to other subordinates because of an understandable (if erroneous) belief that what is appropriate motivation for themselves is appropriate for others. There may be some real justification for this extension. Etzioni explains that mixed compliance systems suffer from dissonance or, dual compliance structures 'result in some waste of power resources through neutralization, and some loss of involvement because of the ambivalence of lower participants exposed to conflicting expectations ... Such ambivalence is generated, for example, when lower participants are expected to be calculatively and morally committed at the same time' (Etzioni 1961 : 55). But, he says, 'organizations tend to move towards congruent types of compliance structure because they are under pressure to be effective and congruence is more effective' (Etzioni 1961 : 12).

A simpler way of putting it is that management will seek to establish its own goals for general pursuit. It does this by adopting a unitary framework, a stance respectfully abandoned by sophisticated managers since it was so heavily criticized by Fox (1966). Whether they will rush back to it now that Fox has recanted remains to be seen. In *Beyond Contract* (1974), Fox argues that the prevalence of economic exchange and the spread of the division of labour have combined to destroy trust relationships and to promote low-trust work in which each side develops a 'suspicious vigilance' towards each other. Unitary notions may have served an integrative function, but in more respectful times than ours. Pluralism is, he says, a more sophisticated attempt to bring about integration but it has suffered damaging radical attacks because it rests on an illusion of equality of power and because it serves to promote efficient management. Unions and collective bargaining are of no use in challenging the power of employers because unions are composed of 'men who have already been socialised, indoctrinated and trained by a multiplicity of influences to accept and legitimize most aspects of the work situation' (Fox 1974 : 284). Fox is distressed at the consequences of low-trust relationships in the organization of work as they result in 'suspicion, jealousy ... inhibitions to co-operation' (1974 : 317). If society remains in this mould 'the consequence might well be to make the existing type of industrial organization unworkable' (1974 : 334).

To avoid disaster, low-trust subordinates must somehow develop high-trust attitudes which allow them to legitimize and endorse their place in the total structure. How can it be done? Fox dismisses the usual paraphernalia of job-enrichment and 'socio-technical manipulation' as irrelevant. The abandonment of the division of labour in favour of handcrafts and local markets is impractical. The only hope, it seems, is in accepting the fact of divided low-discretion, low-trust jobs and in getting the occupants to accept them by a 'matching shift in institutions and ideology which would mitigate the operation of the low-trust dynamic without sacrificing the production methods to which individual and social expectations are increasingly and universally geared' (1974 : 357). There must be greater equality, 'a radical reconstruction which seeks to rally major sections of society behind shared purposes of social justice' (1974 : 358).

The debate following Fox's recantation of his earlier view will continue for some time.[19] It is not clear what form his radical and egalitarian society would take. There are grounds for believing that the changes he would applaud would not be very considerable and that their extent would be determined by what was necessary to make subordinates in divided jobs believe that it was right for them to do what they are told. Fox recommends changes in order to meet the threat of social disturbance which alarms him. Fox has in fact retreated from one untenable position to another in an effort to fend off the disorderly conduct of the proletariat. In 1966 he said the unitary framework must be abandoned because it is no longer appropriate. In 1974 he said the pluralist framework must be abandoned because it no longer work. The purpose remains the same, to promote a degree of social order, it is the methods of achieving it that change. Fox looks with some approval at the Soviet Union where, according to Soviet sociologists, 'the special condition of their society enable those doing even the humblest work to take what is described as a high-trust perspective of the productive system and their own place in it' (Fox 1974 : 90). Fox apparently sees this as an admirable state of affairs.

He acknowledges that success in our own society might be more limited for those with highly divided jobs, but if it could exercise some 'restraint in asserting claims for increased money income and the acceptance of some degree of labour and income planning they would mitigate ... the chronic expression of low trust ... namely inflation' (1974 : 358). He has also acknowledged that nothing can be done about divided work. What we are to prevent, by the appearance of radicalism, is either change in jobs or the demand that dull work should be well paid. The change requires, he says, a coherent radical ideology in order to rally major sections of society behind shared purposes of social justice. But there is nothing radical or coherent about a programme that would keep people in their place while convincing them that it has changed or that it is proper.

Fox has certainly abandoned the advice he once gave to managers, that any partial change in their own authority is likely to be effective. Fox has abandoned the managers to save themselves as best they can while attention turns to wider social issues and adjustment. Management continues to try to establish its own goals for general pursuit. One way is to parallel the approach which Fox recommends for society in the firm. Managers aim to establish the belief that power has been redistributed in order to legitimate their own position. Managers advocate participation.

'Participation' as the term is used by managers is very different from what it means to workers or syndicalists. We could suggest that workers participate in the control of their establishments to the extent that they or their representatives influence management's decisions concerning the enterprise. But this is not always what managers mean when they talk of encouraging worker participation, in fact, they may mean quite the opposite, that 'participation' enables managers to influence the workers more readily to comply with managers' decisions (which have often already been taken).

The distinction between the two uses has been clearly identified by French (in Kahn and Boulding 1964 : 38):

'"Psychological participation" is the extent of influence on a jointly made decision which the participant *thinks* he had. "Objective participation" is the amount of influence on the decision which he *actually* has.' Objective participation implies that the decisions that management takes are different from those that would have been taken had workers not participated in the process. Objective worker participation is likely to impose a set of new constraints on management decision-making and, in many circumstances, management will seek to avoid these constraints. Management, will, on the other hand, seek to create a sense of participation, in order to achieve the commitment of the worker to the organization's goals. Management will, therefore, tend to reduce objective participation to a minimum while seeking to maximize psychological participation. Management will tend to resist attempts to achieve 'participation' when they are launched by employers while itself offering opportunities for greater 'participation' to the employees. One means of achieving this apparent contradiction is by defining the level at which participation takes place. Our typist can decide about her carpet, not about the intensity of effort she is required to expend. Ends are determined by management, the determination of means may be shared with employees.

Managers will also come to regard alienative involvement (associated with coercion) and calculative involvement (associated with a remunerative basis of compliance) both as implying a degree of inevitable resistance and, therefore, of inefficiency and cost. They will tend to attempt to extend their own, much more efficient, moral involvement in the organization.

Management literature is heavy with recommendations for this process to be set in motion. Thus, Likert (1961 : 98) argues that the highest producing managers show

> 'a preponderance of favourable attitudes on the part of each member of the organisation toward all other members, towards superiors, toward the work, toward the organisation — toward all aspects of the job. These favourable attitudes toward others reflect a high level of mutual confidence and trust throughout the organisation. The favourable attitudes toward the organisation and the work are not those of easy complacency, but are the attitudes of identification with the organisation and its objectives and a high sense of involvement in achieving them.'

McGregor (1960 : 49), put the matter in much the same way: 'The central principle which derives from Theory Y, is that of integration: the creation of conditions such that the members of the organisation can achieve their own goals best by directing their efforts towards the success of the enterprise'.

The 'central principle' of a great deal of the social scientist's contribution concerns 'integration' and the subordination of the individual's goals to those of the organization that employs him. We have briefly examined some of the approaches which are designed to bring integration about. They all seem concerned to achieve greater efficiency by promoting the development of organizations that are more humane and less irksome to their inhabitants, by sharing control, by allowing for greater participation, by recognizing the reality of conflict, by acknowledging the needs of employees for responsibility and growth. Both the end, of greater efficiency, and the means, of greater involvement, seem thoroughly benign and deserving of approval. What, then, explains the faint but discernible odour of stinking fish?

Let us say first that the intentions of management and of their social scientist spokesman are open to criticisms from those committed to an ideological attack either on capitalist or on industrial society. From this point of view, the paraphernalia of enhanced control is designed to advance objectives which are not valued by the critics, be they communist or anarchist. Is there anything more to say concerning the intentions and objectives of managements' use of social science techniques? Leaving aside questions of whether these techniques do or do not lead to increased efficiency (and the fact that there is, in some instances, room for considerable debate is increasingly acknowledged by social scientists), how much doubt can there be about the additional claim, that these approaches improve life at work.[20]

The doubts that remain are of three kinds. First, the way in which many of the arguments are developed give rise to the clear impression that human happiness is not the purpose of the changes which are being proposed, but that human happiness will follow from 'directing their efforts toward the success of the organization'. Human work and its reorganization is still being regarded as instrumental to the achievement of other objectives and, while it is perfectly possible to achieve two quite different goals at the same time, it is sufficiently rare to justify one's suspicions about the authenticity of the claim if for no other reason than that the process for achieving them flies in the face of Kant's axiom that people should be treated as ends and not means.

The second reason for suspicion is that unlike more traditional and perfectly respectable programmes for enhancing efficiency and profits (including the 'heartless' advocacy of some pioneers of scientific management) the programme currently under review seems to be deceptive. While efficiency or profit seems to be the aim one has to reach this conclusion by a process of inference from arguments conducted on quite different grounds. This sense of deceptiveness pervades not only the goals to be achieved but the methods that are to be employed to reach them. It involves, in extreme cases, the almost total destruction of meaningful language so that terms of an apparent scientific objectivity are used only for propagandist purposes. It involves the process of terminological exchange (for example; industrial democracy = participation, dismissal = severance,) on a level and at a degree of skill previously seen only in political confrontations. It involves the process of capturing the enormous power of social groups and tethering them to the organization's norms and attitudes so that their power of enforcement over their members' action becomes almost absolute and unchallengeable. It involves the individual's definition of sanity being supplied by his employing organization in a way that closely relates to his 'positive' attitude to his work. It involves defining the rejection of these humane, warm, and loving approaches as deviant, criminal, or lunatic. It involves, finally, the demolition of authority in the name of democracy because the organizations that promote its demolition recognize that authority cannot be resisted unless it is first identified.

None of this would be so entirely regrettable if it were not for the third area of doubt. The human engineering which is advocated by the new science of management is aimed at achieving large scale changes in society in order to facilitate business objectives. It is, in this sense, irresponsible. It contributes to placing or maintaining work at the centre of social life in that its primacy is a justification for the widespread changes in social organization which it proposes to make. The primacy of work is, in this way, exaggerated by managers who have, perhaps a genuine and special preoccupation with its problems. Then, having enlarged its importance in order to justify reforming our lives, we are forced to take the advice of those who are neither expert nor responsible in order to bring about these reforms. Managers, at least in the social science literature which is written for them, are encouraged to treat society by reference to managerial concepts which may be quite inadequate for promoting social changes which the application of those very concepts demand. Management's most recent position, or the one which it has been encouraged to occupy by those social scientists who write for it, is one that is beyond its resources of training and ability and for which it has no representative authority.

12. Management Ideology

What we have called the recruitment of social science in the service of management concerned first the utilization of the psychologist's techniques and expertise. The application of psychology extended from an initial concern to improve methods of selection and training to a much more general concern with the individual's motivation in which, finally, the business organization and the tasks which it requires to be performed are both changed in order to make work become the satisfier of fundamental human needs. Work becomes a much more valued and valuable activity, we are the more likely to regard it as a central life interest, to take its performance requirements seriously, and to become deeply involved in its distribution of rewards when these rewards include our own psychological health.

But, powerful though this new appeal of work is meant to be, it is not yet omnipotent. The individual worker is not the sole determinant of his own behaviour, even when his environment has been controlled in order to encourage his individual decisions to be those of which the organization which controls his environment would approve, there still remains the uncontrolled influence of groups and the informal social structure of the work place. The next extension of control is therefore to exert some influence over the social system. The end result is to be able to propose to the worker that the social system is his in that it, like his work, has been constructed in order to take account of his wishes and his needs so that its objectives become his own. The end result is achieved when the application of authority and power is no longer necessary to assist in the achievement of the organization's goals because the goals have been internalized by those who are to pursue them. While the goals are left untouched (indeed there are instances in management literature when the goals, in terms of production, have been increased) the apparatus of bureaucratic authority is concealed or dismantled. As McGregor (1960 : 31) put it: 'There is nothing inherently wrong or bad about giving an order or making a unilateral decision. There are many circumstances however, when the exercise of authority fails to achieve the desired results. Under such circumstances, the solution does not lie in exerting more authority or less authority; *it lies in using other means of influence'* (McGregors emphasis).

The apparatus can be dismantled because its use is unnecessary or a nuisance, because 'other means' are a more effective substitute for authority in achieving goals about which there is often no real debate. The manager has come to rely more and more heavily on the psychologist and the sociologist for the determination of other means which are appropriate to his own particular situation. The manager's life has become much more complicated as the result of this dependence because he is constantly being told about the unreliability of the old saws, clichés, and principles by which he used to direct his affairs. This new complexity does not necessarily challenge the legitimacy of managerial authority, rather it seeks to point out its limits 'and even to improve its effectiveness by analysing the barriers to managerial control' (Child 1969 : 205).

However, it is not our business to discuss the theory and practice of management except in so far as it influences an ideology of work. In this respect we see a strange departure from the ideological evolution which we have been observing. While, at every previous stage, we have seen improvements in the appeal to work associated with attempts to make the appeal more legitimate, now that legitimacy appears to be more firmly established than ever, the appeals to work seem to diminish in frequency and force. Such appeals as are now directed by managers at workers are much more likely to require their continued presence at work rather than the expenditure of greater effort and enthusiasm while there. Appeals are now normally concerned with the avoidance of disputes or absence.

Is this the end of ideology? In a limited sense, it is. The whole approach which we have been outlining under the heading of the recruitment of the social scientist is essentially to make any managerial exhortation for effort unnecessary and redundant. To continue to appeal *to* the workers *by* managers would indeed be a contradiction of the new understanding that management is now seeking to bring about; the continuation of a process of exhortation would be a confession that the process of social and psychological integration had failed.

The major necessity now is not that workers should be appealed to for greater effort but that their managers should be appealed to to bring about the conditions which will encourage it — to some extent, from workers but, more so, from managers themselves. The ideological onslaught is now almost entirely directed at managers and it is no longer composed of a naive, Smilesian appeal for hard work.

The ideology of work is now essentially a managerial syndrome. It contains several strands, the first of which, concerned with the construction of an environment which the worker will find, in every sense, rewarding, we have examined at some length. A second strand consists of a more direct appeal for managerial effort and hard work. This strand is supported by a whole mass of techniques designed to measure, monitor, control, and reward managers' performance. Despite its apparent technical complexity, this is the element in the managerial appeal which is the most simple and most directly related to the evolution emerging from the protestant ethic to Smiles and beyond; it concerns the motivation of the manager. A third strand consists of the continued search for a legitimate foundation upon which appeals and authority can be based.

This third element takes us very close to a discussion of the whole controversy concerning managerialism. In the sense that this involves a debate about whether or not managers are established as an elite, a group or a class, which has ultra-national similarities, is concerned to advance its own power and influence and to control access to membership and the behaviour of its personnel, in this, macro sense, we can avoid it. But in the more limited sense that we have concluded that it is now managers and managers alone who are concerned with the direction of appeals concerning the commitment to work and are therefore involved in legitimating their own authority in work, in this sense, we are concerned with an aspect of managerialism.

This particular aspect of managerialism has two important characteristics which distinguish it from previous attempts at establishing the legitimacy of authority in industry. The first is the sheer scale of the ideological effort. Previous ideological appeals were often implicit in entrepreneurs' speeches and writings, occasionally they were given explicit and coherent form in the writings of specialist apologists or propagandists like Robert Owen, Andrew Ure, or Samuel Smiles. Currently, ideology plays a very considerable part in the curricula of management courses at universities, polytechnics, technical colleges and industrial staff colleges.

The ideological element is not always instantly recognizable for what it is. We would not identify it as ideology as readily, for example, as we would that part of Chinese educational curricula which are devoted to Marxist-Leninist theory and the contributions of Chairman

Mao. One reason for our difficulty is that much of the ideological element in management education appears to be concerned with objective, scientific, research-based conceptualization of practical managerial problem-solving. Thus Child (1969 : 250), referring to a survey of management teachers which he carried out in 1964, concluded that 'at the time considerable emphasis was given in courses to discussions about increasing the discretionary content of work and employees participation within organizational affairs. This strongly supports the view that neo-human relations has become the new "orthodoxy" in management education.' The continued popularity of courses with titles such as 'A day with Herzberg' suggests that little has happened subsequently to require an amendment of this judgement. The content of these courses has, of course, become more sophisticated in that they are now likely to take account of 'plural frames of reference' and the recognition of the 'reality of conflict' but we have suggested, if not established, that the intention behind these more complex contributions remains the same.

The intention, quite apart from the disguise of scientific language, is twofold: to provide a basis for the control of subordinates by facilitating their integration in work, and to reinforce the integration of managers. A great deal of management education, that part of it concerned with behavioural science, is in fact theocratic, it is designed to establish a sense of unity of purpose and of values largely by providing managers with a common language and a system of concepts. Management education is truly ideological in this sense, that it aims to influence behaviour by inculcating beliefs and expectations. Dissemination of an ideology by way of management training has these two latent functions: it helps to promote the internal solidarity of management and it helps to justify its authority over subordinates. The manufacture and spread of an ideology also gives a more spiritual or cultural appearance — particularly when it emanates from universities — to what would otherwise be a purely money-grubbing and materialist pursuit. This confers a welcome dignity and it helps, as we have noted, to shift the basis of control over managers from a remunerative to a normative base.

An ideological explanation of this element in managerial education also explains the astonishing absence of controversy. Perhaps we have quoted at sufficient length from some of the influential sources in this area to illustrate that much of them are based on uncertain theory applied by questionable logic to unrelated circumstances. Much of the

behavioural sciences do not fulfil the most elementary tests of the
validity of scientific method. This is not an idle accusation. It has been
argued by a number of authoritative analysts of scientific method that
scientific propositions are advanced as the result of a hypothetical-
deductive method in which the resultant theories, although they can
never be proved, continue to stand while the scientist rigorously looks
for evidence to *overthrow* them. The scientist's theories stand for as
long as he fails to upset them. This is the opposite of the way in which
most behavioural scientists go about their work; they advance theories
which they have 'proved' as the result of a singularly hasty search for
evidence that will *support* them.

If there are methodological problems concerning the validity of
behavioural science theory these problems are multiplied by the time
unrealiable theories have been vulgarized by consultants and then
simplified by teachers in order to transmit them to managers, whose
knowledge of basic behavioural science theory may be nil. Perhaps we
can understand why there is no controversy. It would be hard to find
another field of educational activity in which intelligent, and
sometimes educated minds, were so harmoniously disposed. There
may be occasional disagreement about educational methods, never
about doctrine.

On the very rare occasions when a manager, or come to that one of
his teachers, meets someone carrying another set of doctrines based
uon different values, he reacts with bewilderment.

Let me illustrate with two examples, perhaps in this context we
should really call them 'case studies'.

The first example comes from a staff college where industrial
relations specialists had prepared a project report on productivity
bargaining. In the general atmosphere of complete consensus with
which the report was presented, I ventured, as visiting adjudicator, to
say that there was a very different view concerning productivity
bargaining, that Cliff (1970 : 11) had described productivity
bargaining as 'part of a determined offensive by the employing class'
which is 'aimed at finding a *permanent* solution to employers'
problems' and that this view was not without support from workers.
The result was laughter. It seemed that these specialists in labour
relations were so insulated from a view that would be either familiar or
acceptable to their trade union opposite numbers that they thought it
was a joke.

The second example goes some way to explain the sense of cloistered privacy in which those discussions are often conducted. Fox (1971 : 172), in discussing 'New Modes of Joint Regulation' explains that 'only by fully recognizing and accepting the constraints imposed by the aspirations of its subordinates, and working through these constraints towards a new synthesis, can management now enjoy any creative role in its handling of the social organization' and that this recognition was embodied in the growing number of managements who had engaged in productivity bargaining. This new form of bargaining enabled both management and 'employee collectivities' 'to achieve a major reconstruction of the normative system which leaves all the parties conscious of having improved their position' (Fox 1971 : 174). Productivity bargaining offers 'something to the aspirations of all the parties involved. It represents a joint struggle to accommodate conflicting demands to the survival or growth needs of the coalition.' And how does this particular sociologist respond to a counter-view of productivity bargaining, from a party who is *not* conscious of having improved his position? He refuses to discuss any attack upon productivity bargaining (the underlying assumptions of which he so obviously approves) by simply identifying the ideological source of the opposition. Thus: 'Finally, one would predict that the new modes of regulation involving as they do a closer collaborative pattern of relationships would be condemned by those whose anti-management stance is ideological and total. The perspectives and behaviours required for integrative bargaining are incompatible with the class war' (Fox 1971 : 175).

Fox's response suggests an approach that is itself basically ideological. This is illustrated first because, having gone further than most in acknowledging a counter-view, he cannot apparently discuss it but can only discount it by reference to its own ideological commitment — 'one would predict ...'. Second, the identification of the enemy is loose, ambiguous, and general, as it often is in ideological accounts. 'Those whose anti-management stance is ideological' — but who are they? 'Those committed to the class struggle'. Ah, then, the communist party? But communists are demonstrably not anti-management. Indeed Cliff, (1970) making an equally 'predictable' attack on productivity bargaining gives and criticizes many instances of communists who have supported it. Finally, Fox's account illustrates a basic refusal to enter into a discourse. This is a rare departure in the development of European thought, even the most arid schoolmen were prepared to debate the

potential density of angels upon pins. The sociologists' pronouncements are, we are intended to believe, value free, so that their defence
cannot be contaminated by conducting it in terms of the concealed
values on which it rests. But if any attack must always be ideological,
does this not prove, at least, that a conflicting ideology will find values
underlying the sociologists' case to disagree with?

The ideological content of managerialism is illustrated by one other
characteristic, its ambition. We have observed, ever since Tawney
(1925) commented on the 'revolution which was to set a naturalistic
political arithmetic in the place of theology, substitute the categories
of mechanism for those of theology ...', the gradual domination of
economic interests and work-related values. This domination has
reached the point where the values of management culture can be
described as having these three components:

> 'The first is the value system of economic rationality analysed by
> Weber, prominent in which are such principles as the measured
> weighing of utilities and costs; the use of money as the universal
> measure of value, and the importance of maximising-behaviour and
> of capital accounting. The second major component is the value-
> system of economic growth: the philosophy which measures
> national success by performance in the international league-table
> of Gross National Product. This philosophy is now virtually world-
> wide and completely transcends fundamental differences in political
> and social systems. The third component is the closely associated
> notion of technological progress; the philosophy that finds terminal
> as well as instrumental value in extending human control over
> material resources. These three components constitute the dominant
> culture of industrial societies ...' (Fox 1971 : 68)

In this sense, the political, economic, and social lives of
industrialized communities are suffused with managerial values. But
managerial ideology is ambitious in another sense. There are signs that
the transcendence of its values is not enough, that the demand is
emerging for its supremacy to be explicitly acknowledged.

While claims to managerial legitimacy once rested upon analogies
with government and with political democracy, so that management
drew credibility and authority by comparisons with established
political systems the argument and the analogy is now beginning to
run in the opposite direction. Governments and political systems are
now being recommended to model themselves on management. The

expertise, authority, and objectivity of managers is offered to governments and the British government begins to emulate that of the USA in its willingness to give senior ministerial posts to managers who next have to be found Parliamentary seats. Sometimes the offers of assistance are more wholehearted, as when Lord Robens and Sir Paul Chambers advocated government by businessmen as more efficient. There is even support for more managerialism from the politicians; Roszak (1970 : 11) quotes the late President Kennedy: 'What is at stake in our economic decisions today is not some grand warfare of rival ideologies which will sweep the country with passion, but the practical management of a modern economy. What we need are not labels and clichés but more basic discussion of the sophisticated and technical questions involved in keeping a great economic machinery moving ahead.'

Management, meanwhile, makes more modest claims to achieve new influence. It has now become common-place to talk of the management of areas of activities which were previously regarded as the province of professionals. In medicine the nurses have been gradually forced to abandon a close professional attachment to patient care in favour of a typically hierarchical structure in which the superordinate levels are concerned with administration or management of the ward or the hospital and in which the subordinate levels have been subjected to specialism and the recruitment of auxiliary labour. Massive courses of management education are now directed at the nurses, the main ingredients of which are a grounding in the behavioural sciences and the constant attempt to make the nurses see themselves as essentially engaged in managerial activities. Nurses are often accompanied by hospital administrators who are very ready to admit the newcomers to the highly regarded ranks of management in which the administrators, of course, are already well established. This process has the additional advantage that, apart from 'converting' the nurses, it solves the serious status problems of the administrators in an erstwhile professional structure by changing the structure so that administrators can see themselves at its centre, while the old professionals become the newcomers. The process would be even more satisfactory if the doctors could also be persuaded to become claimants for managerial status; the hospital administrators would be delighted to assist them with instruction and advise. The further development of status inversion has, however, not met with the entire approval of the doctors who stubbornly continue to regard themselves as professionals and who, as yet show no great enthusiasm for managerial treatment.

In other professions (apart from the law) there are similar signs of conversion. Headmasters conscientiously attend behavioural science courses on motivation and the management of scarce resources. Architects show signs of having been so thoroughly committed to a process of employment and management by institutions and organizations that there are even signs of a revolt.

All these developments suggest a rampant managerialism that is no longer content to camouflage its values and disguise itself in a society in which other institutions (like the professions) and other activities (like politics) are paid the greatest respect. And apart from overt claims to influence, there is the 'broad power' in

> 'the position that corporate management occupies as task setter or style leader for the society as a whole. Business influence on taste ranges from the direct effects through the design of material goods to the indirect and more subtle effects of the style of language and thought purveyed through the mass media — the school of style at which all of us are in attendance every day. Further, these same business leaders are dominant social models in our society: their achievements and their values are to a large extent the type of the excellent, especially for those strata of society from which leaders in most endeavours are drawn.' (Kaysen in Bendix and Lipset 1967 : 234)

In such a society, the crudities of a straightforward ideology of work are no longer necessary and no longer effective. Economic enterprise, and those who are responsible for its control and whose own value is measured by its results, have virtually succeeded in transforming society so that politics, as well as theology, have been transformed from 'the master interest of mankind into one department of life with boundaries which it is extravagant to overstep'.

Part IV

The New Radical Reaction

13. A Re-examination of Work

Is this process so successful that a challenge is virtually impossible? If it is no longer necessary to make straightforward ideological appeals for work then the appeals can neither be heard nor countered. If the apparatus of capitalist authority based on property has been dismantled both by the left and the right because of its essential inefficiency in eliciting subordinate support, then it hardly makes sense to look for a radical reaction to it. If work is being reconstructed in order to become a satisfying activity which the worker will welcome then how can the same worker be expected to reject it?

Nicholls (1969 : 215), for example, doubts whether business ideology is in any sense a defensive mechanism for, if it is a defence, then 'what is the attack'. He rejects one possible reply, that the attack emerges from

> 'pleas for workers' control, nationalization, and production for social use, which are put forward by some members of the political left — but today such battle cries are rarely heard and seem most unlikely to be accepted and implemented as matters of principle by those who are effectively organised politically. It may be true that by the 1920's two generations of Fabian intellectuals had turned the sacred word "profits" into an obscenity — but a later generation has sought to do just the reverse for the words "productivity" and "efficiency".'

One feels considerably less certain as the result of Nicholls's reassurance. It was followed by the events in Paris, May 1968, the shipyards of Upper Clyde were taken over by their workers, some forty engineering firms were submitted to 'work-ins', the AUEW abandoned the engineering procedure agreement largely as the result of a dispute over managerial rights and the TUC has supported the inclusion of union representatives on directorial boards.

Nicholls goes on to argue that one cannot understand contemporary union-management relationships if one assumes 'that the formal representatives of the employee interest now consistently challenge the right of management to manage or the right of shareholders in the rewards of profit-making' (Nicholls 1969 : 221). The question is these days, not whether employees should be given fair wages, but rather what is a fair wage.

This argument seems to be quite unrealistic. It seems to rest upon the assertion that the only issue over which the foundation of management can be seriously challenged is that of capitalism or private ownership. This is surely not so. The 'right of management to manage' is itself a slogan representing one of the most elemental of managerial ideological claims that Nicholls quotes with a straight face. The 'right to manage' has been, and is constantly, the subject of challenge by unions or by work-shop pressures in the effort bargain. There is, of course, no dispute about whether workers should be given a fair wage. There never has been. There is no record of any management seriously advocating the payment of an *unfair* wage, the dispute has always been over totally different subjective views about what *is* a fair wage. Moral justification is always the accompaniment of any statement of self-interest. It is not in the least surprising, for example, that Nicholls's Northern City directors could not distinguish between their Company's interest and social or ethical responsibilities. No one is ever capable of accepting the immorality of goals which he is publicly seeking — although the process of rational reconciliation may be tortuous. Both Hitler and Himmler believed themselves to be moral men; it is much easier for managers to do so.

We might point out, in passing, that the institution of the new terms 'efficiency' and 'productivity' for the older term 'profit' may be a significant exchange. 'Fabian intellectuals' may have done permanent damage to the term 'profit', just as Galbraith suggests that permanent damage may have been done to the term 'capitalism'. 'Productivity' and 'efficiency' are different concepts; they suggest the substitution of means for ends, means which, if made acceptable, will lead to the very ends (profits) that can no longer be the subject of agreement.

It seems to be the purpose of Nicholls's argument to establish that managers have no consistent ideological position, that they see themselves as co-ordinators, acting for the organization as a whole, that the subordinate posts of the organization are not seen as existing in anything other than a purely temporary state of conflict. Managers have no need of a defensive ideology because there is no attack and no prospect of any attack developing. Is the implication that manage-ments' beliefs are objectively verifiable, that the situation is as management believes it to be, that managers *are* co-ordinators and allocators and that there *is* no long term contradiction between the goals of the organization and those of the society in which they live?

If this is true then it is not evidence of the absence of any managerial ideology but rather, of its extraordinary success. We have already argued that the direct ideological appeal for work may now have been superceded by other and more subtle approaches and that an ideology which has been successful in achieving its 'manifest purpose of influencing the sentiments and actions of others' (Sutton *et al*. 1956 : 2) may become difficult to identify when it ceases to be challenged. And certainly there is now very wide agreement about the desirability of goals closely associated with an ideology of work; economic growth, the accumulation of wealth, efficiency, productivity. There also seems to have been a progressive extension of managerial personnel, techniques, and standards into areas of activity which were previously immune because of a primacy of traditionalistic attitudes or because of professionalism.

But there is also evidence of this triumphal progress having been halted at some points and reversed at others. The first check has been established by penetrating the deceptive subtlety of this new approach. It may be that management distributes benefits, material, psychological, social, and political (that is, benefits of material resources, worker satisfactions, group integration, and participative involvement) but the fact is that these are not terminal values for management; they are not ends but means to the satisfaction of managerial ends. This simply means that management seeks a more total area of influence in the direction of human life and of society, and seeks to achieve it by more insidious means than at any previous time in history. Managers must seek omniscient influence in order to achieve efficiency, as the areas of influence become more personal and significant, so that the attempt at influence becomes more dangerous. It is not that this influence is *necessarily* dangerous but rather that, because psychological involvement or democratic decision-making is sought for managerial ends and is therefore always subordinated to them, it always *may* be dangerous. It is not that managers are wicked but rather that they are neither competent nor representative in the wider areas of influence in which their drive for control leads them to act.

Roszak (1970 : 5) among others, has identified this process as the influence of the technocracy. He defines technocracy as 'that social form in which an industrial society reaches the peak of its organizational integration' in which 'The meticulous systematization Adam Smith once celebrated in his well known pin factory now extends to all areas of life giving us human organization that matches the precision of our mechanistic organization. So we arrive at the era of social engineering in which entrepreneurial talent broadens its province to orchestrate the total human context which surrounds the industrial complex' (1970 : 6).

Roszak (1970 : 19) goes on to remind us that it would be a mistake to associate the technocracy exclusively with 'that old devil capitalism. Rather, it is the product of a mature and accelerating industrialism.' One of his examples of 'technician paternalism' comes, as he puts it, 'from a non-capitalist institution of impeccable idealism: The British National Health Service'. He describes accounts given in a BBC television documentary on the health service, in which professionals complained about lay interference in the expert management of hospitals (a recurrent complaint about them) and in which predictions were made concerning the psychiatric certification of normal behaviour, of NHS administered population planning, including a 'programme of "voluntary euthanasia" for the unproductive and incompetent elderly' (Roszak 1970 : 20).

The advance of managerialism, or of the technocracy, is associated with the application of great expertise and science to the solution of problems. The employment of scientists and engineers at senior levels of management is increasingly apparent and is said to be breaking down the class basis of managerial authority. The further recruitment of the social sciences can be seen not merely as a temporary situation in which social theorists are employed in the solution of managerial problems, but as part of the continuing process in which *all* science is promoted by the industry which it develops. Weber (1967 : 76) provocatively suggested, before rejecting the notion, that capitalism might be 'best understood as part of the development of rationalism as a whole' because 'it is one of the fundamental characteristics of an individualistic capitalist economy that it is rationalized on the basis of rigorous calculation, directed with foresight and caution toward economic success'. Weber rejected this thesis. But there is some contemporary evidence to suggest that although rationalism and science cannot be identified with capitalism in their historical development, rationalism and science may be rejected with capitalism in an association firmly established in the minds of some young people. Giddens has pointed out that the cultural opposition to technocratic rule (the counter-culture) 'can easily lead to a condemnation of these objectives as essentially "irrational", since they seem to represent a protest against reason itself, or rather against the systematic application of reason in the technocratic ethos' (Giddens 1973 : 259).

One of the most poignant slogans in the eruption of slogans in Paris, May, 1968, was 'Nous sommes Marxist, tendence Groucho'. It can stand for a short, sardonic, and untheoretical rejection of the surrounding environment, whether it is labelled capitalist, technocracy, or industrialism. The reaction of the young, in so far as it is syndicalist, communist, or Trotskyist, does not take the objectors outside the industrial environment. Indeed, one could argue that the reaction, in so far as it is politically directed, is inexorably involved in the industrial environment which provokes so much protest and that this association could lead to the further hypothesis that the process of industrialization has been so dominant that it contains and conditions *all* modern political behaviour. The conclusion then would be that not only *is* there no rejection of industrialism but that there can be no rejection of industrialism.

But such an hypothesis would be unprovable and the evidence suggests that a considerable reaction does exist. We might usefully distinguish between a rational and an anti-rational reaction. While it does seem to be the case that rational or theoretical reactions to industrialism concern arguments over control, ownership, and distribution and do not challenge the fundamental assumptions on which industrialism rests, the anti-rational reaction may represent a much more total rejection of industrialism and the values which are associated with it. Unfortunately, this rejection of associated values seems to embrace those values of rationality and intellect so that some parts of the new left represent a return to romanticism carried on by way of drugs, esoteric religion, or mysticism. To this extent, if the rejection of industrialism entails the rejection of science and the whole inheritance of the enlightenment, the outcome may be more sinister than the present condition of triumphant materialism to which it appears as an alternative.

It is not our business to look so far except, perhaps to explain why there is no theoretical challenge to the system of values which maintains and has been supported by an ideology of work. Alternative systems of values have virtually been destroyed. The Christian or classical outlooks from which we set out are archaic and the Christian institutions have constantly adjusted to the modern world so that the independence of their values have been sacrificed to the need to continue to achieve influence over economic drives. We have argued finally that capitalism itself has been abandoned because of its ideological deficiencies in the general pursuit of material advantage. What we have been observing is the emergence of work as the dominant idea in our lives. There is no alternative, in the sense of a coherent challenge based on alternative values, there are, at best, subordinate debates concerning its differential rewards. The institutions and political theories which at first sight appear to offer radical challenges turn out, on close examination to be, like trade unions, essentially economic organizations or like communism, even more pure apostles of the theology of work.

But what about the workers? How far has this transcendent ideology succeeded in dominating their lives?

The focus of the question now shifts to ground heavily trodden over by industrial sociologists in recent years. A great mass of well-known research has sought to establish that work is the most highly valued activity, that it influences perceptions of status and that it deeply involves the satisfaction of the individual. There are, however, formidable questions concerning the value of some of this evidence. There is, for example, a reluctance to confess that one's work is tedious and disliked when there is a general assumption shared by questioner and questioned that one's value is determined by one's work; to admit to hating one's job is to admit to hating one's life.

However, the evidence, although it has often been collected by questionable means, points to the conclusion that most people find their work important and derive satisfaction from it. But several qualifications and refinements have to be introduced to this conclusion. 'What precisely is the source of their satisfaction — the pay, the working conditions, the social relationships, the work itself, the simple fact of being able to conform to a universal social expectation? It is doubtful if more than a small proportion of respondents know themselves ...' (Fox 1971 : 76).

Also, what is the kind of work about which the worker is responding? Several classifications have been made between kinds of work.[21] Two relevant and general conclusions emerge from the mass of evidence available: first, that workers can be related to their jobs essentially by the nature of the task they perform, by their relationship to other workers, or by the remuneration they receive for doing their work;[22] second, 'the higher the individual's position in the occupational hierarchy the greater the evidence, on the whole, of concern with intrisic values in work' (Fox 1971 : 23). The response of the worker to ideological appeals or to changes in his environment which are calculated to make him work more effectively depend, in part, on the kind of work he has to do. For the most part, people seem to take work very seriously and this is no surprise because they have been taught by every means available that, if they do not, they are delinquent.

So, the evidence of the importance attached to work should be treated with suspicion, and there is real evidence to the contrary. Those studies which are sometimes dismissed as 'impressionistic' in which people have been allowed to describe themselves and their work, point to more alarming conclusions.[23] Accounts of the killing, lunatic boredom of what many people have had to do every day for forty years in the factory, on the production line, are familiar. To the people who have to do the jobs the tedium can even be an advantage, it enables one to behave like a machine, to make one's body into a mechanism operating on remote control. 'All the jobs are boring ... so it is better to stay on the one you know and don't have to think about any more' (Toynbee 1971 : 62). 'With a rag wrapped round my eyes I could still do it, and could do dozens before I realized that I had done any at all. But underneath this my mind never stops working. It lives by itself. Some call it dreaming, and if so, I am dreaming all day long, five days a week. The whole bench dreams like this. It is a galley of automatons locked in dreams' (Fraser 1968 : 97). Dennis Johnson admires the women workers in factories for being much happier than men, because they can 'chatter all day long about their homes, their holidays, who is in the family way, and anything else unconnected with work. Women turn their minds from the futility of factory life' (Fraser 1968 : 14).

> 'You dream, you think of things you've done. I drift back continu-ously to when I was a kid and what me and my brothers did ... Lots of times I worked from the time I started to the time of the break and I never realized I had even worked ... It don't stop. It just goes and goes. I bet there's men who have lived and died out there, never seen the end of that line. And they never will — because it's endless.' (Terkel 1975 : 152)

When work is not so mercifully tedious it can be savage. Dulcie, in Toynbee's account (1971 : 66), tells of a serious nervous breakdown that stopped her working for six months. She attributed it to her job at the time, 'I was working on components that had twenty eight parts. It was piecework and you couldn't stop for a moment if you wanted to get your time in.'

If the reader doubts the accuracy of such accounts let him read the training-manual job descriptions for jobs in almost any factory. A job analyst's account of a job in a motor-car factory flatly stated that: 'If protective goggles are worn for any length of time they sweat and steam up, the worker on track rarely has time to stop and wipe the lenses clean'. If the reader still doubts these conclusions let him meet the unanswerable challenge of the average manual worker: 'do my job'.

These conditions are not confined to the man on the line, the factory worker. The clerk who knows he is comparatively fortunate, even in terms of other and worse clerical jobs, can say: 'I'm not ungrateful. The basic fact remains though that in common with the other jobs I've had, it has no value as work. It is drudgery done in congenial surroundings. You feel dispensable, interim: automation will take it over one day, the sooner the better. You are there for the money, no other reason.' Callow describes one of his less lucky clerical jobs: 'We had a pile of stores vouchers, a register, an indelible pencil each. There were numbers in your register which tallied with the vouchers. You had to find the corresponding number, tick a space, turn the voucher from a pile on your right to one on your left. No talking, no contact, nothing unless you counted trips to the bogs. I had to move my legs somehow just to convince myself I was still alive, so my trips became more and more frequent' (Fraser 1968 : 57-9).

There is a general belief that the worst characteristic of work belongs to the modern factory or office and that, until quite recently there was a golden age of natural, agricultural work which was satisfying and in which there was contentment and peace. The accounts in *Akenfeld* present a different picture. Leonard Thompson, a retired farm worker: 'I want to say this simply as a fact, that village people in Suffolk in my day were worked to death. It literally happened. It is not a figure of speech. I was worked mercilessly. I am not complaining about it. It is what happened to me' (Blythe 1972 : 41). For manual workers the nearest thing to a golden age is probably the present when for some, unionization has at least limited the hours of work and has assured them of at least a subsistence wage. Work, for most people, has always been ugly, crippling, and dangerous.

But there is another image, a notion of qualities in work that are attractive and that demand love and affection from workers. This is the other side of the coin, summed up in the craft ethic. George Sturt's wheelwrights 'would sooner have been discharged than work badly, against their own conscience', they demonstrated a respect for perfection not always shared by their employer, they 'exaggerated the respect for good workmanship and material ... The main thing after all ... was to keep the business up to a high level ... To make it pay — that was not their affair' (Burnett 1974 : 326).

Akenfeld again provides some good examples of this quite different relationship with work. Frances Lambert, the forge worker: 'I love work. It would be work all the time if I had my way ... No man should go in at morning to wait for the clock at night. And people who want the money without the work spoil everything' (Blythe 1972 : 140). And his employer, Gregory Gladwell, blacksmith: 'We have our pressures now with bills and bank managers and book-keeping, but I say to myself, this is not the highest thing; this is business. You are a tradesman, this is the highest thing. Making, doing' (Blythe 1972 : 132).

Making things *is* an essential human activity; necessary, enjoyable, inseparable from human existence. Arendt has constructed a richly analyzed distinction between making things, on the one hand, and consuming the products of labour, on the other. The distinction is simply between labour and work. Labouring is engaged in to survive, it leaves nothing behind it, its results are consumed almost as quickly as the effort that created them. Work on the other hand, 'the work of our hands, as distinguished from the labour of our bodies ... fabricates the sheer unending variety of thing whose sum total constitutes the human artifact' (Arendt 1958 : 136). The things made by work stabilize life and give it objectivity. Labour has to be carried on out of necessity, it is part of a natural cycle, which has to be sustained through consumption, which is made possible by labour. The closeness of labouring to the natural elemental cycle of life is what makes labour pleasurable: 'The "blessing or the joy" of labour is the human way to experience the sheer bliss of being alive which we share with all living creatures, and it is even the only way men, too, can remain and swing contentedly in nature's prescribed cycle, toiling and resting, labouring and consuming, with the same happy and purposeless regularity with which day and night life and death follow each other' (Arendt 1958 : 106).

Arendt argues, contrary to most proponents of the craft ethic, that the joy in life as a whole, which is 'inherent in labour, can never be found in work and should not be mistaken for the inevitably brief spell of relief and joy which follows and attends achievement' (Arendt 1958 : 107). Whether we follow her in the distinctions between the forms of pleasure which attend these different activities, or not, the distinction between labouring and work is an important one. Labouring may be part of an elemental cycle but it is work, the making of things for use, that appears to be the more satisfying activity, and, if it gives man a sense of objective permanence in his transitory experience of the world, it is surely understandable that he should experience from it more than a 'brief spell of relief and joy which follows and attends achievement'.

Craft work has often been associated with the two characteristic features of pleasure and use. Mills (1956 : 220) catalogued the features of craft work as containing pleasure in work itself, establishing a real relationship between the producer and the thing produced (either in owning it or 'investing' sweat, skill, or material in it), allowing the craftsman freedom to plan his work and to modify his plan, enabling the craftsman to develop his skill and himself (so that 'he lives in and through his work' (222)). The craftsman, says Mills, does not separate his work from the rest of his life, he does not experience a split between work and play, 'he is at work and play in the same act'. This means that the craftsman does not seek to escape from work. The craftsman's work is the mainspring of the only life he knows: he does not flee from work into a separate sphere of leisure; he brings to his non-working hours the values and qualities developed and employed in his working time' (1956 : 223). Mills concludes, after this affectionate description, that none of these characteristics are relevant to modern work, that 'the model of craftsmanship has become an anachronism' (Mills 1956 : 224).

For one of the purest statements of the meaning and pleasure of craft work we must turn to a craftsman, to William Morris. Morris joined the Democratic Federation in 1883, when he was forty-nine. He had, he claimed, never heard of Adam Smith or Ricardo or Marx; he became a socialist out of disgust with the vulgarity of capitalism and the ugliness of industrialism. This disgust was associated, he said, with a religious feeling based on a sense of injustice and personal guilt.

Morris believed that he was lucky and that he ought to do something to pay for his luck. He was lucky in two senses, because he was independent and because he enjoyed his work. He expressed this feeling in a letter to the Manchester Examiner of 1883:

'I could never forget that in spite of all drawbacks my work is little else than pleasure to me; that under no conceivable circumstances would I give it up even if I could. Over and over again I have asked myself why should not my lot be the common lot. My work is simple enough — much of it, not that the least any man of decent intelligence could do if he could but get to care about the work and its results. Indeed I have been ashamed when I have thought of the contrast between my happy working hours and the unpraised, unrewarded, monotonous drudgery which most men are condemned to.' (Briggs 1962 : 139)

Morris is more interested than most social critics in the actual content of work, perhaps because he was a worker. He was bitterly hostile to the work involved in machine production because it would destroy art, civilization itself, and because it degraded work. Machinery did not save labour, he said, it reduced the skilled worker to the ranks of the unskilled. Machine production was an evil that produced ugliness and degraded life. But he could be ambivalent about it, in *News from Nowhere*, Guest, the writer, is told: 'All work which would be irksome to do by hand is done by immensely improved machinery; and in all work which it is a pleasure to do by hand machinery is done without' (Briggs 1962 : 267).

Morris was hostile to repetitive, over-specialized work, not to work itself. He did not accept the protestant view that all work should be venerated: 'we have seen that the semi-theological dogma that all labour is a blessing to the labourer is hypocritical and false, that on the other hand, labour is good when due hope of rest and pleasure accompanies it' (Briggs 1962 : 135).

Work is devalued by its social context — 'the first characteristic of civilized work is that it presses unequally and heavily on the working class so that it makes them worse off than the beast of the field' (Briggs 1962 : 119). The rich are kept at the expense of the poor. This is an old and an elementary criticism. But the system de-humanized work in a more specific manner. It was self-perpetuating and there was little hope of remission. Assurances that hard work would lead to an increasing degree of material prosperity which could be shared in order to lead to a reduction in the need for hard work, assurances of ultimate salvation by way of the use of machines to undertake all drudgery, all those comforting beliefs were delusions. We were operating an ever-accelerating treadmill, all the 'devices for cheapening labour simply resulted in increasing the burden of labour' (Briggs 1962 : 117). World markets demanded the creation of artificial necessities, work became 'the ceaseless endeavour to expand the least possible amount of labour on any article made, and yet at the same time to make as many articles as possible ... everything was sacrificed to the cheap production of things not worth producing at all.' Articles of appalling quality were produced to be sold, not used. Paradoxically, the only exception was the machines themselves, 'wonders of invention, quite perfect pieces of workmanship, admirably adapted to the end in view' (Briggs 1962 : 266).

There are two kinds of work, one a curse, such that 'it would be better for the community and for the worker if the latter were to fold his hands and refuse to work, and either die or let us pack him off to the workhouse or prison' (Briggs 1962 : 117), the other a blessing associated with the hope of rest, with a use for the product and with pleasure in its accomplishment. Unless work is directed at producing something that is truly useful and wanted, then it is 'slaves work — mere toiling to live that we may live to toil'. Work should be pleasurable, Morris defined art itself as 'the expression by man of his pleasure in labour' (Briggs 1962 : 119). Pleasure and work can be associated only when work is accompanied by sufficient leisure and when it is freed from subordination. Morris believed that we must achieve a more simple life in which work must cease to be a curse because no society could be happy unless daily work was happy.

Morris's solutions often demand sardonic questions. Who is to perform those tasks which it would be farcical to regard as pleasant? What are we to do about work which, by its nature, is irksome, dull, and degrading? Morris's uncertainty is revealed by the variety of the answers he provides. Hammond, in *News from Nowhere* says that irksome work in the new society is done by machinery. But Morris warns us specifically that one cannot expect this solution to emerge from present-day industrialized society. Machines will not ease men's burdens by accident or as a by-product of the commercial society that employs them; this beneficial result can only be achieved by making its achievement the object of the organization of work, that is, it can come about only when a true society has been constructed in which machines are employed only in order to reduce work.

In *Useful Work versus Useless Toil* (1885) Morris faced the question again and produced an alternative answer: 'those who did the roughest work shall work for the shortest spells' (Briggs 1962 : 134) and 'if the rougher work were of any special kind we may suppose that special volunteers would be called on to perform it' (Briggs 1962 : 135). So, irksome work will be organized as it would be in a Boy Scout camp, with every one taking his stint at washing up and doing latrine duties. In a reformed society there would also be a good deal of exchange of work. In *News from Nowhere*, a Yorkshire weaver, rather paler than most of Guest's companions, has come down to London to seek temporary outdoor work; he becomes a boatman on the river Thames (quite unpolluted).

Yet a third answer to the same question is more uncompromising.

'And yet if there be any work which cannot be made other than repulsive, either by the shortness of its duration ... or by the sense of special and peculiar usefulness (and therefore honour) in the mind of the man who performs it freely — if there be any work which cannot but be a torment to the worker, what then? Well, then, let us see if the heavens will fall on us if we leave it undone, for it were better that they should. The produce of such work cannot by worth the price of it.' (Briggs 1962 : 135)

Hammond confesses that there is only one worry remaining after all these changes have been made, the possibility of a work famine. This is unlikely for some time however because, he says, of conditions in what we would call the underdeveloped countries and because of the appalling plight of the USA which 'suffered so terribly from the full force of the last days of civilization, and became such horrible places to live in, that they are now very backward in all that makes life pleasant. Indeed ... for nearly a hundred years the people of the northern parts of America have been engaged in gradually making a dwelling-place out of a stinking dust-heap' (Briggs 1962 : 268).

We have spent some time in this exposition of Morris's view because it makes a clear distinction between craft work and the rest and because Morris is a truly independent critic of industrial society, perhaps the only independent critic. Professor Asa Briggs has called Morris one of the most searching critics of British society in the nineteenth century because he cared nothing for its institutions, questioned its achievements, and scorned its values. He goes on to suggest that Morris is particularly relevant in the twentieth century because his views 'provide the materials for a critique of twentieth century socialism (and communism) as much as for a critique of nineteenth century capitalism' (Briggs 1962 : 17).

This is because Morris came to capitalism from a position outside the economic system altogether. He was not a particularly clear thinker and he abominated systems; much of what he wrote consists of what Raymond Williams has called 'generalised swearing'. But the values which he brought to politics were not those to which society had become conditioned, they remained paramount and enabled him to regard with a contempt, rare since the middle ages, the vulgar atrocities of capitalist industrialization. His view of work serves as a platform for an absolute attack upon a society based upon economic values.

We have previously commented upon the closeness of capitalism and communism. In one sense, all that Morris retains of communism is his outraged sense of justice, otherwise he seems to be totally outside the tradition which we have seen developing since the seventeenth century and in which thesis and antithesis are both founded in the same structure of economic values. Morris is different.

Morris's attacks on repetitive, specialized work, also serve to remind us of the distinction between the work that most men have to do and craft work. Making and doing *is*, perhaps, the highest thing, but it is an activity that few of us are given to share in. It is also an activity which, as Mills says, may be declining in extent and importance. Looking at the transformation of work as the result of the application of the division of labour, Arendt (1958 : 124) concludes that 'The industrial revolution has replaced all workmanship with labour, and the result has been that the things of the modern world have become labour products whose natural fate is to be consumed, instead of work products which are there to be used'. The ideal of work, she continues, which was associated with making a more permanent world, has been sacrificed to the ideal of labour, to abundance, 'we live in a labourers' society ... and we have changed work into labouring ... Whatever we do, we are supposed to do for the sake of ''making a living'', such is the verdict of society, and the number of people, especially in the professions who might challenge it has decreased rapidly' (Arendt 1958 : 126-7).

The distinction between 'work' and 'labour' is a difficult one. Has work been changed into labour? Industrial society certainly seems trapped in a cycle of work and expanding consumption but as Russell said, 'the desire for commodities, when separated from power and glory, is finite and can be fully satisfied by a moderate competence. The really expensive desires are not dictated by a love of material comfort' (Russell 1975 : 9). The drive for consumption in industrial society is often a disguise for a drive for status, a demand for things that are not needed, are not used, and that will not last. 'Labouring', in Arendt's sense, is not for consumption, it is certainly not for 'making a living', it is to show things rather than to use them. One of the explanations of the current reaction against the work ethic is that both work and labour have lost identifiable purpose. The relationship of labour to the natural cycle, the dignity conferred by its relationship to survival, is not apparent on the assembly line or in the office. The physical content which could obscure the severance of labour from the natural world has often been removed. Labour remains as a series of activities, obscurely or mysteriously related to survival and lacking even the natural characteristics of fatigue and exhaustion. Labour, the most elemental of activities, has become unreal.

Work, the production of artifacts, the construction of man's world, is said to have declined. Craft work has certainly declined but the man-made environment has not been noticeably reduced. Work, the making of things, was believed to be a satisfying activity when it made satisfying things. But if meaninglessness is a characteristic of alienation and work creates an increasingly meaningless world, then work begins to seem more alienating than labour which retains, however tenuously, some purpose.

It is the world that has changed rather than the content of jobs. What once conferred dignity on labour and pleasure in work was not the activity that they involved but the purpose for which it was performed. It is a mistake simply to imagine that jobs have been de-skilled, made routine, and robbed of interest. In fact, the proportion of skilled jobs (or of managerial, professional, and scientific jobs) has never been higher. The phenomenon of the middle class drop-out is of a man in interesting and demanding work seeking to exchange it for labour, of an industrial designer saying, 'I'll stop existing in this society. I'll work on a road crew. I'll cut lumber or whatever the hell it'll be' (Terkel 1975 : 427). Even if few members of the middle-class actually do begin to work on the roads (some, including Oscar Wilde, were persuaded by Ruskin to do so) the popularity of the idea of self-sufficiency is sufficient to sustain two television series, 'The Good Life' and 'The Survivors'. The middle-classes may once have dreamed of treasure islands, now they dream of back-breaking work down on the farm. The fantasy is a search for purpose, to recreate meaning in life by repairing the link between work, use and survival, between work and life.

If it is the setting and purpose of work rather than its content that is important, it suggests that changes to increase self-actualization by enriching, enlarging, or rotating jobs, are not likely to achieve their end. Improvement in the content of jobs is of little account if the job itself is seen as a detached activity, unrelated to reality. The demand that work should be provided with more significance cannot be fulfilled because it cannot be met by simply changing work. The differences between extrinsic and intrinsic rewards in work, between instrumental and self-fulfilling attitudes are extraordinarily complicated,[24] and are almost impossible to disentangle even on a conceptual basis, leaving aside the further problems of empirical enquiry. There is no doubt that work, even when carried on to satisfy economic needs, can be satisfying in itself and there is no doubt that this satisfaction is not necessarily confined to craft work or creative work. Even the mindless, simple rhythm of labouring, in Arendt's sense of the term, is satisfying because, perhaps, as she says, it is so closely associated with life itself and because 'the protection and preservation of the world against natural processes are among the toils which need the monotonous performance of daily repeated chores' (Arendt 1958 : 100). She goes on to suggest that the struggle can achieve heroic proportions as in Hercules' task of cleaning the Augean stables. But, she concludes, the human labour of keeping the world clean and free from decay is hardly heroic because the Augean stables were, after all, unique in that they were mythical and they stayed clean. These differences, however, would not necessarily remove the characteristics of heroism which cling to some kinds of labour. The primary labouring activities like mining and fishing are often invested with heroic qualities. The endless nature of the task adds to the heroism; like the Dutchman forever battling to round the Horn the final blessing is the release of death. The heroism of labour is also associated with strength and endurance in the face of danger.

These associations may help to explain some of the inherent satisfactions in work but they cannot explain why a man should find pleasure in it unless he is peculiarly masochistic. The distinction between pleasure and satisfaction may be an important one because accounts of the inherent satisfaction of work often stress characteristics which are the opposite of pleasurable. An ambivalent character has always been present in work, and was observed clearly by Ruskin in *Time and Tide*: 'on the whole simply manual operations *are* degrading' (Ruskin 1905 : XVII, 423). Ruskin observed that many of his working readers had disputed this conclusion, 'feeling the good effect of work in themselves'. Ruskin acknowledged that within limits manual labour could be refreshing, wholesome, and necessary but that totally, manual work was degrading; it was as necessary and wholesome to eat sometimes as it was degrading to eat all day. One suspects that a great deal of the intelligentsia's cant about work has been occasioned by the pleasurable experience of an hour's labour in the garden being projected to labour as an activity in itself. Ruskin was under no illusion about the character of labour but he saw that its menial character and its discipline contributed moral virtue; servile work, under certain conditions 'might be a holy undertaking' (he therefore recommended it to the clergy). He took a classical Christian view that the disciplined necessity of work made its undertaking virtuous and educational. The ability to undertake purposeful work is seen as lending a certain *gravitas* and dignity to the worker, whose head is bloody but unbowed. He is responsible for his own affairs, for the upkeep of his family, for conducting himself in a disciplined fashion. Work is associated with maturity and experience. It is important because it is not fun, it is a portion of the burden of the world.

It is significant that once we begin to talk in this way we are describing not work so much as the worker. All the characteristics that are ascribed in this kind of account, dignity, courage, maturity, experience, are human characteristics, not characteristics of work. Work is certainly supposed to produce them by some magical process which cannot be explained, and, because the characteristics are highly esteemed, esteem flows backwards to the circumstances that produced it. It is as though, admiring the qualities produced in war, we advocated a continuous state of war so that they could be manifested.

It may be this association, between labouring and the response to it by labourers that has helped society to confer some importance upon tasks which are brutish and upon which it places so low a value in economic terms. Even those whose wage, status, working conditions and tasks provide with continuous evidence of degradation and failure, can still believe that their work is important to them and to others, and that it is interesting and worthwhile. But we found also that in the worst imaginable conditions in sub-arctic Russian labour camps, men on starvation diets will struggle to do the best job they can, will take some pathetic pride in their work. Is this evidence of the natural, intrinsic importance of work to man or is it evidence of man's reaction to inhuman conditions. Solzhenitsyn implies that it is evidence of the heroism of the human spirit. It seems that if we are asked to engage in any continual and exhausting activity, no matter how tedious, our survival and our sanity may depend upon our conferring some dignity on it and, thence, upon ourselves.

The question of what is intrinsic satisfaction thus becomes a difficult one. Are workers on the assembly line related to their work by a 'bond based on the need for cash from which all moral commitment is absent and which can be easily broken?' (Beynon 1973 : 239). To some extent intrinsic satisfaction may truly reside 'in' the job itself. But it may also reside in the worker as a necessary reaction to the disabling characteristics of the work he has to do. In these circumstances he may be more conscious of working 'for the money' but he can rarely withdraw himself from the job. Its pressures and its dangers may produce a perverse pride in it and his vulnerability may force him into close collective association with his fellows so that it is not the job so much as the community involved in it that commands his loyalties and his affection. Writing of Hull trawlermen Salaman says:

> 'to say that fishermen must be involved in their work is certainly not to say that they find it satisfying or enjoyable, but to suggest that it has considerable emotional significance for them. The nature of this emotional importance is difficult to establish, it probably varies over time. The involvement of a deckie-learner differs from that of a veteran trawlerman. The trawlermen are committed by their work to a view of themselves and their mates, a definition of the world and their position in it, which cannot be simply sloughed off. They are enmeshed in a work-based world which, for all implications, constitutes their world — their only one.' (Salaman 1974 : 19)

Similarly, the work of coalmining, however dirty, dangerous, or degrading has in a real sense created the community in which miners live, and through it, to a large extent, their world. Salaman suggests that involvement in work depends upon features in it which include danger, skill, the existence of extreme conditions, and the feeling that the work is important to society.

No doubt the combination of intrinsic and extrinsic satisfaction varies from job to job but it is complications like these which make them difficult to separate one from the other and which explain why, as Fox says, the worker himself often cannot tell you what he gets out of his work.[25]

Whatever the proportions of the particular mixture, even if we could allow for the inextricable relationship between worker (and his subjective reaction) and work (and its objective content), it seems fairly certain that a great deal of the self-actualizing school's energy has been directed at the achievement of managerial ends and that its appearance of reformist zeal has been the more dangerous as the result of its subordination to an interest group different from that which attracts its public sympathy.[26] We argued that, even in the case of that most respectable radical, Karl Marx, the result of a concern with work and the worker had been a theoretical structure which was the most suitable of any yet constructed for the pursuit of managerial ends. The very confusion over the ingredients of different kinds of work, over the complex relationship between the worker and his job, over his association with his fellows, his pride in strength or survival, his need for self-deception about the importance of tasks which occupy the whole of his life, all these complications provide a foundation for the view that work itself is or should be 'rewarding'. The complexity of the matter, in fact, always helps to give a kind of credibility to formulations of an ideology of work. If it were not for the complexity it might be impossible to convince workers that the nonsense to which they are subjected should be taken seriously.

A concern with the worker's happiness, with the need for him to find inherent satisfaction in his job leads to considerable ambiguities. The confusions help to explain why William Morris, for example, has been classed as an antecedent in the development of self-actualizing theory. But Morris *is* different. It is not only a question of feeling, it is a question of ends, of terminal values. Whatever Morris argues is in the interest of workers themselves, not as producers, or consumers, or employees. Happy people, he says, means people happy in work, it means happy work. The distinction between Morris and those self-actualizers with whom he has been falsely associated (like Herzberg) is both simple and subtle. Their concern is with efficiency, for which committed workers are necessary. His concern is with people, to whose happiness work is severely subordinated. One cannot, after all, imagine Herzberg and his colleagues advising workers 'to fold their hands' and refuse to do the kind of work which is a curse.

Their unions, it must be said, do not often give them this advice either, unless as a tactic in the effort bargain, in which case the refusal to work is part of an economic strategy rather than the result of revulsion from the work itself. There is little evidence of workers 'folding their hands' or being instructed to do so by their unions. Unions, even at their most militant, find it hard to escape from the charge of 'economism' and the implication that the work required of their members is perfectly acceptable as long as the price is right. There is little evidence either of industrial employees, either in East or West, rejecting the demands of the industrial environment. This may be because the demands are essentially acceptable, or because the workers see their work as instrumental to other satisfactions, or because the environment of work has been changed by a process of human engineering, so that the appeal is internalized. It begins to appear, certainly, that human engineering has been successful enough to make the continuation of simple ideological appeals for hard work unnecessary. Perhaps it also explains the singular absence of any co-ordinated opposition and the fact that the trade unions no longer operate as vehicles of criticisms of the economic environment. The workers themselves show no sign of moving towards any more revolutionary situation or towards any more thoroughgoing questioning of the relationships of work and authority.

Although there is no opposition from the worker there seems to be a great deal of sympathy for his lot. It seems that the failure of unions and workers to follow the 'proctor-intellectuals' and students to the barricades may be the result of fundamental differences of perception in which the intellectuals' sympathy for the workers is not reflected by the workers' view of themselves. One response to inconvenient evidence of worker passivity is to explain it at a level of criticism which accounts for it without accepting it as objectively valid. In one version or another, this sort of explanation amounts to saying that workers have been so deceived by the system in which they are trapped that statements of their satisfaction with it can no longer be accepted. These statements should be ignored while an accurate or objective analysis of the workers' 'real' situation reveals them as unwilling victims.

This is roughly the position of Herbert Marcuse. In *One Dimensional Man* he argues that technical progress has been extended to the whole of society in the form of systems of power, domination, and influence so effective that no criticism outside this system is possible. Opposition is assimilated partly because it is bought off by the largesse which technology can dispense, partly because its protests are reconciled with the ultimate goals at which the system is aimed. Men's material needs are made the instruments by which they are dominated. As such, they are incapable of independent judgement; they must be the final judge of what are their true and their false needs, but they cannot make this judgement unless they are free and they cannot be free in a society like ours. The population has been conditioned and the working class has been domesticated so that it is no longer a threat. As Professor MacIntyre puts it (1970 : 88): 'The human nature of those who inhabit advanced industrial societies has been moulded so that their very wants, needs and aspirations have become conformist — except for a minority which includes Marcuse. The majority cannot voice their true needs for they cannot perceive or feel them. The minority must therefore voice their needs for them and this active minority must preserve the necessarily passive majority.'

MacIntyre's criticisms of Marcuse's theories are very damaging. The theory of the militant minority or the revolutionary student élite is dismissed as 'idealized students who have produced the first parent-financed revolts in what is more like a new version of the children's crusade than a revolutionary movement' (MacIntyre 1970 : 89). Proctor-intellectualism, as we have noted before, will not do. The appearance of a minority claiming to act as surrogate for an absent majority must always be regarded with suspicion.

In any case, the refusal of workers to follow a few disgruntled intellectuals and importunate students to the barricades may result from the workers' cynical but realistic refusal to take such a serious view of work. with which they are much better acquainted. It has become the fashion among the educated, while it was always a truism among the rest, to assert that workers work for the money. Perhaps they always did. Evidence of such an instrumental attachment to work, which subordinates it to other ends and values, is shocking only to those who regard it as evidence of alienation from what should be a central life-interest. But, we have argued, those who take this view are the last survivors of those propounding a work-based ideology, the communists and, like all last survivors, they maintain the purity of the doctrine with the greatest zeal.

Workers know better. They know that it may be farcical to be asked to take seriously the circus tricks which they are asked to perform, for longer and more assiduously than a performing animal would tolerate. One of the many characteristics of outlook and attitude which serve to distinguish subordinate workers from their managers may be the contempt that the former feel for the managers who seem to take their work seriously. It is one explanation for the continued echoes of an ideology of work that, in some quarters, managers are still pathetically trying to get the subordinates to share their concern, perhaps in order to reinforce the realism of the managers' delusions.

Are managers deluded in their apparent devotion to a work ethic? They have good reasons for idealizing it. Managers and professional people are commonly believed to have enjoyable jobs which are intrinsically rewarding. They are encouraged to generalize from their own experience and the view that all work is or ought to be satisfying, is useful for them when they have to co-ordinate and control subordinate labour. That work is satisfying and important must be both a necessary and a realistic view. When they are confronted with evidence of incongruence between their view of work and reality as experienced by other people, managers will often conclude that it is the content of work that must be changed rather than their view of it. It is as thought they wished to change their surroundings rather than adjust their own defective vision. We have noticed that the latest versions of an ideology of work have been formulated by managers or by their more literate spokesmen. We have noticed also that the object of ideological attack or environmental reconstruction has been managers themselves. It is time now that we looked at managers' work.

14. Managerial Work

The nature of the manager's job and of his relationship to it begins to seem particularly important if we identify the manager as the author of the appeals concerning its performance and as the reason for continuing attention to its ideology. If we conclude also that managers are increasingly becoming the object for attention in terms of exhortation, restructuring, and control, then it would seem that all roads converge on the manager as the essential point of attention in any analysis of work.

But if managers are becoming the object of attack, who is launching it? Who is doing what and to whom? The dangers of becoming engaged in a spiralling process of semantic confusion are great and they suggest, as is often the case in such puzzles, that the category or class with which we are dealing is too crude. It is altogether too simple to talk of 'managers' as a single homogeneous group. It is probably too simple, also, to hit upon an easy hierarchical division between higher managers and lower managers or directors and managers. In the first place the terms have no precise connotation and are, therefore, virtually useless and, in the second place, little is known about the respective functions of these two groups, even if we knew how to classify them. Directors, in so far as they are members of the boards of limited liability companies, may carry legal responsibilities for their companies' affairs, but we certainly could not say of them, as a group, how far they were actively engaged in the control and co-ordination of managers' activities and behaviour. Some directors may be actively concerned in the management of managers, others in the broad determination of the commercial objectives and responses of their companies, still others in the arrangement of personal payments in the Cayman Islands.

Managers can be divided in a variety of ways, by education, career progression, function, status and position, but in the particular respect with which we are concerned they can most usefully be divided between those whose special responsibility it is to commit the activity of colleagues and subordinates to the pursuit of corporate aims, and those whose activity is so committed and directed. They can be divided, in short, between those 'who see managers primarily as "a resource" and those managers who are seen as the resource.

The division is a complex one and it is probably not associated with any levels of the hierarchical structure. Those who see managers as a resource may be lower down the hierarchy of authority than some of the managers who are used as a resource. A management-development specialist may, for example, have a lower salary, less responsibility, and a lower status than the production or sales manager whose career he is attempting to plan and control. The division between resource planners and resources, between human engineers and machines, between manipulators and manipulated, is apparent in the growing literature devoted to the techniques of management training and motivation. It is evidence of a much wider shift of attention to managers and professionals as objects for the intensification of work. While it was once assumed that all managers had like jobs and like attitudes, and were responsible for the control of subordinate manual labour, it was also conveniently, perhaps accurately, assumed that they shared in the work ethic which they were earnestly peddling to their subordinates. Now that they are recipients of similar, if more sophisticated treatment, evidence is beginning to emerge that they do not always share the primitively simple ideology that still pervades some management literature.[27]

Once we begin to pay attention to managerial jobs some peculiar conclusions and questions begin to emerge; peculiar, that is, in the light of managerial formulations and requirements of an ideology of work. J.M. and R.E. Pahl (1971 : 99) conclude that: 'A firm commitment to achieve success is not typical of our managers and they quote Riesemann, W.E. Moore and Cyril Sofer in support of the view that their own "Mr. Newington" was not a totally eccentric manager when he said: "My career in terms of commerce is really a means to an end. I'd like to mentally turn my back on the job and get on with something worthwhile".' Williams and Guest (1971) produced several similar examples to support a mildly affirmative answer to their question, 'Are the middle classes becoming workshy?' The managerial drop-out, running a country pub, pottering in the harbour, keeping a chicken-farm, is, they said, becoming an increasingly familiar figure.

Even so, most managers are still at work and, no doubt, have no intention of leaving it prematurely. Even these, however, seem to be describing their work in more cynical terms than would seem to be appropriate to the close relationship that was believed to exist between the manager and his job. Mr Newington's distinction between his job on the one hand and 'something worthwhile' on the other, is relatively novel because the manager was supposed to share at least one characteristic of the craft ethic; he did not make a clear distinction between being at work and being at play. This was in part because his work was supposed to provide many of the fulfilments which alienated, subordinated, manual labour so notoriously failed to do. The manager, unlike the labourer, was a lucky man, enjoying all the advantages of high status, high pay, and rewarding work. 'Top management', in particular 'is in a privileged position inasmuch as its role is so diffusely defined that, given its command over resources, it has wide scope for shaping the normative system to accommodate its own aspirations' (Fox 1971 : 83). This may be so of 'top managers', but given our assumption of a more significant distinction between resource planners and resources, even some of those top managers may find themselves with less command over resources than is comfortable for them. For the rest, the extent to which a manager's job is satisfying in terms of helping him to achieve a sense of identity (Nef 1968 : 140) is, once again, not only determined by the content of his job but also by his relationship to it. And this in turn is partly a question of the prevailing ideology of management work for, as Argyris (1964 : 41) told us, incongruence between what the worker wants out of work and what work can provide him with will not arise where 'the individual has decided not to aspire toward psychological success, where it is a cultural norm not to be involved in work'. And however ambiguous, confused, and misdirected the ideology of work has been for the manual labourer, for the manager himself its statements have been clear and dominant. Work, managerial work, has mattered more than anything in the world. If the individual manager has been able to survive a career-long process of selection, appraisal, training, education, reward, promotion, development, transfer, counselling, sensitivity-training, group-goal-determination, and human resource auditing without believing that his job is of central importance then the constant day-to-day influence of his work environment at least ensures that he keeps his private scepticisms to himself. What evidence there is suggests that the manager has been convinced of the paramount importance of his job at least insofar that he is often willing to subjugate other important considerations to its demands. He is more likely to move house frequently, with or without the full approval of his wife, and to cause upheavals to his education of his children by doing so: 'for most managers frequent mobility is an inescapable part of their way of life'

(J.M. and R.E. Pahl 1971 : 67). For many managers 'the challenges presented at work were irresistable, whatever sacrifices might have to be made at home' (J.M. and R.E. Pahl 1971 : 235). Practically everything that has been written about the manager, whether it is anecdotal, fictional, or academic, seems to agree that it is 'the cultural norm' for the manager, at least, to be involved in his work.

Whether the work has always justified or deserved this involvement is another question, although anyone who has observed the Napoleonic grand strategy of a retail-store manager in deploying his display material or the autocratic decisiveness of an office manager in ordering his forces must have sometimes doubted it. We know little about managerial work because the managers, until very recently, have concentrated their attention upon their subordinates and, for reasons we have mentioned, managers' interests seem to have largely defined the curiosities of social scientists. If it were possible to judge the objective interest inherent in managerial work it might turn out that much of it was tedious, demanding in time and attention without being stimulating to the intelligence. The close association that has often been supposed to exist between managerial work and intelligence might also be exposed as largely inaccurate. But we do not know and a measure of objective interest may be unattainable. All we do know is that managers seem to have behaved as though they found their work the most rewarding and important thing in their lives. This would seem to suggest the extraordinary success of an ideological appeal directed at establishing the importance of work to the manager, if not to his subordinate.

The different receptions given to the message by the different recipients can be readily explained. The workers have been protected by well practised 'strategies of independence' reinforced by class boundaries, values, and traditions which work-based ideologies have been unable to penetrate. Labour institutions like the trade unions, perhaps because of the very ideological poverty which we have noticed as characteristic, have also preserved their members from indoctrination. The incongruence between the nature of much of manual work and the importance that the worker was supposed to attach to it may have been greater than in the case of managerial work. Manual workers are also, in a sense, recruits to a work environment while managers are, to a greater extent, volunteers or aspirants to a set of values and goals that do not have to be imposed on them.

These differences may have contributed to the existence, as we observed earlier, of two cultures concerning work. The culture of the workers sees it in cynical or humorous terms, work is a joke, to be avoided, cheated at. It may have close similarities to the soldiers' culture concerning war. The soldiers' attitude, the British soldiers' attitude, at least, towards authority, his job and the dangers and privations associated with it is one of sullen, cynical, humorous resignation, a combination of realism and self-denegration. It is summed up in descriptions like the 'poor bloody infantry' and almost any soldiers' song.[28] The second is the official culture, the one adopted by superordinates and which incorporates themselves and the relationship to be maintained with their subordinates. It is in this culture that ideological statements about work reside and again there is a similarity with the official, military attitude represented by statements about our gallant soliders, regimental traditions, the importance of courage and discipline. The analogy between the two work cultures and the two military cultures breaks down in time of war because the existence of an enemy and the need to beat him gives the official statements a measure of general support that promotes a convergence rare in the field of work.

A collapse of the official military culture in war time would certainly be a serious matter, associated with a general state of demoralization. War time convergence normally presupposes the ascendence, at least temporarily, of the official view. Convergence, in the field of work, seems to involve the growing popularity of the unofficial view so that convergence seems to be the result of demoralization amongst the managers. To speak of it in these terms is to exaggerate the process but there is a growing belief that managerial work is less highly favoured both among potential recruits and current occupants of posts. Managers, or rather, those managers whose role is to plan and co-ordinate the resources which comprise other managers, are more and more frequently reporting concern about managerial moral, about the shrinking commitment of managers to their work and their employing organizations. The evidence which supports these conclusions is entirely impressionistic but it is based on the impressions of many managers of managers who report considerable change in the managerial environment. The evidence as to why this has come about is, unfortunately, easier to find than the evidence that it is so.

That most expert of management consultants, John Humble has told us (1973 : 21) that 'if middle managers are confused there is likely to be a significant loss in the sense of entrepreneurial spirit and competitive edge so important for success'. There seems to be good reason for a

degree of 'middle' management confusion at the present time. Peter
Watson (in Williams 1973 : 9) quotes another consultant, McKinsey
and Company, to the effect that 'the current rate of organisational
change among large industrial corporations is one major restructuring
every two years'. It is not unknown, in large organizations, for managers
to be still implementing one enormous organizational change while
another one overtakes them (indeed, on McKinsey's evidence, this state
of affairs is almost inevitable because it is probably impossible to carry
through these very big organizational changes within a period of two
years so that the next *must* begin before the last has been completed.
The big industrial organizations must, like Chairman Mao's China, be
in a state of constant revolution). So, the fashionable passion for
reorganization is added to technical development, mergers, rationaliza-
tions, take-overs, and bankruptcies as a promoter of redundancy,
uncertainty, or unemployment among managers. In a special study of
the treatment of scientists, technologists, and engineers in industry,
Robins (1973 : 5) commented that at 40 + ,

> 'often without realising it, the individual is frequently specialised,
> institutionalized, expensive and pension-tied. For many the day of
> reckoning comes out of the blue and the effect is traumatic. His skills
> seem unmarketable, mobility may be at its lowest and he feels
> rejected both by the employer and the community in an apparent
> overnight change of values. In fact, his chances of similar employ-
> ment are slender and the self-appraisal of what he has to offer, and
> what he is worth, is not quickly achieved. Some hard knocks have to
> be taken before he realises his personal market value, and that there
> are many others like him.'

There are so many like him, according to Watson (in Williams, 1973 :
10), that 'the whole idea of the conventional career is beginning to
collapse'. Although the engineer is likely to be a victim of redundancy
because half of what he knows is likely to be obsolete within ten years,
'the most likely casualties are ... the men without special skills who have
allowed themselves to get stuck in one particular company'. This
tendency reverses traditional virtues to the extent that 'an individual's
past lack of loyalty to any one firm often, in the case of mergers at least,
brings benefit rather than harm' (Williams 1973 : 11). There are good
grounds for a degree of bewilderment among managers and industrial
technologists. The latter, it is now commonly agreed, is becoming
unemployable in his mid-forties or later.[29] A middle-aged and

redundant technologist can turn for help to the Professional and Executive Recruitment Service and, says (Robins 1973 : 7), 'His qualifications, experience and requirements can be matched daily against opportunities in the Runcorn computer. However, if he is a 53 year old Research Scientist the chances are that the memory bank will store no more opportunities for him than for hansom-cab drivers.' So, the industrial scientist, in particular, is likely to find himself in the position in which he has spent longer in the educational process of acquiring knowledge and skills than in the period of employment in which he can utilize them and this state of affairs arises, apparently, because the demands of industry were so highly specialized in the first place that their satisfaction leads to the production of scientists whose useful employment becomes shorter and shorter. In other words, it is the demand for more intensive scientific specialization, allied to and associated with the speed of technological change, which produces unemployable scientists.

One cannot help but notice a certain Marxian contradiction in these developments. The 'crippled monstrosities' which were produced by the division of labour now seem to have their counterparts in the managerial sector, for they seem to be crippled to the extent that they have been made unemployable by the very forces that produced them.

It is, in a similarly paradoxical fashion, the managers themselves, or the managers of the managers, who seem to be wreaking the most considerable havoc among assumptions and values which have been so carefully cherished in the managerial environment. For these reasons Fletcher (1973 : 135) has predicted that 'management is about to end; the masters are making new hirelings'. 'By attrition, redundancy or revolution, management will be finished and managers themselves are facilitating their own end' (Fletcher 1973 : 156). Whether we will see the demise of managers or not, it seems very likely that we may be witnessing the destruction of the managerial ethos. It is destroyed as soon as the managers, who were recruited partly to apply it in the control of their subordinates, begin to see it applied to themselves. As their work becomes more specialized, more intensively controlled or totally redundant they are forced to reject the assumptions and values which their recruitment and careers have taught them to adopt. Their reaction may take a number of forms. They may seek their satisfactions elsewhere in leisure pursuits, they may turn to their families, they may drop out into jobs which are less intensely demanding and the withdrawal of which is less intensely painful. They may begin to learn that their rejection by the work-world they have been taught to believe in is only serious if they continue to take the demands of their work seriously. The survivors may begin to be pitied, rather than envied for their commitment to a way of life that demands their involvement for seventy hours a week, their 'being worn out, literally, by work and worry — by trying to adjust to a disequilibrating momentum' (Fletcher 1973 : 135).

Managers' discoveries of the inconsistencies between the commitments expected of them and the responsibilities shown to them may also be complicated by attacks from the world outside the managerial culture. Their children often seem to regard their values with contempt and are less likely, even in the United States, to opt for careers in business management. The ethics of production and profit are under constant attack by a commitment to conservation and the protection of the environment against industry which has reached the level of unassailable cliché. Even their wives, those most patient subordinates of the managerial world, are beginning to exert some pressure on managements' commitment to their work. J.M. and R.E. Pahl conclude (1971 : 261) that the changing role and attitudes of women is beginning to have influence on managers as husbands.

> 'Even if the men do not question their work-dominated lives, their wives are likely to demand more *time*. Money is not necessarily an adequate compensation for time. Already the indications from our study suggest that wives are more sensitive to ambiguities in their situation. Those who have been contemporaries with their husbands at school, college or university or who have shared a similar pattern of life before marriage in some other way are unlikely to be so ready to lose their husbands to the demands of the system. It is significant that both in our pilot studies and in the extended interviews with our managers there is an emphasis on ensuring that offsprings should either marry or train to be a *professional* ... the professional was perhaps seen as someone who could hold his own against the system.'

The belief in the impregnability of the professions, may, in fact, be pathetically old-fashioned because they are themselves subject to considerable managerial infiltration and attack, but as the Pahls say, it is the implication of this belief rather than its accuracy which is interesting. They put the implication in significant terms: 'what we may be detecting is the beginning of a middle class reaction against competition' (J.M. and R.E. Pahl 1971 : 262).

We have previously argued that competition, in the sense of capitalist market competition, may have been superceded and is, in any case, not as significant as the work-based industrial economic culture to the development of which it has contributed. Indeed, capitalism, in its pure form, made relatively few and restricted demands upon the individual's commitment to his work because it was seen as instrumental to his self-interest measured in economic terms. A middle-class reaction against competition would not, by now, be in the least surprising but what in fact we may be observing is a middle-class reaction against work.

This is not to say that work will end or that anyone seriously contemplates its demise. 'Work has to be done', but the inherent pessimism of that statement, that work is inescapable, stresses an element in our attitude to it which has not been fashionable for several hundred years. It may be that workers have always known it but if the middle-classes are coming to take an instrumental view of it then the work ethic may, at last, have run its course. The instrumental necessity of work may be seen in different lights, as instrumental to survival, to luxury, to status or (for Newington) 'to preserving natural country life and wild life', but all these attitudes to work, in that they subordinate it, remove it from its established pinnacle.

It may be the final Marxian contradiction, the last paradox in the development of the protestant ethic, that the shabby inadequacies of an ideology of work are exposed only when the ideological attack is turned, at last, upon the bourgeoisie itself. The crafts, as significant areas of human activity, have been submerged long ago by the tide of managerial attention. The managers have now turned upon themselves, and the professions, those last citadels of independence and humanity, are now subjected to continuous erosion. When everything has been corrupted we may then be able to see the consequences of the development of a special view which would have us all believe in the exaggerated value of work. At least, it seems that the prevailing assumptions are more likely to be questioned when the very core of the system that produced them is under attack from within. If the managers are in disarray, who is to persuade us to take the tasks they have set us seriously?

These questions can be levelled, not because of a new and radical scepticism which suddenly presents itself in opposition to the protestant ethic. Work has always been important, but its organization, motivation, and control in conditions of industrialization demanded a wholesale commitment to its values and a concerted attempt to achieve it by ideological and other means. The fact that these conditions of massive industrialization may now be coming to an end is suggested by the confused and contradictory treatment which even the managers are receiving at the hand of their employing organizations. The total commitment to work is no longer necessary to the large organizations, it can even be an embarrassment to it. Peter Watson (in Williams 1973 : 10) suggests that 'temporary work ... will occupy nearly two-thirds of the work force by the year 2000'. This new notion of temporary work will mean frequent intervals between jobs, 'at the moment we call it unemployment, but we shall probably need a new word ... what we will have to get used to, however, is the fact that a person's job will no longer be the central factor in his or her life' (in Williams 1973 : 12).

It becomes not merely likely, but imperative that we find new words. The changing demands of work make it possible, at last, to re-examine the work ethic and our attachments to our jobs. It may have become not only possible but necessary to carry out this examination.

15. Conclusion

We set out, at the beginning of this book, with a brief historical excursion in order to suggest some of the origins of current attitudes and ideas about work. A more important intention, however, was to propose that our present attitudes are in some senses modern, that is, that they are not axiomatic, not the result of some innate disposition of the human mind and body, not universal. We meant to suggest that our outlook upon work was characteristic of a period in which it formed part of a particular economic environment and where certain characteristics of performance and commitment became associated with particular kinds of manufacturing process. The expectation of consistent and dependable performance among workers was part of a framework in which economic values had attained the highest regard, economic goals had displaced other social or spiritual objectives, and industrial requirements had become more demanding in terms of the requisite behaviour of subordinates.

This is none too contentious a position from which to set off. The manufacturing and consuming world has observably become more complex, its parts more interdependent, the whole requiring more sophisticated orchestration. Industrialized countries are particularly aware of the influence that industry and its successful direction has on other aspects of their corporate lives. In Great Britain, few would disagree that industry appears to have permanently occupied the field of politics. It is no surprise to be told, therefore, that our outlook upon work has been conditioned and produced by the industrial environment in which we have grown up. But there are those who still maintain, despite the attractive coincidence between public attitudes to work and industrial demands for such attitudes to be forthcoming, that work, nevertheless, occupies a timeless position of importance in human life, that it is a persisting and unchanging want experienced by all men and women, concerned with basic needs for self-expression and fulfilment.

We suggested that it did not appear to be always so and that even today, some men and some workers seemed singularly exempt from such an instinctive and universally characteristic feeling. Everyone would agree, though, that work has to be done.

Individuals may escape from it, some of those most frequently regarded as most fortunate seem able to escape most regularly, but, even so, someone has to do it. There is no argument about this much at least, whatever value we put upon work as human activity, it has to be done by someone. If its performance (by many rather than by some) becomes associated with rigorous standards concerning output to be accomplished, hours and positions to be attended, techniques to be acquired, tasks to be shared, co-operation to be extended, co-ordination to be achieved, judgement to be exercised, then, in these circumstances, the grudging acceptance that work has to be done will not get us very far. In those circumstances, that is, in the circumstances of machine production in factories, work has to be done by volunteers.

The necessity for some measure of voluntary effort, for skill, care or dexterity in work and for some degree of commitment to its object, required the various statements expressing forms of what we have called the ideology of work. At the same time, the maintenance of a labour market and the necessary mobility of the labour that supplied it presented the possibility of some form of withdrawal of co-operative effort. The employee, unlike the slave, can leave and as the market becomes more highly developed, his opportunity for expressing choice between employers may increase. His opportunity for taking protective action with his fellows also increases. As his tasks become more specialized, or more skilled, or, simply, more interdependent, so the employers' dependence upon his co-operation appears to increase. The relative importance of the industrial worker, his growing associative strength and the increasing awareness of the costs and dangers of his withdrawal of co-operation begins to focus the employer's attention upon the fragility of the relationship of dependence which binds him to the employee. He begins to see the worker as a threat. The higher the expectations of performance the employer has of the worker the greater the potential threat the worker is seen to represent.

In order to achieve his co-operation the employer contributes to the production of various statements which set out the worker's duty in religious terms, or in terms of self-interest ('you too can succeed by effort') or in terms of the worthiness of the employer and the appropriateness of his commands. If the industrial employee occupies a sufficiently important position in the political society and if the potential threat which he offers is sufficiently damaging to the fabric of the state, then the process of communicating an ideology of work, in one form or another, becomes a part of the business of government and finds expression in various formulations of political policy. In the mildest form these are inseparable from the government of any industrialized country but there are circumstances in which the government of industrial workers becomes (or is believed to have become) so urgent a problem that it dominates political life. One form of this domination by an ideology of work is to be found in communist countries where the government is inextricably involved in the management of workers because:

1. the state has been founded on the most consistent work ideology (from Marx);
2. the government is directly involved as employer and manager of substantial numbers of workers; and
3. the foundation of the state on an ideology of work means that the state perceives evidence of lack of zeal among workers as treachery, so reinforcing the association between work and politics.

The relationship between communist coércion and Marxist theory thus begins to appear not so much as an accidental aberration as a logical consequence. A reviewer in *The Times Literary Supplement* (11 January 1974) asked 'how it came about that the great man's theory ended in the Soviet straightjacket' and listed a number of scapegoat explanations often advanced (Engels, Lenin, the condition of Russia). We have suggested that the Soviet government is simply involved, one way and another, in a heavy dependence upon an ideology of work and in bridging the chasms of alienation and political withdrawal which its unreality creates.

The peculiar fragility of emphasizing the importance of work and workers in the government of the state illustrates another contradiction which is inherent in the exaggerated view often taken of work in ideological expression concerned to achieve its satisfactory performance. Much of the attention given either at a political or at a managerial level is directed at overcoming the so-called alienation of the industrial worker. In one form or another the 'problem' of the industrial worker haunts the administration of the industrial state from the level of direct worker supervision to the level of general politics. The whole concept of alienation has become so loose and general in its meaning that its use in social analysis has been widely criticized, but its ambiguity is probably an indication of the extent to which it has entered general usage. It is, by now, a popular concept. It is most certainly a popular term among managers because a great deal of the extensive literature devoted to aspects of labour management is concerned to overcome the alienation of the employee. Now this managerial preoccupation with what is essentially a Marxist concept is, on the face of it, odd.

The oddity is only superficial because the notion of alienation is a very useful formulation of what managers identify as one of the most important problems which confronts them in work, the obstacle to the realization of their own objectives which is presented by their subordinates' withdrawal of co-operation. One of the most appealing paradoxes to emerge from an area particularly full of contradiction is that alienation is not simply a concept which is useful for managers, it is, in essence, a managerial conception. The essential paradox of alienation is that it emerges with any meaning only as the result of an over-emphasis on a work ethic and work-based values. Man can be regarded as alienated from his work only when he has been subjected to an ideology of work which requires him to be devoted to it.

There are strict limits to the extent which capitalism can produce alienated workers. Capitalism, we argued earlier, can only require that employees will work 'for the money', any deeper commitment or involvement by the worker goes beyond any requirement which is consistent with the capitalist rule book. The question immediately arises that if the worker's involvement in his work is never called for in a capitalist system, if he enjoys a plainly calculative attachment to his job, then it becomes difficult to speak of him as ever having become alienated from it: the worker cannot be alienated from work which he has never been closely attached to. But this remote and calculative relationship between the worker and his job is not only a characteristic of capitalism, it is also a weakness because it provides a motive to work which is insufficient to overcome bounds set by reality (insatiable economic needs in a dustman can only lead to despair) and insufficient to encourage work of sufficient energy and enterprise to meet the capitalist's own interest. In some occupations, notably the crafts, the professions, and managerial jobs, straightforward capitalist, economic motivation (what Etzioni calls a 'remunerative basis of compliance') may be positively dysfunctional. It is not that capitalism alienates labour, it is simply that it does not succeed in synthesizing labour and yet its appetites lead to the perception that it requires synthesized labour, particularly in those areas where it is least likely to produce it.

The capitalist's need for synthesized labour leads him to break out of his own conceptual system.

The practical illustration of the capitalist shedding the capitalist framework is to be found in the discussion of the controversy over 'ownership and control', over the asserted evolution of capitalism to managerialism. Whether the change has taken place or not the belief in it overcomes the ideological disadvantages of capitalism. This is not to say simply that the innovation of managerialism is a conspiracy or a myth deliberately engaged in by groups of deceptive capitalists lying doggo until they can safely re-emerge. The foundation of a new ideological appeal outside the framework of capitalism is laid by those who need it, by the managers. The need becomes more urgent as a special group of managers is created which is given the specific function of managing labour. These are the agents who are most dramatically confronted by the problem, who are likely to see the ideological shortcomings of capitalism simply as a special problem concerning the co-ordination of labour, a problem which they must somehow overcome in their own managerial work. Alienated labour is simply an obstacle to the achievement of managerial objectives; alienation is a managerial problem.

Alienation also emerges as a concept in the process of development which leads to industrialization. Marx argued that capitalist industrialization exposed the impersonality of employment relation-ships. But the same process of industrialization requires the construction of an effective ethic of work. The construction of such an ethic by ideological means is, however, inseparably related to the notion of alienation which is both entailed by it and which contradicts it. Alienation is a mirror-image of a work ethic: it reflects what is projected into it but the image is reversed. The concept of alienation emerges from a work ethic because of an inevitable recognition that men are not as involved in their work as the ethic demands; there is a recurrent managerial problem of imperfect commitment which has to be overcome. Alienation is a concept produced by an ideology of work, it demands a more effective ideology of work, but refinements in the ideology merely re-emphasize the problem of alienation.

Alienation is a concept that is essentially incompatible with capitalism. The ideological limitations of capitalism, the impoverish-ment of its appeals for effort and co-operation and the bleak explanations which it offers for the situation of the worker are all impediments to the complete development of industrialism and to the achievement of the capitalist's own goals. Marx proposed the removal of the impediments to industrialism, although at some cost to the capitalist. Marx also helped the capitalist to see the difficulties which surround him and certainly developed a concern with the problem of alienation as the consequence of a conception of a degree of commitment which the capitalist could never claim but which he began to see as an ideal.

The capitalist employer's promotion of an ideological appeal for work had, because of the incomplete structure upon which it was founded, always been elementary and ineffective. The most complete expressions of such statements, to be found perhaps in Ure and Smiles, now seem ridiculous. The very notion of launching a direct appeal for committed work on behalf of the owner now runs the risk, in a mature industrial community, of arousing a cynical response from those at whom it is directed. We rarely observe examples of such appeals, unless they are launched from the wider premise of concern with the national economy and refer to a necessary infusion of the Dunkirk spirit; although, perhaps, in younger industrial communities, the direct ideological appeal from the employer may still be effective (or, rather, the employer may still believe in it). It is 'the end of ideology'. It might be more correct to call it the end of communicated ideology because the attempt continues to inculcate beliefs and attitudes among workers which are intended to influence their behaviour in a favourable way. We suggested that the attempt has taken two forms.

The first follows from the discovery of the ideological disadvantages of appeals based upon a capitalist framework. The most complete reaction to this discovery is to set about the actual dismantling of a capitalist structure by constructing an economy which is freed from its disadvantages and which facilitates a more effective ideological exhortation. Communism takes the place of capitalism partly because of the belief that 'capitalism will not work', that is, that it cannot engage that work will be done. An intermediary position, less extreme but emerging from the same conviction, is that capitalism need not be destroyed because it has evolved into a state which no longer requires the advent of communism because it has removed the greatest ideological obstacle to the appeal for work and co-operation. In this situation ownership, although not destroyed, has become so diffuse as to disappear or to be imperceptible in its influence. This is the case for managerialism and it has two advantages, it seems to offer at least some of the ideological advantages which accompany the overthrow of capitalism and it offers them at the least possible cost and disturbance to the *status quo*. Its value as a strategy of defence or conservation is so obvious that one ought, perhaps, to be wary of its appeal on this ground alone. It seems admirably suited to the needs of capitalists in convincing the rest of us that we need no longer fear them because they are no longer there.

The case for a managerial revolution is given great credence by the new prominence which the managers seem to have achieved in recent years. They *have* emerged as a recognizable group, sharing habits of dress and opinion, exhibiting the same restless mobility, often exceeding the old owners in their devotion to their work. They have also emerged as the single focus of attention in all discussions of industrial and economic progress and control. Whether these discussions are trivial or learned they always concern the ability and intentions of managers, not owners, so that, practically, managers seem to be seen as the controllers of industry and commerce. It is the managers, we are told, who must improve productive performance, conduct industrial relations more effectively, develop a sense of public responsibility and ethics, or do whatever else is to be done in the industrial world. So there is some evidence to support the appealing contention that the managers have taken over from the capitalists. It is an argument which is both attractive and convenient, not least for the capitalists.

Managers emerged, we said, partly as better exponents of an ideology of work because the authority of their appeals seemed more legitimate and because the division of interest separating them from the workers whom they addressed seemed less enormous. But the division persisted and it was part of our argument that no ideological appeal could succeed in achieving its objective partly because of the empirical difficulties involved in applying unrealistic descriptions to most industrial tasks and partly because of the logical difficulties in solving problems of alienation which have been created by the very ideology intended to overcome it. The difficulties were recognized: while the logical paradox went unnoticed the opposition of workers to the appeals directed at them could hardly be missed. This prompted, or at least, explained, the second attempt to favourably influence the behaviour of subordinates.

This we described as the attempt to create an industrial

environment which would either make for a receptive response from
its inhabitants to managerial appeals or would make appeals
unnecessary because the response would be conditioned. The attempt
to create a favourable environment may emerge from a fairly simple
concern to be a good and enlightened manager. It may, on the other
hand, involve the sophisticated application of all the resources of the
psychologist and the sociologist in an attempt to reconstruct both the
content of work and its surroundings, relationships, and organization.
The end, whatever the participative, integrative, enriched, group-
centred, and co-operative means employed, is to produce a response
from the worker which recruits his unhindered energy to the
performance of his tasks for his employing organization. The most
important ingredient in 'releasing the co-operative potential' of the
worker is not the worker himself, because the complex amalgam of
human qualities which he is to contribute in this process is to be
tapped rather than consulted. The vital element in bringing about this
change is the manager, no longer as the transmitter of an ideology of
work but as the essential agent who can change the worker's
environment in a favourable manner. The manager must now act
rather than talk. More than that, he must act and he must believe.

Countless instructions and exhortations to managers on the
necessary steps to achieve the 'new style' of management are, for this
reason, devotional in character. They emphasize, whether the
particular changes concern the introduction of management by
objectives, productivity bargaining, performance appraisal, group-
target setting, human resource accounting, personnel development, or
whatever else, that what matters more than doing it right is that 'the
philosophy' should be accepted. When managers speak about a
philosophy in this way they invariably do *not* mean any rigorously
related chain of conceptual propositions, they simply mean that their
assumptions should be accepted, that their ideology should not be
questioned. The ideological content concerning the direction of work
is, therefore, as important as it ever was but it is now directed at
managers rather than their subordinates. We suggested in passing that
the content of ideology, its careful concealment, and the need to
achieve the unquestioning commitment of managers to the restructuring of work which they have to undertake, all explain the
singular characteristic of much management training, that it is
designed to discourage thought.

Managers now begin to receive ideological attention because it is they who have to bring changes about which, it is hoped, will achieve the commitment of the once alienated worker. But, as this process is taken forward with every hope of having, at last, squared the logical circle, we begin to see that, in many parts of productive industry, the worker is less important than he was and that his commitment may not matter any more. The comforting belief begins to grow that, in the circumstances of many process and automatic industries, human effort is no longer necessary to production so that our ideological apparatus constructed over two hundred years for the better direction of work can be dismantled. We also perceive, however, that the worker is displaced not by the machine or the computer but by the manager, the scientist, and the technologist. A second and compelling reason emerges for making the manager the focus of attention for ideological appeal; in many respects he is likely to replace the manual worker as the determinant of productivity.

At least, we can surely suppose that the lessons learnt in the painful process of developing an ideology of work for application to the shop floor will be remembered in its redirection to the managers and the engineers. We will, one imagines, go straight to the latest development which we have seen emerge and prefer to structure the managers jobs and their organization rather than make crude and unrealistic appeals based on fractured foundations. It may be so. There is considerable evidence to suggest that the management of managers is receiving careful attention and refined treatment. In many organizations their importance to the productive and profit making process is recognized by the generous salaries they receive and by the expansion in the level of fringe benefits which can include cars, provision for hospital treatment and for the private education of their children. There is great demand for their services, specialist companies set out to recruit and select them and some 'executive search' agencies exist solely to provide intelligence upon the whereabouts of individual managers who are likely to meet the requirements of a particular employer. In every respect they seem to be the most cosseted inhabitants of industrial organizations.

It is generally acknowledged, however, that they have to earn such treatment and that means that their total commitment is required. It is often obtained by a high level of reward and by a steady stream of communication aimed at establishing the importance of the company, its products or service and of the managers' importance to both. In many organizations, managers are expected to establish a particular sense of identity with the company, to see themselves as company men, to believe that the world centres around the activities for which they are responsible, to believe in their products and to subordinate all other activities to the company's ends. Such a description must look like an exaggeration to anyone who has not experienced the peculiar expectations demanded of a manager in a private company. Most people who have been in this situation may acknowledge, particularly if they have been able to resist such appeals, the requirements of loyalty, faith, and good works which are the normal expectation of the behaviour of managers. Even nationalized industries (which are both exempt from some of the grosser delusions about their own unique importance to the human race and which, because of their size, are less capable of commanding person loyalty) can expect and get the attention of managers and administrators for one hundred hours per week, week after week, for colliery maintenance work not carried out by mineworkers in their ban on overtime. They did it because it was expected of them and, like the Russian infantry at Borodino, they were rewarded by a sight of their — chairman.[30]

But these are surely the very expectations which were to be met by the direction of ideological appeals at manual workers. The basis already exists for the transmission of direct appeals to managers. Far from by-passing that unsuccessful stage (as we argued) in the development of ideology of work, when it comes to be applied to managers there would appear to be every expectation of success. A degree of commitment appears already to exist, alienation is unknown, there is nothing like the same defensive apparatus of class hostility and trade-union opposition as has been created on the manual front and the manager's work *is* more inherently satisfying and rewarding so that ideological appeals do not run the same risks of cognitive dissonance, of patently misrepresenting the facts. It seems likely then that managers are to become the objects of ideological attention, because their work is important and because, unlike manual workers, they are likely to be receptive. This is hardly a prediction, evidence for the continuous transmission of the message that managerial work is important is impossible to avoid.

Predictions arise over the response. We cannot avoid the disquieting suspicion that, if managerial work is identified as of critical importance to the productive process, it will be subjected to the same attention that important operations have always received. Marx, whatever his standing as political and economic theorist, deserves an unrivalled reputation as analyst of the production process and Marx asserted that the worker's hours of work would be extended to the limits allowed by nature and society and that, thereafter, his work would be intensified by specialization, division, and mechanization. Managers may already have reached the limits by way of extension and we see signs of the continued application of intensification to their jobs by much the same methods. So, we see them as likely to occupy the classic position, as it is being vacated by their manual subordinates, a position in which they are subjected to job intensification and ideological appeal at the same time and despite the mutual inconsistency of such approaches.

Managers receive generous salaries but there is, in fact, little evidence that they are being treated in the advanced and sophisticated way which they have been persuaded to adopt toward their subordinates. They are not often consulted about the design of their organization and the structure of their jobs. They are more likely to be the unwitting victims of reorganization (more and more frequently); transferred, retrained or dismissed at the behest of organizational plans drawn up by distant consultants; regarded as human resources, shuffled and distributed by specialists in management develop- ment and planning; encouraged to become more highly trained and specialized. The most strategically significant of them all, the scientists and the technologists, must endure all this concentration of expert attention in addition to the prevailing myth that they are unemployable at over forty. For these and other reasons they contribute to a peculiar problem, professional redundancy, when they begin to be told that their jobs and the infinitely specialized skills which they demanded were, after all, not so important to the conduct of a full life. The final predictions must concern the possible reactions of a group of people who are apparently of vital importance to the production process, who are often ill-used by it in consequence of their importance and who, because of it, are subjected to exhortations concerning the nature of their work, exhortations which are made to appear increasingly irrelevant by the intensification of their jobs. It would seem inevitable that the next problem on the agenda will be that of alienation amongst managers and the steps that must be taken to produce an ideological appeal likely to combat it.

The cycle through which we see the ideology of work develop seems complete when we see managers facing the same problems of inconsistency and inappropriateness in expressions about the importance of their own work as we saw produced by ideological expressions concerning manual work at a time when that, too, was important. There is nothing more likely to release managers from their illusory beliefs about the significance of work in their lives than for their work to become truly important to the productive process. When the managers are bewildered or, as they will then be described, alienated, we may all be able to return to a more cynical, a more realistic view, that work has to be done, that its performance often produces rugged and admirable qualities but that the search for deeper satisfactions must be conducted in other directions.

If these developments take place the process will be confused and difficult to perceive. Confusion will exist because it is the nature and the purpose of ideology to produce it. Ideological appeals to the manual worker become easier to disentangle when the need for their transmission is reduced, when his crucial importance to the productive process is lessened, and when technical improvement has advanced to overcome his resistance to subordination.

There is another and partly contrary reason for confusion in understanding the ideology of work. It succeeds in communicating its imperatives because they are acceptable to the audience it addresses. But ideology would be ineffective if there were not some readiness to be convinced. If there is one thing that emerges from this study it is that work is a thing of such richness and complexity that it defies analysis. At the risk of another contradiction, let us end by looking at some of the elements contributing to its complexity.

Work is a co-operative process. However 'imperatively co-ordinated' it is, it always rests upon voluntary co-operation. In the most coercive forms of organization, prisons, or labour camps, there is always some sort of negotiated accommodation between those who command and those who obey which carries co-operation beyond the point of the sullen, minimal performance necessary to avoid punishment. In capitalist enterprise, trust and co-operation have to go beyond the minimal performance of the obligations of a control, either between businessmen or between employer and employed. Whether the basis of co-operation is innate or acquired, psychological or social, natural or conditional in man, without it, organized work would constantly border on insurrection and breakdown. The immediate impression any observer of a factory has is of a degree of order and co-operation. The impulse to co-operate has done much to legitimize ideological appeals for the requisite performance of work.

Work is a necessary activity. It has always been necessary for the survival of the worker and those who have sought to avoid the necessity, criminals, the indigent and in past times, sailors and soldiers[31] have been subjected to considerable social pressure. Idleness, except in the rich, has been associated with deviance and so work has come to mean self-respect, even psychological health. 'Prolonged unemployment is for most people, a profoundly corrosive experience, undermining personality and atrophying work capacities' (Harrison 1976). Such effects are the result of conditioning, no doubt, but the conditioning has gone on for a very long time. Work has also been thought necessary for social progress, for 'making a better life'. Growing uncertainty about progress and about what makes a better life has contributed to the examination of accepted shibboleths but all these strands have contributed to the conviction of the necessity of work.

Work is a satisfying activity. The self-fulfilling nature of work has usually been reserved for craft work but, in ths· respect, the distinction between craft work and the rest is extraordinarily difficult to maintain. Skilled work, which is not the same, is a satisfying activity. Unskilled work is a satisfying activity, shown in the pride in cleaning the boiler of a steam locomotive remembered by Bill Morgan (Morgan and Meyrick 1973). Work commonly believed to be without skill or status, is satisfying. 'To be a waitress, it's an art' (Terkel 1975 : 252). The satisfying quality in work is itself complex. Dolores, the waitress, obviously believes that her work is important, 'professional', as she says. By any 'objective' standards, the job is not professional, not difficult, not rewarding, but it can be done well or it can be done badly and doing it well contributes to the sanity of the worker. Believing it to be important contributes to her self-respect. Some parts of Dolores's account of her work smacks of pure fantasy. 'I get to be almost Oriental in the serving ... I feel like a ballerina', but it may be a necessary fantasy. Things are invested in the job which an observer might say are not there, in order to make it difficult, thence rewarding. Work is a mixture of skills which are difficult to acquire and apply, of demands in the job and delusions in the worker necessary to his self-regard. It is not only the job but the worker that makes work rewarding and it is not necessarily 'good' workers who are rewarded; mentally deficient workers will find deficient work rewarding. There is no simple relationship here, however, because men can find things in their work or in their environment however brutal, to enable them to survive it. What they find and how they react to it may be influenced by their personality; confronted with routine work some men may 'fold their hands', some may fight, some make it into a joke and some create a fantasy of it.

Work is a respected activity. The dignity of labour was not discovered by Marxists. Work has always been associated with maturity and responsibility, as much in industrial as in agricultural societies, a boy became a man when he began to work. Work has always been invested with moral qualities, to engage in responsibility towards oneself, the family or the community, is a moral act. The drudgery of work and its acceptance is part of its moral character, work is discipline willingly accepted.

This incomplete list of characteristics suggests that ideological appeals for hard work were disguised and difficult to identify because they met a ready response, a resonance in the worker to whom work was and is important. Ideology has sought to use qualities inherent in work but it is a deliberate, partial, and manipulative use. The imperative 'work hard in your calling' was a command by God necessary to social order, but it was available to the employer for use in his own interest. Ideology has sought literally to employ and subordinate qualities inherent in work.

The ideology of work is a necessary characteristic of a divided society. Many observers have seen it as a characteristic of divided work but this is very doubtful. Machine production and the intense division of labour has produced boring, repetitive, and undemanding work but there is no means of knowing whether the work is worse 'than it was in, say, the seventeenth century, or whether men are more or less alienated by it. The complaint about divided labour is that it has destroyed work, made it worse than some ideal image demands that it should be. But the qualities of work are composed of negative as well as positive characteristics; work is a dialectic in itself. Many of the traditional virtues in work depend upon its unpleasantness, upon work that is 'hard'. It may be the case that ideological appeals about work begin to fail, to become more easily identified as emanating from the self-interest of a group or class, when work becomes *easier*, when it is no longer associated with the traditional qualities.

The setting of work is as important as its content. If work has been impoverished by changes following industrialization it may be the setting more than the content that has been damaged. If work is to be rehabilitated it may be the setting rather than the content that must be restored. A change in the setting may have to wait upon the end of ideology, at least of the ideology of work. The ideology has used work for purposes other than the workers', has employed it for the sake of economic ends. If there is to be a change in the setting of work then values will have to be changed. The need for a new spiritual or moral foundation has been emphasized often enough but it is a most pathetic and mechanistic fallacy to believe that the need will be met because it exists.

The radical critiques of society and of the organization of work have done nothing to expose the values of economic society to criticism, they have entrenched them rather than replaced them. Real criticism, has come from outsiders like Ruskin and Morris. Ruskin told Victorian England what was necessary to restore spiritual values; that education should concern compassion, gentleness, justice and truth, and that wealth constituted these things valuable in themselves; that work should produce useful things and should not entail ill-health; that economics should be a branch of morals. Victorian England did not and could not listen because a change in moral values cannot be planned or manufactured. But a change in material circumstances may make it possible for new values to emerge.

If work has become meaningless it is because it is less important, because it is less important it is less the subject of ideological bombardment. If the obfuscations of ideology are removed from work it may become possible to restore to it its original virtues, to regard it more realistically. If work has become purposeless it is because, although it is still necessary, the immanent connection between work and survival has become obscure, at least in complex industrial societies. But if that is so, purpose may be restored by turning (in the terms used by Hannah Arendt) from labour to work, to making things. Making things is also likely to be seen as a purposeless activity if the things made are vulgar, trivial, or dangerous. Are we likely to begin to ask what men should be employed for rather than that they should simply be employed? It may be that the question can be put when the simple equation between effort and output has broken down, when production does not depend upon employment. It may be that the question can be answered when the monetary and psychological costs of unemployment (or of a lower level of employment, a 20 rather than a 40 hour week) have been reduced by a preparedness to face a non-labour intensive society. Partial work for all, rather than full employment, may become a practical possibility. If it does it may be possible to choose what is to be done. The choice may even concern what should be done or what should be made. If work is ever directed at the production of good and useful objects and at meeting important needs it may be restored in some sense to meaning.

But it is time to stop, for to talk of restoring the meaning of work is to come dangerously close to re-establishing an ideology.

'for God's sake, when we have demolished all *a priori* dogmas, do not let us think of indoctrinating the people in our turn ... Let us not make further work for humanity by creating another shambles.'

Notes

1 One estimate suggests that 1200 square miles of agricultural land were enclosed from 1455 to 1637, resulting in the dispossession and possible unemployment of 35,000 families (Jordan 1959 : 62).

2 This is still a modern management problem. It is said to have been solved recently by an academic acting as consultant in a plant where the workers were reported to be 'insufficiently economically motivated'. He recommended the introduction of consumer attractions in the plant which would reduce workers net spending power and so make them work harder. A return to the Tommy shop would presumably also have this effect.

3 Paternalism cannot be dismissed as outmoded or irrelevant, however, as the recent interest in corporatism shows. The relationship of dependence and responsibility may return when the final authority of the State is substituted for the authority of God with the employer, once again in an intermediate position. Paternalism returns with a concern for the maintenance of social order; it re-emerges when the employer, having 'taught' labour independence, discovers that it must be controlled.

4 There is a close similarity between the theories of Saint-Simon and Auguste Comte. Gide and Riste suggest that 'textual evidence, however precise, cannot decide the question of the reciprocal influence which these two Messiahs exercised upon one another'. (Gide and Riste 1948 : 233, footnote).

5 It probably really did surprise many social scientists; managers on the other hand, have always believed that men worked primarily for money. Many social science teachers have spent their lives unsuccessfully trying to convince managers of the opposite.

6 The circumstances which will make association along one axis appear to be more appropriate than another (that is, association within the firm, with other workers outside it, or with a professional group) is an interesting field for study and is particularly important in the development of collective bargaining. There is a discussion of some aspects in relation to white-collar employees by Ray Loveridge, BJIR, November, 1972.

7 As Will Paynter (1970 : 168) puts it: 'A dispute that affects a very
   small number of men can affect the employment of thousands
   who are remote and unconnected with the issue or the settlement.
   In fact, as distinct from the inter-war years, a sectional strike in a
   key industry can be almost as extensive in its effects as was the
   General Strike in 1926.'

8 The proportion of post-graduate students is to be reduced and,
   still further following Marx's predictions concerning the shortening of training periods, two-year diploma courses are to be introduced. Universities are to take more of their students from the
   surrounding localities. The Labour Party's spokesman on
   education, Mr Short, has proposed the consideration of two-year
   degree courses.

9 In *The Dissenting Academy* (Roszak : 1969) there are several acrid
   discussions leading to the conclusion that this critical heritage
   has been abandoned, at least in American universities. Unfortunately the discussion also seems to point to the contradictory
   conclusions that universities are both engaged in quite useless
   activities and that they are entirely devoted to serving the interests
   of government, military establishments, and business corporations.

10 To the extent that throughout Europe, Britain, and America, it
   now claims 'professional' prestige.

11 This comment should not be regarded as critical. The lack of a
   consistent ideology is no disadvantage to the governors and is
   likely to be of great benefit to the governed. There is little doubt
   that consistency of ideology often accompanies an oppressive
   regime and that the absence of ideology may be associated with a
   civilized administration. This point is more fully and persuasively
   argued by Popper in *The Open Society and its Enemies*.

12 This exposition of Michels closely follows the account given by
   Lipsett in *Revolution and Counter-Revolution* (1970).

13 *See also* Orwell, 1970 : Vol.2, 130 and Vol.3, 178).

14 It is important to acknowledge that paternalism is not dead yet.
   Some of the leading employers in this field, IBM, Marks and
   Spencer, Kodak, Texas Instruments, can be fairly described as
   paternalist. If the managers are truly becoming separate from the
   owners and even, as we shall see, 'alienated' in the same way as
   the workers, a revival of paternalist ideology may be expected not
   least in order to recapture the loyalty of the managers. Fox's

recantation of his attack on the unitary outlook may be very significant (1974).

15 T.P. Kenny (1975) has made a powerful appeal to personnel managers to return to an enlightened concern with employee welfare, arguing that to focus on 'the place of work as a point of contact for solving the problems of citizenship in the larger society ... is the essence of personnel management'. There has been little sign of a widespread or favourable reaction to Mr. Kenny's case in the audience he was addressing.

16 Harris seems effectively to have disposed of the myth of a property-owning democracy — even to the extent of the Conservative Party's commitment to it as a slogan (Harris 1972 : 172-3).

17 This is not to suggest that the radical aim has been abandoned, it has not. It is encouraged by the Institute of Workers' Control. There are similarities between Clydeside 1972 and Clydeside 1917. The major difference is that in 1972 the workers succeeded; in 1917 they failed.

18 The preservation of managerial rights or 'managerial functions' has been a specific cause of controversy in the British Engineering Industry and led, more than any other single issue, to the termination of the Engineering Procedure agreement in September 1971. The employers have always insisted upon management's right to impose changed conditions which, if disputed, operate while they are the subject of consultation. The Union has always wanted the status quo to prevail, that is, that the changed conditions should be removed, so that the original established conditions are restored while the innovation becomes the subject of consultation. The controversy neatly illustrates the difficulty of reconciling participation with management rights.

19 Clegg responded with a defence of pluralism in industrial relations (Clegg 1975).

20 This is to put the claim in a comparatively modest form. There are many more grandiose versions which claim that 'group-centred leadership' will meet a new challenge, 'For man throughout the world is on the march to acquire for himself a new dignity, increased worth, and greater respect' (Gordon 1955 : 5). McGregor, one of the most managerially quoted authorities, puts the matter simply: '... if we can learn how to realise the potential for collaboration inherent in the human resources of industry, we will provide a model for governments and nations which mankind sorely needs' (1960 : 246).

21 For example, on the basis of the degree of discretion and prescrip-
    tion in its performance (Jaques 1961), on the basis of technology
    (Trist *et al*. 1963; Woodward 1963; Blauner 1964); on the basis of
    characteristic work groups (Sayles 1958); on differences in com-
    pliance (Etzioni 1961); on the degree of and type of bureaucracy
    (Lockwood 1958; Gouldner 1964); on the characteristic attitude
    of workers (Goldthorpe *et al*. 1968); on differences in structure
    (Burns and Stalker 1961).

22 This is based on the Goldthorpe *et al*. (1968) distinction between
    instrumental, bureaucratic, or solidaristic orientations.

23 The label 'impressionistic' presumably refers to the fact that the
    studies contain no attempt at measurement and qualification. As
    it is precisely the attempt to measure and quantify that has done
    much to discredit aspects of social science, the values of these
    surveys seem likely to increase as those of attitude surveys
    diminish. 'Impressionistic' studies of the kind carried out by
    Blythe, Toynbee, and Fraser have almost reached the level of
    insight achieved by creative writers like Dickens: they far exceed
    that of most social scientists.

24 As Fox has pointed out in an excellent summary in *A Sociology
    of Work in Industry* (1971 : 4-9).

25 The difficulties may also explain a certain ambivalence which has
    crept into the academic debate about the relative importance of
    instrumental and intrinsic attachments, a debate which, itself
    begins to seem more and more arid. The proponents of instru-
    mentalism ('people work for the money, and why shouldn't
    they') were first associated with an economist's view which was
    not popular among 'pure' sociologists. It was then taken up by
    sociologists of a radical disposition as helping to expose mystifi-
    cations in the employment relationship. It was next extended
    (Goldthorpe *et al*. 1968) to an argument concerning the
    worker's attachment to his union, which became included in the
    'instrumental' network. Instrumentalism thus begins to cut both
    ways, against the boss and against the union. Hence radical ambi-
    valence, thus Beynon (1973 : 101): 'Some sociologists have
    maintained, for example, that this sector of the working class, has
    during the 1960s, been increasingly concerned about money to
    the neglect of "traditional" brotherhood with their workmates.
    While these responses appear superficially to be indicative of
    some form of "pure" instrumentalism, a concern for money and

nothing else, it should be noted that, for the stewards, the question of premium payments was a moral question.'

26 An excellent example of managerial prescriptions, disguised to some extent under a false prospectus, is to be found in *New Perspectives in Job Enrichment* (Maher 1971). It contains a chapter entitled 'Job Enrichment "Cleans Up" at Texas Instruments' in which the 'matrons' who did the lavatory cleaning were described as being trained in 'T.I. philosophy and personnel policies to create an attitude of pride through an understanding of the importance of clean restrooms to the success of Texax Instruments and to illustrate the need for and value of everyone being creative and innovative in improving their operations' (1971 : 69).

27 *See*, for example, *The Experienced Manager*, British Institute of Management, 1969.

28 That is, a song popular with soldiers rather than a song about soldiers. For example:
'Send out my mother,
Send out my sister and my brother,
But for Gawd's sake don't send me.'
(Brophy and Partridge 1969 : 51)

29 There seems to be no evidence at all to suggest that this is a result of ageing, that it follows from inability to carry out necessary tasks or to solve problems or that it is simply a widely held belief among the managers of scientists and technologists. One can, however, often notice two characteristics of such beliefs among managers: when they are held they are held unanimously (so that solidarity gives the appearance of validity) and they often turn out to be quite wrong.

30 Derek Ezra, Chairman of the National Coal Board toured collieries in the Lancashire coalfield on January 12 1974 to give his personal thanks to managers, marketing officers, and others who had been working for several weeks to the limit of endurance in manning pumps and carrying out maintenance work.

31 Kipling's 'Tommy' illustrates society's contempt for the soldier in peacetime. The old sailor's contempt for the organized work of the landsman is shown in Dana's 'Two Years Before the Mast'.

References

Allen, V.L. 1966. *Militant Trade Unionism*. London: Merlin Press.

Amalrik, A. 1971. *Involuntary Journey to Siberia*. Newton Abbot: Readers Union.

Arendt, H. 1958. *The Human Condition*. Chicago: The University of Chicago Press.

_____1970. *On Violence*. London: Allen Lane.

Argyris, C. 1964. *Integrating the Individual and the Organization*. New York: John Wiley.

Aristotle, 1912. *Politics*. London: J.M. Dent and Sons.

Barber, D. 1970. *The Practice of Personnel Management*. London: Institute of Personnel Management.

Baritz, L. 1965. *The Servants of Power*. New York: John Wiley.

Barry, E.E. 1965. *Nationalisation in British Politics*. London: Jonathan Cape.

Bautier, R.H. 1971. *The Economic Development of Medieval Europe*. London: Thames and Hudson.

Beichmann, A. 1970. Beware of the Proctors. *Encounter* XXXV (2).

Belloc, H. 1912. *The Servile State*. London and Edinburgh: Foulis.

Bendix, R. 1966. *Work and Authority in Industry*. New York: John Wiley.

_____ 1970. *Embattled Reason*. New York: Oxford University Press.

Berliner, J.S. 1957. *Factory and Manager in the U.S.S.R.* Cambridge: Harvard.

Berle, A. and Means, G. 1932. *The Modern Corporation and Private Property*. New York: Macmillan.

Best, G. 1971. *Mid-Victorian Britain, 1851-75*. London: Weidenfeld and Nicolson.

Beynon, H. 1973. *Working for Ford*. Harmondsworth: Penguin.

Blake, R.R. and Mouton, J.S. 1964. *The Managerial Grid*: Houston: Gulf Publishing.

Blauner, R. 1964. *Alienation and Freedom*. London: University of Chicago Press.

Blythe, R. 1972. *Akenfeld*. Harmondsworth: Penguin.

Bowle, J. 1963. *Politics and Opinion in the Nineteenth Century*. London: Jonathan Cape.

British Institute of Management. 1969. *The Experienced Manager*. London: British Institute of Management.

Brophy, J. and Partridge, E. 1969. *The Long Trail*. London: Sphere.

Briggs, J. (ed.) 1962. *William Morris, Selected Writings and Designs*. Harmondsworth: Penguin.

Briggs, A. 1972. *The Guardian*. February 6.

Bukharin, N. and Preobrazhensky, E. 1969. *The A.B.C. of Communism*. Harmondsworth: Penguin.

Burnett, J. 1974. *Useful Toil*. London: Allen Lane.

Burnham, J. 1941. *The Managerial Revolution*. London: Putnam.

Burns, E.M. 1963. *Ideas in Conflict*. London: Methuen.

Burns, T. and Stalker, G.M. 1961. *The Management of Innovation*. London: Tavistock.

Calhoon, R.P. 1967. *Personnel Management and Supervision*. New York: Appleton Century Crofts.

Carr, E.H. 1952. *The Bolshevik Revolution, 1917-1923*, Vol.2. London: Macmillan.

Carter, M. 1966. *Into Work*. Harmondsworth: Penguin.

Child, J. 1969. *British Management Thought*. London: Allen and Unwin.

Clapham, L.H. and Power, E. *See* Nabholtz.

Clayre, A. 1974. *Work and Play*. London: Weidenfeld and Nicolson.

Clegg, H.A. 1975. Pluralism in Industrial Relations. *British Journal of Industrial Relations* XIII (3).

Cliff, T. 1970. *The Employers Offensive*. London: Pluto Press.

Cohn, N. 1962. *The Pursuit of the Millenium*. London: Mercury Books.

Cohn-Bendit, D. 1969. *Obsolete Communism the Left-Wing Alternative*. Harmondsworth: Penguin.

Cole, G.D.H. 1954. *Socialist Thought*, Vol.2. London: Macmillan.

———1948. *Communist Manifesto, Socialist Landmark*. London: Allen and Unwin.

Comte, A. undated. *Early Essays on Social Philosophy*. London: Routledge.

Conquest, R. 1967. *Industrial Workers in the U.S.S.R.* London: Bodley Head.

——— 1971. *The Great Terror*. Harmondsworth: Penguin.

Cook, E.T. and Wedderburn, A. (eds.) 1905. *The Works of John Ruskin*. London: George Allen.

Coser, L. 1956. *The Functions of Social Conflict*. London: Routledge and Kegan Paul.

Crichton, A. 1968. *Personnel Management in Context*. London: Batsford.

Dahrendorf, R. 1959. *Class and Class Conflict in Industrial Society*. London: Routledge and Kegan Paul.

D'Entrèves, A.P.D. 1970. *Aquinas Selected Political Writings*. Oxford: Blackwell.

Dickinson, J.W. 1971. What's in a Job. *Personnel Management*, 3 (6): 40.

Du Boulay, F.R.H. 1970. *An Age of Ambition*. London: Nelson.

Durkheim, E. 1959. *Socialism and Saint Simon*. London: Routledge and Kegan Paul.

_____ 1960. *The Division of Labour in Society*. New York: Free Press of Glencoe.

Edwards, S. and Fraser, E. 1970. *Selected Writings of Pierre Joseph Proudhon*. London: Macmillan.

Emmet, D. 1966. *Rules, Roles and Relations*. London: Macmillan.

Engels, F. 1969. *The Condition of the Working-Class in England*. London: Panther.

Etzioni, A. 1961. *A Comparative Analysis of Complex Organizations*. New York: Free Press of Glencoe.

Fanfani, A. 1935. *Catholicism, Protestantism and Capitalism*. London: Sheed and Ward.

Femia, J. 1975. Hegemony and Consciousness in the Thought of Antonia Gramsci. *Political Studies*, 23 (1)

Fidlon, D. (translator) 1973. *Outline History of the Soviet Working Class*. Moscow: Progress Publishers.

Fletcher, C. 1973. The End of Management. In J. Child (ed.) *Man and Organisation*. London: Allen and Unwin.

Fletcher, R. 1974. *The Crisis of Industrial Civilization, the Early Essays of Auguste Comte*. London: Heinemann.

Ford, H. 1922. *My Life and Work*. London: Heinemann.

Fox, A. 1966. *Industrial Sociology and Industrial Relations*, London: HMSO.

_____ 1971. *A Sociology of Work in Industry*. London: Collier-Macmillan.

_____ 1974. *Beyond Contract*. London: Faber and Faber.

Fraser, R. (ed.) 1968. *Work*. Harmondsworth: Penguin.

French, J. 1964. In R.L. Kahn and E. Boulding (eds.) Power and

Conflict In Organizations. London: Tavistock.

Friedman, G. 1961. *The Anatomy of Work*. London: Heinemann.

Fromm, E. 1956. *The Sane Society*. London: Routledge and Kegan Paul

Galbraith, J.K. 1970. *American Capitalism*. Harmondswoth: Penguin.

Gaskell, P. (1836) 1968. *Artisans and Machinery*. London: Frank Cass.

Genovese, E.D. 1975. *Roll Jordan Roll*. London: André Deutsch.

Gibb, M.A. 1947. *John Lilburne the Leveller*. London: Lindsay Drummond.

Gide, C. and Rist, C. 1948. *A History of Economic Doctrines*. London: Harrap.

Gissing, G. 1968. *New Grub Street*. Harmondsworth: Penguin.

Goldthorpe, J.H., Lockwood, D., Bechofer, F., and Platt, J. 1968. *The Affluent Worker: Industrial Attitudes and Behaviour*. London: Cambridge University Press.

Gouldner, A.W. 1964. *Patterns of Industrial Bureaucracy*. New York: Free Press.

Granick, D. 1954. *Management of the Industrial Firm in the U.S.S.R.* New York: Columbia.

—————— 1960. *The Red Executive*. London: Macmillan.

Grant, M. 1960. *The World of Rome*. London: Weidenfeld and Nicolson.

Groethuysen, B. 1968. *The Bourgeois: Catholicism vs. Capitalism in Eighteenth Century France*. London: Barrie and Rochliff.

Hanson, A.H. 1954. Labour and the Public Corporation. *Public Administration* 23 (2).

Harris, N. 1972. *Competition and the Corporate State*. London: Methuen.

Harrison, J.F.C. 1971. *The Early Victorians, 1832-51*. London. Weidenfeld and Nicolson.

Harrison, R. 1976. The Demoralising Experience of Prolonged Unemployment, *Department of Employment Gazette*, XIII (3).

Hayek, F.A. 1944. *The Road to Serfdom*. London: Routledge and Kegan Paul.

Heilbroner, R.L. 1968. *The Making of Economic Society*. New Jersey: Prentice Hall.

Herzberg, F. 1968. *Work and the Nature of Man*. St Albans: Staples.

Herzen, A. 1968. *My Past and Thoughts*. London: Chatto and Windus.

Hill, C. 1964. *Society and Puritanism in Pre-Revolutionary England*. London: Secker and Warburg.

Humble, J. 1973. *Social Responsibility Audit, a Management Tool for*

Survival. London: Foundation for Business Responsibilities.

Inglis, B. 1971. *Poverty and the Industrial Revolution*. London: Hodder and Stoughton.

Institute of Personnel Management. 1972. *Digest*, May.

Jaques, E. 1961. *Equitable Payment*. London: Heinemann.

Joll, J. 1964. *The Anarchists*. London: Eyre and Spottiswood.

Jordan, W.K. 1959. *Philanthropic England, 1480-1660*. London: Allen and Unwin.

Kaysen, C. 1967. The Corporation: How Much Power. In Bendix and Lipsett (eds.) *Class, Status and Power*. London: Routledge and Kegan Paul.

Kendall, W. 1969. *The Revolutionary Movement in Britain, 1900-1921*. London: Weidenfeld and Nicolson.

Kenny, T.P. 1975. Stating the Case for Welfare. *Personnel Management*, 7 (9).

Kolaja, J. 1965. *Workers' Councils, the Yugoslav Experience*. London: Tavistock.

Kornhauser, A., Dubin, R., and Ross, A. (eds.) 1954. *Industrial Conflict*. New York: McGraw Hill.

Krausnick, H. and Broszat, M. 1970. *The Anatomy of the S.S. State*. London: Paladin.

Laidler, H.W. 1949. *Social-Economic Movements*. London: Routledge and Kegan Paul.

Lane, T. 1974. *The Union Makes Us Strong*. London: Arrow Books.

Laski, H.J. (ed.) 1948. *Communist Manifesto: Socialist Landmark*. London: Allen and Unwin.

Lawrence, S. 1971. Putting People on the Balance Sheet. *Personnel Management* 3 (1).

Le Chêne, E. 1971. *Mauthausen, the History of a Death Camp*. London: Methuen.

Lenin, V.I. 1969. *Selected Works*. London: Lawrence and Wishart.

Lichteim, G. 1966a. *Marxism in Modern France*. New York: Columbia University Press.

———— 1966b. The Transmutations of a Doctrine. *Problems of Communism* 15 (4) : 14. July/August.

Likert, R. 1961. *New Patterns of Management*. New York: McGraw Hill.

Lipsett, S.M. 1969. *Revolution and Counter Revolution: Change and Persistence in Social Structure*. New York: Doubleday.

Lockwood, D. 1958. *The Blackcoated Worker*. London: Allen and Unwin.

Loveridge, R. 1972. Occupational Change and the Development of Interest Groups among White-Collar Workers in the United Kingdom. *British Journal of Industrial Relations* 10 (3): 340. November.

Lupton, T. 1964. *Industrial Behaviour and Personnel Management*. London: Institute of Personnel Management.

McGregor, D. 1960. *The Human Side of Enterprise*. New York: McGraw Hill.

MacIntyre, A. 1970. *Marcuse*. London: Fontana/Collins.

McLellan, D. (ed.) 1971a. *Karl Marx : Early Texts*. Oxford: Blackwell.

———— 1971b. *Marx's Grundrisse*. London: Macmillan.

Maher, J.R. 1971. *New Perspectives in Job Enrichment*. New York: Van Nos Reinhold.

Malthus, T. 1914. *An Essay on Population*. London: Dent.

Mantoux, P. 1948. *The Industrial Revolution in the Eighteenth Century*. London: Jonathan Cape.

Marcuse, H. 1964. *One Dimensional Man*. Boston: Beacon Press.

Manuel, F.E. 1956. *The New World of Henri Saint-Simon*. Cambridge, Mass: Harvard University Press.

Marx, K. 1901. *Capital*. London: Swan Sonnenschein.

Marx, K. and Engels, F. 1965. *The German Ideology*. London: Lawrence and Wishart.

Mayo, G.E. 1940. *The Human Problems of an Industrial Civilization*. Boston: Harvard Business School.

Meszaros, I. 1970. *Marx's Theory of Alienation*. London: Merlin Press.

Meun, J. de 1971. *Roman de la Rose*. Princeton: Princeton University Press.

Mills, C.W. 1956. *White Collar*. New York: Oxford University Press.

Mill J.S. 1946. *Essay on Liberty*. Oxford: Blackwell.

Miner, J.B. 1963. *The Management of Ineffective Performance*. New York: McGraw Hill.

Miners' Unofficial Reform Committee. 1912. *The Miners' Next Step*. Tonypandy.

Moonman, E. 1965. *The Manager and the Organization*. London: Pan.

More, T. 1910. *Utopia*. London: Dent.

Morgan, B. and Meyrick, B. 1973. *Behind the Steam*. London: Hutchinson.

Morrison, H. 1954. *Government and Parliament*. London: Oxford University Press.

Mossé, C. 1969. *The Ancient World at Work*. London: Chatto and Windus.

Nabholtz, H. 1941. Medieval Agrarian Society in Transition. In J.H. Clapham and E. Power (eds.) *The Cambridge Economic History of Europe*. London: Cambridge University Press.

Nagy, K. 1966. Hungary's Alienated Workers. *Problems of Communism*, July/August.

National Institute of Industrial Psychology. 1952. *Joint Consultation in British Industry*. London: Staples Press.

Nicholls, T. 1969. *Ownership, Control and Ideology*. London: Allen and Unwin.

Nicolaus, M. 1973. Foreword. *Grundrisse*. Harmondsworth: Penguin.

Nove, A. 1972. *An Economic History of the U.S.S.R.* Harmondsworth: Penguin.

Orwell, G. 1970. *The Collected Essays, Journalism and Letters*. Harmondsworth: Penguin.

Ovid 1966. *Metamorphoses*. London: Heinemann.

Owen, R. 1920. *The Life of Robert Owen by Himself*. London: Bell.

Pahl, J.M. and Pahl, R.E. 1971. *Managers and their Wives*. London: Allen Lane.

Parry, A. 1966. *The New Class Divided*. New York: Macmillan.

Paynter, W. 1970. *British Trade Unions and the Problems of Change*. London: Allen and Unwin.

Plato, 1970. *The Republic*. London: Sphere.

Polanyi, D. 1944. *The Great Transformation*. New York: Holt, Rinehart and Winston.

Pollard, S. 1965. *The Genesis of Modern Management*. London: Edward Arnold.

Popper, R.K. 1962. *The Open Society and its Enemies*. London: Routledge and Kegan Paul.

Pratt, V. 1973. Mrs. Thatcher's White Paper : Some Unstated Principles. *Communication* 2 (1).

Pribićević, B. 1959. *The Stop Stewards' Movement and Workers' Control, 1910-1922*. Oxford: Blackwell.

Rawls, J. 1972. *A Theory of Justice*. London: Oxford University Press.

Robins, W. 1973. Privately circulated paper on executive redundancy.

Roszak, T. 1969. *The Dissenting Academy*. Harmondsworth: Penguin.

———— 1970. *The Making of a Counter Culture*. London: Faber and Faber.

Russell, B. 1946. *History of Western Philosophy*. London: Allen and Unwin.

———— 1975. *Power*. London: Unwin.

St Augustine 1945. *The City of God*. London: J.M. Dent and Sons.

Sabine, G.H. 1941. *The Works of Gerard Winstanley*. Ithaca: Cornell University.

———— 1951. *A History of Political Theory*. London: Harrap.

Salaman, G. 1974. *Community and Occupation*. London: Oxford University Press.

Sayles, L. 1958. *Behaviour of Industrial Work Groups*. London: Chapman and Hall.

Schact, R. 1971. *Alienation*. London: Allen and Unwin.

Schonfield, A. 1965. *Modern Capitalism*. London: Oxford University Press.

Sheppard, H.L. 1954. Approaches to Conflict in American Industrial Society. *British Journal of Sociology* V.

Smiles, S. 1862. *Lives of the Engineers*. London: John Murray.

———— 1907. *Life and Labour*. London: John Murray.

———— 1908 *Self-help*. London: John Murray.

Smith, A. 1845. *An Inquiry into the Nature and Causes of the Wealth of Nations*. Edinburgh: Thomas Nelson.

Solzhenitsyn, A. 1970. *The First Circle*. London: Fontana.

———— 1973. *One Day in the Life of Ivan Denisovitch*. Harmondsworth: Penguin.

Southern, R.W. 1970. *Western Society and the Church in the Middle Ages*. Harmondsworth: Penguin.

Spearman, D. 1939. *Modern Dictatorship*. London: Jonathan Cape.

Sturmthal, A. 1964. *Workers' Councils: A Study of Workplace Organization on Both Sides of the Iron Curtain*. Cambridge, Mass. Harvard University Press.

Sutton, F.X., Harris, S.E., Kayson, C. and Tobin, J. 1956. *The American Business Creed*. Cambridge, Mass.: Harvard University Press.

Tannenbaum, A.S. 1968. *Control in Organizations*. New York: McGraw Hill.

Tawney, R.H. 1912. *The Agrarian Problem of the Sixteenth Century*. London: Longmans Green.

———— 1925. *Thomas Wilson, A discourse upon usury*. London: Bell.

———— 1948. *Religion and the Rise of Capitalism*. Harmondsworth: Penguin.

Terkel, S. 1975. *Working*. London: Wildwood House.

The Times Literary Supplement. January 11, 1974.

Thompson, E.P. 1968. *The Making of the English Working Class*. Harmondsworth: Penguin.

_____ (ed.) 1970 *Warwick University Limited*. Harmondsworth: Penguin.

Toynbee, P. 1971. *A Working Life*. London: Hodder and Stoughton.

Trevelyan, G.M. 1944. *English Social History*. London: Longmans.

Trist, E.L., Higgin, G.W., Murray, H., and Pollock, A.B. 1963. *Organizational Choice*. London: Tavistock.

Tucker, R.C. 1964. *Philosophy and Myth in Karl Marx*. London: Cambridge University Press.

Ure, A. 1965. *Philosophy of Manufacturers*. New York: Harper and Row.

Walzer, M. 1966. *The Revolution of the Saints, a Study in the Origins of Radical Politics*. London: Weidenfeld and Nicolson.

Ward, J.T. 1970. The Factory Movement. In J.T. Ward (ed.) *Popular Movements c 1830-1850*. London: Macmillan.

Waugh, E. 1947. *Scott-King's Modern Europe*. London: Chapman and Hall.

Webb, S. and Webb, B. 1920. *The History of Trade Unionism*. London: Longmans.

Weber, M. 1967. *The Protestant Ethic and the Spirit of Capitalism*. London: Allen and Unwin.

Whisler, T. and Harper, S. 1962. *Performance Appraisal, Research and Practice*. New York: Holt, Rinehart and Winston.

White, G.E. and Roberts, K. 1972. A Question of Character. *Personnel Management* 4 (4).

Williams, R. (ed.) 1973. *Tomorrow at Work*. London: British Broadcasting Corporation Publications.

Williams, R. and Guest, D. 1973. Work Content and Environment. In R. Williams (ed.) *Tomorrow at Work*. London: British Broadcasting Corporation Publications.

Wohl, R.R. 1967. The Rags to Riches Story. In R. Bendix and S.M. Lipsett *Class, Status and Power*. London: Routledge and Kegan Paul.

Woodcock, G. 1963 *Anarchism*. Harmondsworth: Penguin.

Woodward, J. 1963. *Industrial Organization*. London: Oxford University Press.

Woolf, S.J. 1968. *The Nature of Fascism*. London: Weidenfeld and Nicolson.

Yovchuk, M.T. 1966. Improvement of the Cultural and Technical Standards of Workers. In G.V. Osipov (ed.) *Industry and Labour in U.S.S.R.*. London: Tavistock.

Zimmern, A.W. 1915. *The Greek Commonwealth*. London: Oxford University Press.

Authors Index

Subject Index